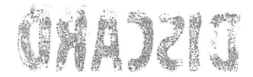

Cardiovascular Disorders
SOURCEBOOK

Sixth Edition

Health Reference Series

Sixth Edition

Cardiovascular Disorders

SOURCEBOOK

Basic Consumer Health Information about Heart and Blood Vessel Disorders, Such as Cardiomyopathy, Heart Attack, Heart Failure, Heart Rhythm Disorders, Heart Valve Disease, Aneurysm, Atherosclerosis, Stroke, Peripheral Arterial Disease, Varicose Veins, and Deep Vein Thrombosis, with Details about Risk Factors, Prevention, Diagnosis, and Treatment

Along with Information about Cardiovascular Concerns of Special Significance to Children, Men, Women, and Minority Populations, a Glossary of Related Medical Terms, and a Directory of Resources for Further Help and Information

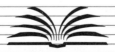

OMNIGRAPHICS

615 Griswold, Ste. 901, Detroit, MI 48226

Bibliographic Note
Because this page cannot legibly accommodate all the copyright notices, the Bibliographic Note portion of the Preface constitutes an extension of the copyright notice.

* * *

Health Reference Series
Keith Jones, *Managing Editor*
***

OMNIGRAPHICS
A PART OF RELEVANT INFORMATION
***

Copyright © 2016 Omnigraphics
ISBN 978-0-7808-1526-1
E-ISBN 978-0-7808-1527-8

Library of Congress Cataloging-in-Publication Data

Names: Omnigraphics, Inc.

Title: Cardiovascular disorders sourcebook: basic consumer health information about heart and blood vessel disorders, such as cardiomyopathy, heart attack, heart failure, heart rhythm disorders, heart valve disease, aneurysms, atherosclerosis, stroke, peripheral arterial disease, varicose veins, and deep vein thrombosis, with details about risk factors, prevention, diagnosis, and treatment; along with information about cardiovascular concerns of special significance to children, men, women, and minority populations, a glossary of related medical terms, and a directory of resources for further help and information.

Description: Sixth edition. | Detroit, MI: Omnigraphics, [2016] | Series: Health reference series | Includes bibliographical references and index.

Identifiers: LCCN 2016021250 (print) | LCCN 2016022275 (ebook) | ISBN 9780780815261 (hardcover: alk. paper) | ISBN 9780780815278 (ebook: alk. paper) | ISBN 9780780815278 (eBook)

Subjects: LCSH: Cardiovascular system--Diseases--Popular works.

Classification: LCC RC672 .C35 2016 (print) | LCC RC672 (ebook) | DDC 616.1--dc23

LC record available at https://lccn.loc.gov/2016021250

Table of Contents

Part II: Heart Disorders

Part V: Diagnosing Cardiovascular Disorders

Part VI: Treating Cardiovascular Disorders

Part VII: Preventing Cardiovascular Disorders

Part VIII: Additional Help and Information

Preface

About This Book

Cardiovascular disease is the leading cause of death in the United States. According to the Centers for Disease Control and Prevention, 735,000 Americans suffer a heart attack and 614,000 people die of heart disease in the United States every year. Additionally, stroke kills almost 133,000 Americans annually and is a leading cause of long-term disability. Yet cardiovascular disease is often preventable. With careful attention to diet, an active lifestyle, and control of contributing factors such as diabetes, cholesterol levels, blood pressure, tobacco use, and weight, Americans can reduce their chances of facing heart disease, stroke, or other blood vessel disorders. Furthermore, advances in our understanding of how to treat cardiovascular conditions make it possible to reduce the disabling health consequences frequently associated with these disorders.

Cardiovascular Disorders Sourcebook, Sixth Edition, provides information about the symptoms, diagnosis, and treatment of disorders of the heart and blood vessels, including cardiomyopathy, heart attack, heart rhythm disorders, heart valve disease, atherosclerosis, stroke, peripheral arterial disease, and deep vein thrombosis. It offers details about the conditions associated with increased risks, explains the methods used to diagnose and treat them, and offers suggestions for steps men and women can take to decrease their likelihood of developing these disorders. The book also includes a discussion of cardiovascular concerns specific to men, women, children, and minority populations, and it concludes with a glossary and a directory of resources for further help and information.

How to Use This Book

This book is divided into parts and chapters. Parts focus on broad areas of interest. Chapters are devoted to single topics within a part.

Part I: Understanding Cardiovascular Risks and Emergencies describes how the heart works, explains the known risk factors for cardiovascular disease, and offers details about the conditions that make it more likely that a person will develop a cardiovascular disorder. It describes recent research on the genetic links associated with cardiovascular disease, and it explains how to recognize a cardiac emergency and what to do when one occurs.

Part II: Heart Disorders provides basic information about the types of disorders that affect the heart. These include problems with the heart's blood supply, problems with the heart's rhythm, heart valve disease, and certain infectious diseases, as well as heart attack, sudden cardiac arrest, cardiomyopathy, and heart failure. Individual chapters include information about the development, symptoms, diagnosis, and treatment of each disorder.

Part III: Blood Vessel Disorders discusses the types of disorders that affect the arteries and veins, including atherosclerosis, carotid artery disease, stroke, disorders of the peripheral arteries and veins, and aortic disorders. It explains how these disorders arise, what their symptoms are, how they are diagnosed, and how they are treated.

Part IV: Cardiovascular Disorders in Specific Populations describes the unique ways that cardiovascular disease affects men, women, and children. It also offers some statistics on the occurrence of cardiovascular disorders in each of these populations, and it concludes with a discussion of cardiovascular disease among minority populations in the United States.

Part V: Diagnosing Cardiovascular Disorders explains the methods used to diagnose disorders of the heart and blood vessels. It describes diagnostic tests, including blood tests, electrocardiogram and echocardiography, coronary angiography, stress testing, and Holter and event monitors, and it explains how to prepare, what to expect, and which risks are associated with each test.

Part VI: Treating Cardiovascular Disorders discusses medications and procedures used to treat these disorders, including catheterization, coronary artery bypass grafting, stenting, and pacemakers. It also includes a discussion of stem cell therapy, aneurysm and heart defect repair, heart transplant, and the use of the total artificial heart. The section concludes with a discussion of cardiac and stroke rehabilitation techniques.

Part VII: Preventing Cardiovascular Disorders describes the things that can be done to help prevent heart and blood vessel disease. It explains how to control risk factors such as high blood pressure, high cholesterol, diabetes, and stress, and it offers suggestions for increasing healthy behaviors, such as maintaining a heart-healthy diet, incorporating physical activity into a daily routine, and quitting smoking.

Part VIII: Additional Help and Information includes a glossary of terms related to cardiovascular disease and a directory of resources offering additional help and support.

Bibliographic Note

This volume contains documents and excerpts from publications issued by the following U.S. government agencies: Agricultural Research Service (ARS); Agency for Heathcare Research and Quality (AHRQ); AIDS.gov; Centers for Disease Control and Prevention (CDC); Centers for Medicare and Medicaid Services (CMS); Federal Occupational Health (FOH); Genetic and Rare Diseases (GARD) Information Center; Genetics Home Reference (GHR); Military Health System (MHS); National Center for Complementary and Integrative Health (NCCIH); National Heart, Lung, and Blood Institute (NHLBI); National Institute on Aging (NIA); National Institute of Arthritis and Musculoskeletal and Skin Diseases (NIAMS); National Institute of Diabetes and Digestive and Kidney Diseases (NIDDK); National Institutes of Health (NIH); National Institute of Mental Health (NIMH); National Institute of Neurological Disorders and Stroke (NINDS); National Organization for Rare Disorders (NORD); Office of Dietary Supplements (ODS); Office of Minority Health (OMH); Office on Women's Health (OWH); U.S. Food and Drug Administration (FDA); U.S. Department of Veterans Affairs (VA); and the and the U.S. Preventive Services Task Force (USPSTF).

In addition, this volume contains copyrighted documents from the following organization: The Nemours Foundation

It may also contain original material produced by Omnigraphics and reviewed by medical consultants.

About the Health Reference Series

The *Health Reference Series* is designed to provide basic medical information for patients, families, caregivers, and the general public. Each volume takes a particular topic and provides comprehensive coverage. This is especially important for people who may be dealing with a newly diagnosed disease or a chronic disorder in themselves or in a family member. People looking for preventive guidance, information about disease warning signs, medical statistics, and risk factors for health problems will also find answers to their questions in the *Health Reference Series*. The *Series*, however, is not intended to serve as a tool for diagnosing illness, in prescribing treatments, or as a substitute for the physician/patient relationship. All people concerned about medical symptoms or the possibility of disease are encouraged to seek professional care from an appropriate health care provider.

A Note about Spelling and Style

Health Reference Series editors use *Stedman's Medical Dictionary* as an authority for questions related to the spelling of medical terms and the *Chicago Manual of Style* for questions related to grammatical structures, punctuation, and other editorial concerns. Consistent adherence is not always possible, however, because the individual volumes within the *Series* include many documents from a wide variety of different producers, and the editor's primary goal is to present material from each source as accurately as is possible. This sometimes means that information in different chapters or sections may follow other guidelines and alternate spelling authorities.

Medical Review

Omnigraphics contracts with a team of qualified, senior medical professionals who serve as medical consultants for the *Health Reference Series*. As necessary, medical consultants review reprinted and originally written material for currency and accuracy. Citations including the phrase, "Reviewed (month, year)" indicate material reviewed by this team. Medical consultation services are provided to the *Health Reference Series* editors by:

Dr. Vijayalakshmi, MBBS, DGO, MD
Dr. Senthil Selvan, MBBS, DCH, MD
Dr. K. Sivanandham, MBBS, DCH, MS (Research), PhD

Our Advisory Board

We would like to thank the following board members for providing initial guidance on the development of this series:

- Dr. Lynda Baker, Associate Professor of Library and Information Science, Wayne State University, Detroit, MI

- Nancy Bulgarelli, William Beaumont Hospital Library, Royal Oak, MI

- Karen Imarisio, Bloomfield Township Public Library, Bloomfield Township, MI

- Karen Morgan, Mardigian Library, University of Michigan-Dearborn, Dearborn, MI

- Rosemary Orlando, St. Clair Shores Public Library, St. Clair Shores, MI

Health Reference Series *Update Policy*

The inaugural book in the *Health Reference Series* was the first edition of *Cancer Sourcebook* published in 1989. Since then, the *Series* has been enthusiastically received by librarians and in the medical community. In order to maintain the standard of providing high-quality health information for the layperson the editorial staff at Omnigraphics felt it was necessary to implement a policy of updating volumes when warranted.

Medical researchers have been making tremendous strides, and it is the purpose of the *Health Reference Series* to stay current with the most recent advances. Each decision to update a volume is made on an individual basis. Some of the considerations include how much new information is available and the feedback we receive from people who use the books. If there is a topic you would like to see added to the update list, or an area of medical concern you feel has not been adequately addressed, please write to:

Managing Editor
Health Reference Series
Omnigraphics
615 Griswold, Ste. 901
Detroit, MI 48226

Part One

Understanding Cardiovascular Risks and Emergencies

Chapter 1

How the Heart Works

About the Cardiovascular System

The heart and circulatory system (also called the **cardiovascular system**) make up the network that delivers blood to the body's tissues. With each heartbeat, blood is sent throughout our bodies, carrying oxygen and nutrients to all of our cells.

Every day, the approximately 10 pints (5 liters) of blood in your body travel many times through about 60,000 miles (96,560 kilometers) of blood vessels that branch and cross, linking the cells of our organs and body parts. From the hard-working heart, to our thickest arteries, to capillaries so thin that they can only be seen through a microscope, the cardiovascular system is our body's lifeline.

The circulatory system is composed of the heart and blood vessels, including arteries, veins, and capillaries. Our bodies actually have two circulatory systems: The **pulmonary circulation** is a short loop from the heart to the lungs and back again, and the **systemic circulation** (the system we usually think of as our circulatory system) sends blood from the heart to all the other parts of our bodies and back again.

The Heart

The heart is the key organ in the circulatory system. As a hollow, muscular pump, its main function is to propel blood throughout the body. It usually beats from 60 to 100 times per minute, but can go much faster when it needs to. It beats about 100,000 times a day, more than 30 million times per year, and about 2.5 billion times in a 70-year lifetime.

The heart gets messages from the body that tell it when to pump more or less blood depending on a person's needs. When we're sleeping, it pumps just enough to provide for the lower amounts of oxygen needed by our bodies at rest. When we're exercising or frightened, the heart pumps faster to get more oxygen to our bodies.

The heart has four chambers that are enclosed by thick, muscular walls. It lies between the lungs and just to the left of the middle of the chest cavity. The bottom part of the heart is divided into two chambers called the **right** and **left ventricles**, which pump blood out of the heart. A wall called the **interventricular septum** divides the ventricles.

The upper part of the heart is made up of the other two chambers of the heart, called the right and left atria. The **right** and **left atria** receive the blood entering the heart. A wall called the **interatrial septum** divides the atria, and they're separated from the ventricles by the **atrioventricular valves**. The **tricuspid valve** separates the right atrium from the right ventricle, and the **mitral valve** separates the left atrium and the left ventricle.

Two other heart valves separate the ventricles and the large blood vessels that carry blood leaving the heart. These valves are called the **pulmonic valve**, which separates the right ventricle from the **pulmonary artery** leading to the lungs, and the **aortic valve**, which separates the left ventricle from the **aorta**, the body's largest blood vessel.

The Role of Blood Vessels

Blood vessels carrying blood away from the heart are called **arteries**. They are the thickest blood vessels, with muscular walls that contract to keep the blood moving away from the heart and through the body. In the systemic circulation, oxygen-rich blood is pumped from the heart into the aorta. This huge artery curves up and back from the left ventricle, then heads down in front of the spinal column into the abdomen. Two **coronary arteries** branch off at the beginning of the aorta and divide into a network of smaller arteries that provide oxygen and nourishment to the muscles of the heart.

Unlike the aorta, the body's other main artery, the pulmonary artery, carries oxygen-poor blood. From the right ventricle, the

pulmonary artery divides into right and left branches, on the way to the lungs where blood picks up oxygen.

Arterial walls have three layers:

- The **endothelium** is on the inside and provides a smooth lining for blood to flow over as it moves through the artery.

- The **media** is the middle part of the artery, made up of a layer of muscle and elastic tissue.

- The **adventitia** is the tough covering that protects the outside of the artery.

As they get farther from the heart, the arteries branch out into **arterioles**, which are smaller and less flexible.

Blood vessels that carry blood back to the heart are called veins. They are not as muscular as arteries, but they contain valves that prevent blood from flowing backward. Veins have the same three layers that arteries do, but they are thinner and less flexible. The two largest veins are the **superior** and **inferior vena cavae**. The terms superior and inferior do not mean that one vein is better than the other, but that they are located above (superior) and below (inferior) the heart.

A network of tiny **capillaries** connects the arteries and veins. Even though they're tiny, the capillaries are one of the most important parts of the circulatory system because it is through them that nutrients and oxygen are delivered to the cells. In addition, waste products such as carbon dioxide are also removed by the capillaries.

What the Heart and Circulatory System Do

The circulatory system works closely with other systems in our bodies. It supplies oxygen and nutrients to our bodies by working with the respiratory system. At the same time, the circulatory system helps carry waste and carbon dioxide out of the body. Hormones—produced by the endocrine system—are also transported through the blood in our circulatory system. As the body's chemical messengers, hormones transfer information and instructions from one set of cells to another.

Did you ever wonder about the process behind your beating heart? A healthy heart makes a "lub-dub" sound with each beat. Here's what happens to make that sound: One complete heartbeat makes up a cardiac cycle, which consists of two phases. In the first phase, the ventricles contract (this is called **systole**), sending blood into the pulmonary and systemic circulation. To prevent the flow of blood backwards into the atria during systole, the atrioventricular valves close, creating the first ("lub") sound.

When the ventricles finish contracting, the aortic and pulmonic valves close to prevent blood from flowing back into the ventricles. This is what creates the second sound (the "dub"). Then the ventricles relax (this is called **diastole**) and fill with blood from the atria, which makes up the second phase of the cardiac cycle.

A unique electrical system in the heart causes it to beat in its regular rhythm. The **sinoatrial** or **SA node**, a small area of tissue in the wall of the right atrium, sends out an electrical signal to start the contracting of the heart muscle. These electrical impulses cause the atria to contract first; they then travel down to the **atrioventricular** or **AV node**, which acts as a kind of relay station. From here the electrical signal travels through the right and left ventricles, causing them to contract and force blood out into the major arteries.

In the systemic circulation, blood travels out of the left ventricle, to the aorta, to every organ and tissue in the body, and then back to the right atrium. The arteries, capillaries, and veins of the systemic circulatory system are the channels through which this long journey takes place. Once in the arteries, blood flows to smaller arterioles and then to capillaries.

While in the capillaries, the bloodstream delivers oxygen and nutrients to the body's cells and picks up waste materials. Blood then goes back through the capillaries into venules, and then to larger veins until it reaches the vena cavae. Blood from the head and arms returns to the heart through the superior vena cava, and blood from the lower parts of the body returns through the inferior vena cava. Both vena cavae deliver this oxygen-depleted blood into the right atrium. From here the blood exits to fill the right ventricle, ready to be pumped into the pulmonary circulation for more oxygen.

In the pulmonary circulation, blood low in oxygen but high in carbon dioxide is pumped out the right ventricle into the pulmonary artery, which branches off in two directions. The right branch goes to the right lung, and vice versa. In the lungs, the branches divide further into capillaries. Blood flows more slowly through these tiny vessels, allowing time for gases to be exchanged between the capillary walls and the millions of **alveoli**, the tiny air sacs in the lung.

During the process called oxygenation, oxygen is taken up by the bloodstream. Oxygen locks onto a molecule called hemoglobin in the red blood cells. The newly oxygenated blood leaves the lungs through the pulmonary veins and heads back to the heart. It enters the heart in the left atrium, then fills the left ventricle so it can be pumped into the systemic circulation.

Things That Can Go Wrong

Problems with the cardiovascular system are common—more than 64 million Americans have some type of cardiac problem. But cardiovascular problems don't just affect older people—many heart and circulatory system problems affect teens, too.

Heart and circulatory problems are grouped into two categories: congenital, which means the problems were present at birth, and acquired, which means that the problems developed some time after birth.

Congenital heart defects. Congenital heart defects are heart problems that babies have at birth. Congenital heart defects occur while a baby is developing in the mother's uterus. Doctors don't always know why congenital heart defects occur—some congenital heart defects are caused by genetic disorders, but most are not. A common sign of a congenital heart defect is a **heart murmur.** A heart murmur is an abnormal sound (like a blowing or whooshing sound) that's heard when listening to the heart. Lots of kids and teens have heart murmurs, which can be caused by congenital heart defects or other heart conditions.

Arrhythmia. Cardiac arrhythmias, which are also called dysrhythmias or rhythm disorders, are problems in the rhythm of the heartbeat. Arrhythmias may be caused by a congenital heart defect or a person may develop this condition later. An arrhythmia may cause the heart's rhythm to be irregular, abnormally fast, or abnormally slow. But, some arrhythmias are not harmful. Arrhythmias can happen at any age and may be discovered when a teen has a checkup.

Cardiomyopathy. Cardiomyopathy is a long-lasting disease that causes the heart muscle (the myocardium) to become weakened. Usually, the disease first affects the lower chambers of the heart, the ventricles, and then progresses and damages the muscle cells and even the tissues surrounding the heart. Some kids and teens with cardiomyopathy may receive heart transplants to treat their condition.

Coronary artery disease. Coronary artery disease is the most common heart disorder in adults, and it's caused by atherosclerosis. Deposits of fat, calcium, and dead cells form on the inner walls and clog up the body's arteries—in this case, the coronary arteries (the blood vessels that supply the heart)—and get in the way of the smooth flow of blood. A clot of blood may even form, which can lead to a heart attack. Heart attacks are very rare in kids and teens.

Hypercholesterolemia (high cholesterol). Cholesterol is a waxy substance that is found in the body's cells, in the blood, and in some of the foods we eat. Having too much cholesterol in the blood, also known as hypercholesterolemia or hyperlipidemia, is a major risk factor for heart disease and can lead to a heart attack.

Hypertension (high blood pressure). Hypertension is when a person has blood pressure that's significantly higher than normal. Over time, it can cause damage to the heart and arteries and other body organs. Teens can have high blood pressure, which may be caused by genetic factors, excess body weight, diet, lack of exercise, and diseases such as heart disease or kidney disease.

Rheumatic heart disease. Teens who have had strep throat infection may develop rheumatic fever. This type of infection can cause permanent heart problems, mostly in kids and teens between 5 and 15 years of age. People who've had strep throat and received antibiotics right away are unlikely to develop this problem.

So what can you do to halt heart and circulatory problems before they start? Getting plenty of exercise, eating a nutritious diet, maintaining a healthy weight, and seeing your doctor regularly for medical checkups are the best ways to help keep the heart healthy and avoid long-term problems like high blood pressure, high cholesterol, and heart disease.

Chapter 2

Risk Factors for Cardiovascular Disorders

Chapter Contents

Section 2.1

Coronary Heart Disease Risk Factors

This section includes text excerpted from "Coronary Heart Disease Risk Factors," National Heart, Lung, and Blood Institute (NHLBI), October 23, 2015.

What Are Coronary Heart Disease Risk Factors?

Coronary heart disease risk factors are conditions or habits that raise your risk of coronary heart disease (CHD) and heart attack. These risk factors also increase the chance that existing CHD will worsen.

CHD, also called coronary artery disease, is a condition in which a waxy substance called plaque builds up on the inner walls of the coronary arteries. These arteries supply oxygen-rich blood to your heart muscle.

Plaque narrows the arteries and reduces blood flow to your heart muscle. Reduced blood flow can cause chest pain, especially when you're active. Eventually, an area of plaque can rupture (break open). This causes a blood clot to form on the surface of the plaque.

If the clot becomes large enough, it can block the flow of oxygen-rich blood to the portion of heart muscle fed by the artery. Blocked blood flow to the heart muscle causes a heart attack.

Coronary Heart Disease Risk Factors

High Blood Cholesterol and Triglyceride Levels

Cholesterol

High blood cholesterol is a condition in which your blood has too much cholesterol—a waxy, fat-like substance. The higher your blood cholesterol level, the greater your risk of coronary heart disease (CHD) and heart attack.

Cholesterol travels through the bloodstream in small packages called lipoproteins. Two major kinds of lipoproteins carry cholesterol throughout your body:

- Low-density lipoproteins (LDL). LDL cholesterol sometimes is called "bad" cholesterol. This is because it carries cholesterol to tissues, including your heart arteries. A high LDL cholesterol level raises your risk of CHD.

- High-density lipoproteins (HDL). HDL cholesterol sometimes is called "good" cholesterol. This is because it helps remove cholesterol from your arteries. A low HDL cholesterol level raises your risk of CHD.

Many factors affect your cholesterol levels. For example, after menopause, women's LDL cholesterol levels tend to rise, and their HDL cholesterol levels tend to fall. Other factors—such as age, gender, diet, and physical activity—also affect your cholesterol levels.

Healthy levels of both LDL and HDL cholesterol will prevent plaque from building up in your arteries. Routine blood tests can show whether your blood cholesterol levels are healthy. Talk with your doctor about having your cholesterol tested and what the results mean.

Children also can have unhealthy cholesterol levels, especially if they're overweight or their parents have high blood cholesterol. Talk with your child's doctor about testing your child' cholesterol levels.

Triglycerides

Triglycerides are a type of fat found in the blood. Some studies suggest that a high level of triglycerides in the blood may raise the risk of CHD, especially in women.

High Blood Pressure

"Blood pressure" is the force of blood pushing against the walls of your arteries as your heart pumps blood. If this pressure rises and stays high over time, it can damage your heart and lead to plaque buildup. All levels above 120/80 mmHg raise your risk of CHD. This risk grows as blood pressure levels rise. Only one of the two blood pressure numbers has to be above normal to put you at greater risk of CHD and heart attack.

Most adults should have their blood pressure checked at least once a year. If you have high blood pressure, you'll likely need to be checked more often. Talk with your doctor about how often you should have your blood pressure checked.

11

Children also can develop high blood pressure, especially if they're overweight. Your child's doctor should check your child's blood pressure at each routine checkup.

Both children and adults are more likely to develop high blood pressure if they're overweight or have diabetes.

Diabetes and Prediabetes

Diabetes is a disease in which the body's blood sugar level is too high. The two types of diabetes are type 1 and type 2.

In type 1 diabetes, the body's blood sugar level is high because the body doesn't make enough insulin. Insulin is a hormone that helps move blood sugar into cells, where it's used for energy. In type 2 diabetes, the body's blood sugar level is high mainly because the body doesn't use its insulin properly.

Over time, a high blood sugar level can lead to increased plaque buildup in your arteries. Having diabetes doubles your risk of CHD.

Prediabetes is a condition in which your blood sugar level is higher than normal, but not as high as it is in diabetes. If you have prediabetes and don't take steps to manage it, you'll likely develop type 2 diabetes within 10 years. You're also at higher risk of CHD.

Being overweight or obese raises your risk of type 2 diabetes. With modest weight loss and moderate physical activity, people who have prediabetes may be able to delay or prevent type 2 diabetes. They also may be able to lower their risk of CHD and heart attack. Weight loss and physical activity also can help control diabetes.

Even children can develop type 2 diabetes. Most children who have type 2 diabetes are overweight.

Type 2 diabetes develops over time and sometimes has no symptoms. Go to your doctor or local clinic to have your blood sugar levels tested regularly to check for diabetes and prediabetes.

Overweight and Obesity

The terms "overweight" and "obesity" refer to body weight that's greater than what is considered healthy for a certain height. More than two-thirds of American adults are overweight, and almost one-third of these adults are obese.

The most useful measure of overweight and obesity is body mass index (BMI).

Overweight is defined differently for children and teens than it is for adults. Children are still growing, and boys and girls mature at different rates. Thus, BMIs for children and teens compare their heights and weights against growth charts that take age and gender into account. This is called BMI-for-age percentile.

Being overweight or obese can raise your risk of CHD and heart attack. This is mainly because overweight and obesity are linked to other CHD risk factors, such as high blood cholesterol and triglyceride levels, high blood pressure, and diabetes.

Smoking

Smoking tobacco or long-term exposure to secondhand smoke raises your risk of CHD and heart attack.

Smoking triggers a buildup of plaque in your arteries. Smoking also increases the risk of blood clots forming in your arteries. Blood clots can block plaque-narrowed arteries and cause a heart attack. Some research shows that smoking raises your risk of CHD in part by lowering HDL cholesterol levels.

The more you smoke, the greater your risk of heart attack. The benefits of quitting smoking occur no matter how long or how much you've smoked. Heart disease risk associated with smoking begins to decrease soon after you quit, and for many people it continues to decrease over time.

Most people who smoke start when they're teens. Parents can help prevent their children from smoking by not smoking themselves. Talk with your child about the health dangers of smoking and ways to overcome peer pressure to smoke.

Lack of Physical Activity

Inactive people are nearly twice as likely to develop CHD as those who are active. A lack of physical activity can worsen other CHD risk factors, such as high blood cholesterol and triglyceride levels, high blood pressure, diabetes and prediabetes, and overweight and obesity.

It's important for children and adults to make physical activity part of their daily routines. One reason many Americans aren't active enough is because of hours spent in front of TVs and computers doing work, schoolwork, and leisure activities.

Some experts advise that children and teens should reduce screen time because it limits time for physical activity. They recommend that children aged 2 and older should spend no more than 2 hours a day watching TV or using a computer (except for school work).

Being physically active is one of the most important things you can do to keep your heart healthy. The good news is that even modest amounts of physical activity are good for your health. The more active you are, the more you will benefit.

Unhealthy Diet

An unhealthy diet can raise your risk of CHD. For example, foods that are high in saturated and trans fats and cholesterol raise LDL cholesterol. Thus, you should try to limit these foods.

It's also important to limit foods that are high in sodium (salt) and added sugars. A high-salt diet can raise your risk of high blood pressure.

Added sugars will give you extra calories without nutrients like vitamins and minerals. This can cause you to gain weight, which raises your risk of CHD. Added sugars are found in many desserts, canned fruits packed in syrup, fruit drinks, and nondiet sodas.

Stress

Stress and anxiety may play a role in causing CHD. Stress and anxiety also can trigger your arteries to tighten. This can raise your blood pressure and your risk of heart attack.

The most commonly reported trigger for a heart attack is an emotionally upsetting event, especially one involving anger. Stress also may indirectly raise your risk of CHD if it makes you more likely to smoke or overeat foods high in fat and sugar.

Age

In men, the risk for coronary heart disease (CHD) increases starting around age 45. In women, the risk for CHD increases starting around age 55. Most people have some plaque buildup in their heart arteries by the time they're in their 70s. However, only about 25 percent of those people have chest pain, heart attacks, or other signs of CHD.

Gender

Some risk factors may affect CHD risk differently in women than in men. For example, estrogen provides women some protection against CHD, whereas diabetes raises the risk of CHD more in women than in men.

Also, some risk factors for heart disease only affect women, such as preeclampsia, a condition that can develop during pregnancy.

Preeclampsia is linked to an increased lifetime risk of heart disease, including CHD, heart attack, heart failure, and high blood pressure. (Likewise, having heart disease risk factors, such as diabetes or obesity, increases a woman's risk of preeclampsia.)

Family History

A family history of early CHD is a risk factor for developing CHD, specifically if a father or brother is diagnosed before age 55, or a mother or sister is diagnosed before age 65.

Section 2.2

Risk Factors for Stroke

This section includes text excerpted from "Stroke," National Heart, Lung, and Blood Institute (NHLBI), October 28, 2015.

Who Is at Risk for a Stroke?

Certain traits, conditions, and habits can raise your risk of having a stroke or transient ischemic attack (TIA). These traits, conditions, and habits are known as risk factors.

The more risk factors you have, the more likely you are to have a stroke. You can treat or control some risk factors, such as high blood pressure and smoking. Other risk factors, such as age and gender, you can't control.

The major risk factors for stroke include:

- **High blood pressure.** High blood pressure is the main risk factor for stroke. Blood pressure is considered high if it stays at or above 140/90 millimeters of mercury (mmHg) over time. If you have diabetes or chronic kidney disease, high blood pressure is defined as 130/80 mmHg or higher.

- **Diabetes.** Diabetes is a disease in which the blood sugar level is high because the body doesn't make enough insulin or doesn't use its insulin properly. Insulin is a hormone that helps move blood sugar into 5 cells where it's used for energy.

- **Heart diseases.** Coronary heart disease, cardiomyopathy, heart failure, and atrial fibrillation can cause blood clots that can lead to a stroke.

- **Smoking.** Smoking can damage blood vessels and raise blood pressure. Smoking also may reduce the amount of oxygen that reaches your body's tissues. Exposure to secondhand smoke also can damage the blood vessels.

- **Age and gender.** Your risk of stroke increases as you get older. At younger ages, men are more likely than women to have strokes. However, women are more likely to die from strokes. Women who take birth control pills also are at slightly higher risk of stroke.

- **Race and ethnicity.** Strokes occur more often in African American, Alaska Native, and American Indian adults than in white, Hispanic, or Asian American adults.

- **Personal or family history of stroke or TIA.** If you've had a stroke, you're at higher risk for another one. Your risk of having a repeat stroke is the highest right after a stroke. A TIA also increases your risk of having a stroke, as does having a family history of stroke.

- **Brain aneurysms or arteriovenous malformations (AVMs).** Aneurysms are balloon-like bulges in an artery that can stretch and burst. AVMs are tangles of faulty arteries and veins that can rupture (break open) within the brain. AVMs may be present at birth but often aren't diagnosed until they rupture.

Other risk factors for stroke, many of which of you can control, include:

- Alcohol and illegal drug use, including cocaine, amphetamines, and other drugs

- Certain medical conditions, such as sickle cell disease, vasculitis (inflammation of the blood vessels), and bleeding disorders

- Lack of physical activity

- Overweight and Obesity

- Stress and depression

- Unhealthy cholesterol levels

- Unhealthy diet

- Use of nonsteroidal anti-inflammatory drugs (NSAIDs), but not aspirin, may increase the risk of heart attack or stroke, particularly in patients who have had a heart attack or cardiac bypass surgery. The risk may increase the longer NSAIDs are used. Common NSAIDs include ibuprofen and naproxen.

Following a healthy lifestyle can lower the risk of stroke. Some people also may need to take medicines to lower their risk. Sometimes strokes can occur in people who don't have any known risk factors.

Section 2.3

Smoking and Cardiovascular Disease

This section includes text excerpted from "Smoking and Cardiovascular Disease," Centers for Disease Control and Prevention (CDC), October 15, 2014.

What You Need to Know about Smoking and Cardiovascular Disease

Smoking is a major cause of cardiovascular disease (CVD) and causes one of every three deaths from CVD, according to the 2014 Surgeon General's Report on smoking and health. CVD is the single largest cause of death in the United States, killing more than 800,000 people a year. More than 16 million Americans have heart disease. Almost 8 million have had a heart attack and 7 million have had a stroke.

Even people who smoke fewer than five cigarettes a day may show signs of early CVD. The risk of CVD increases with the number of cigarettes smoked per day, and when smoking continues for many years. Smoking cigarettes with lower levels of tar or nicotine does not reduce the risk for cardiovascular disease.

Exposure to secondhand smoke causes heart disease in nonsmokers. More than 33,000 nonsmokers die every year in the United States from coronary heart disease caused by exposure to secondhand smoke. Exposure to secondhand smoke can also cause heart attacks and strokes in nonsmokers.

How Smoking Harms the Cardiovascular System

Chemicals in cigarette smoke cause the cells that line blood vessels to become swollen and inflamed. This can narrow the blood vessels and can lead to many cardiovascular conditions.

- **Atherosclerosis,** in which arteries narrow and become less flexible, occurs when fat, cholesterol, and other substances in the blood form plaque that builds up in the walls of arteries. The opening inside the arteries narrows as plaque builds up, and blood can no longer flow properly to various parts of the body. Smoking increases the formation of plaque in blood vessels.

- **Coronary Heart Disease** occurs when arteries that carry blood to the heart muscle are narrowed by plaque or blocked by clots. Chemicals in cigarette smoke cause the blood to thicken and form clots inside veins and arteries. Blockage from a clot can lead to a heart attack and sudden death.

- **Stroke** is a loss of brain function caused when blood flow within the brain is interrupted. Strokes can cause permanent brain damage and death. Smoking increases the risk for strokes. Deaths from strokes are more likely among smokers than among former smokers or people who have never smoked.

- **Peripheral Arterial Disease (PAD)** and **peripheral vascular disease** occur when blood vessels become narrower and the flow of blood to arms, legs, hands and feet is reduced. Cells and tissue are deprived of needed oxygen when blood flow is reduced. In extreme cases, an infected limb must be removed. Smoking is the most common preventable cause of PAD.

- **Abdominal Aortic Aneurysm** is a bulge or weakened area that occurs in the portion of the aorta that is in the abdomen. The aorta is the main artery that carries oxygen-rich blood throughout the body. Smoking is a known cause of early damage to the abdominal aorta, which can lead to an aneurysm. A ruptured abdominal aortic aneurysm is life-threatening; almost all deaths from abdominal aortic aneurysms are caused by smoking. Women smokers have a higher risk of dying from an aortic aneurysm than men who smoke. Autopsies have shown early narrowing of the abdominal aorta in young adults who smoked as adolescents.

Quitting Smoking Cuts CVD Risks

Even though we don't know exactly which smokers will develop CVD from smoking, the best thing all smokers can do for their hearts is to quit. Smokers who quit start to improve their heart health and reduce their risk for CVD immediately. Within a year, the risk of heart attack drops dramatically, and even people who have already had a heart attack can cut their risk of having another if they quit smoking. Within five years of quitting, smokers lower their risk of stroke to about that of a person who has never smoked.

Chapter 3

Conditions That Increase the Risk of Cardiovascular Disorders

Chapter Contents

Section 3.1

Depression and Heart Disease

This section includes text excerpted from "Depression and Heart Disease," National Institute of Mental Health (NIMH), 2011. Reviewed June 2016.

What Is Depression?

Major depressive disorder, or depression, is a serious mental illness. Depression interferes with your daily life and routine and reduces your quality of life. About 6.7 percent of U.S. adults ages 18 and older have depression.

Signs and Symptoms of Depression

- Ongoing sad, anxious, or empty feelings

- Feeling hopeless

- Feeling guilty, worthless, or helpless

- Feeling irritable or restless

- Loss of interest in activities or hobbies once enjoyable, including sex

- Feeling tired all the time

- Difficulty concentrating, remembering details, or making decisions

- Difficulty falling asleep or staying asleep, a condition called insomnia, or sleeping all the time

- Overeating or loss of appetite

- Thoughts of death and suicide or suicide attempts

- Ongoing aches and pains, headaches, cramps, or digestive problems that do not ease with treatment.

What Is Heart Disease?

Heart disease refers to a number of illnesses that affect your heart and nearby blood vessels. Your heart is a muscle that pumps blood through your body. Like any muscle, your heart needs a constant supply of oxygen and nutrients, which it gets from blood pumped from the lungs and other parts of the body. Blood vessels carry this oxygen- and nutrient-rich blood to the heart.

If not enough blood reaches your heart, you may feel a pain in your chest called angina. You may also feel angina pain in the left arm and shoulder, neck, or jaw. You may not always feel angina when your heart is not getting enough blood. A heart attack occurs when the blood supply to your heart is cut off completely. If blood flow isn't quickly restored, the part of your heart that does not receive oxygen begins to die. While some heart muscle may be permanently damaged, quick treatment can limit the harm and save your life.

How Are Depression and Heart Disease Linked?

People with heart disease are more likely to suffer from depression than otherwise healthy people. Angina and heart attacks are closely linked with depression. Researchers are unsure exactly why this occurs. They do know that some symptoms of depression may reduce your overall physical and mental health, increasing your risk for heart disease or making symptoms of heart disease worse. Fatigue or feelings of worthlessness may cause you to ignore your medication plan and avoid treatment for heart disease. Having depression increases your risk of death after a heart attack.

How Is Depression Treated in People Who Have Heart Disease?

Depression is diagnosed and treated by a healthcare provider. Treating depression can help you manage heart disease and improve your overall health. Recovery from depression takes time but treatments are effective.

At present, the most common treatments for depression include:

- Cognitive behavioral therapy (CBT), a type of psychotherapy, or talk therapy, that helps people change negative thinking styles and behaviors that may contribute to their depression

- Selective serotonin reuptake inhibitor (SSRI), a type of antidepressant medication that includes citalopram (Celexa), sertraline (Zoloft), and fluoxetine (Prozac)

- Serotonin and norepinephrine reuptake inhibitor (SNRI), a type of antidepressant medication similar to SSRI that includes venlafaxine (Effexor) and duloxetine (Cymbalta).

While currently available depression treatments are generally well tolerated and safe, talk with your healthcare provider about side effects, possible drug interactions, and other treatment options. Medications can take several weeks to work, may need to be combined with ongoing talk therapy, or may need to be changed or adjusted to minimize side effects and achieve the best results.

Treating your depression may make it easier for you to follow a longterm heart disease treatment plan and make the lifestyle changes required to manage your heart disease, including:

- Eating healthy foods

- Exercising regularly

- Drinking less alcohol, or none at all

- Quitting smoking.

Some people may also need to take heart medications or have surgery to treat heart disease.

Regular exercise not only protects you against heart disease, it may also help reduce depression. One study found that an exercise training program was as effective as an SSRI in improving the symptoms of depression among older adults diagnosed with the disease. Your healthcare provider can recommend safe exercises and activities suitable for you.

Section 3.2

Diabetes and Cardiovascular Disease

This section contains text excerpted from the following
sources: Text beginning with the heading "How Can Diabetes
Affect Cardiovascular Health?" is excerpted from "Managing
Diabetes," Centers for Disease Control and Prevention (CDC),
September 25, 2015; Text beginning with the heading "Reduce
Cardiovascular Disease Risk" is excerpted from "Principle 7: Reduce
Cardiovascular Disease Risk," National Institute of Diabetes and
Digestive and Kidney Diseases (NIDDK), November 9, 2014.

How Can Diabetes Affect Cardiovascular Health?

Cardiovascular disease is the leading cause of early death among
people with diabetes. Adults with diabetes are two to four times more
likely than people without diabetes to die of heart disease or experience a stroke. Also, about 70% of people with diabetes have high blood
pressure, a risk factor for cardiovascular disease.

How Are Cholesterol, Triglyceride, Weight, and Blood Pressure Problems Related to Diabetes

People with type 2 diabetes have high rates of cholesterol and triglyceride abnormalities, obesity, and high blood pressure, all of which
are major contributors to higher rates of cardiovascular disease. Many
people with diabetes have several of these conditions at the same time.
This combination of problems is often called metabolic syndrome (for-
merly known as Syndrome X). The metabolic syndrome is often defined
as the presence of any three of the following conditions:

1. excess weight around the waist;

2. high levels of triglycerides;

3. low levels of HDL, or "good," cholesterol;

4. high blood pressure; and

5. high fasting blood glucose levels.

If you have one or more of these conditions, you are at an increased risk for having one or more of the others. The more conditions that you have, the greater the risk to your health.

How Can I Be "Heart Healthy" and Avoid Cardiovascular Disease If I Have Diabetes?

To protect your heart and blood vessels, eat right, get physical activity, don't smoke, and maintain healthy blood glucose, blood pressure, and cholesterol levels. Choose a healthy diet, low in salt. Work with a dietitian to plan healthy meals. If you're overweight, talk about how to safely lose weight. Ask about a physical activity or exercise program. Quit smoking if you currently do. Get a hemoglobin A1C test at least twice a year to determine what your average blood glucose level was for the past 2 to 3 months. Get your blood pressure checked at every doctor's visit, and get your cholesterol checked at least once a year. Take medications if prescribed by your doctor.

Reduce Cardiovascular Disease Risk

Hypertension and dyslipidemia commonly coexist with type 2 diabetes and are clear risk factors for cardiovascular disease (CVD), and diabetes itself confers independent risk. Because of their increased CVD risk, management of hypertension and cholesterol is particularly important for people with type 2 diabetes.Increased CVD risk also increases the importance of lifestyle modification, including abstinence from smoking. Extensive trial evidence shows the efficacy of targeted treatment of hypertension and statin therapy in the prevention and management of CVD in people with type 2 diabetes.

Although clinical trials to address blood pressure targets and statin therapy have not been conducted in people with type 1 diabetes, attention to CVD risk factors may be particularly important in people with type 1 diabetes because of their high CVD risk.

Evidence for Blood Pressure Control

Although epidemiologic studies suggest that blood pressure higher than 115/75 mmHg is associated with progressive increases in CVD events and mortality in people with diabetes, randomized clinical trials have not demonstrated that lowering blood pressure to less than 140/80 mmHg provides a significant clinical benefit in type 2 diabetes. The United Kingdom Prospective Diabetes Study (UKPDS) found that blood pressure control that targeted less than 150/85 mmHg (achieved 144/82 mmHg) significantly reduced risk for diabetes-related deaths, stroke, heart failure, microvascular disease, retinopathy progression, and deterioration of vision in people with type 2 diabetes compared to a target of 180/105 mmHg.The Hypertension Optimal Treatment (HOT) trial found a 51 percent reduction in major CVD events in people with diabetes at a diastolic goal of 80 mmHg compared with 90 mmHg.

The Action to Control Cardiovascular Risk in Diabetes (ACCORD) trial found no substantial advantage in lowering systolic blood pressure to less than 120 mmHg compared to less than 140 mmHg in people with type 2 diabetes, and found a higher risk of serious adverse events with lower blood pressure targets.A meta-analysis of randomized trials in adults with type 2 diabetes found that the use of intensive blood pressure targets (upper limit of 130 mmHg systolic and 80 mmHg diastolic) was associated with a small but significant reduction in stroke but no significant decrease in mortality or myocardial infarction.

The Systolic Hypertension in the Elderly Program (SHEP) study found that diuretics reduced CVD death in people with diabetes by 31x converting enzyme (ACE) inhibitors have been shown to provide substantial benefits, including reduced risk of heart attack, stroke, and CVD death,and prevention of progression of nephropathy.The Action in Diabetes and Vascular Disease: Preterax and Diamicron MR Controlled Evaluation (ADVANCE) study assessed the effects of the routine administration of an ACE inhibitor-diuretic combination in people with diabetes and found a significant reduction in relative risk of major macrovascular or microvascular events, death from CVD, and death from any cause.

Blood Pressure Management

- Blood pressure should be measured at every routine medical visit.

- Consider home blood pressure monitoring when office/clinic measurements are borderline or elevated.

- The following strategies may have antihypertensive effects similar to pharmacologic monotherapy:

  - Reduce sodium intake by selecting low-sodium foods, not adding sodium to food, and limiting processed foods.

  - Reduce excess body weight by increasing consumption of fruits, vegetables, and low-fat dairy products; avoiding excessive alcohol consumption; and increasing activity levels.

- Follow the Dietary Approaches to Stop Hypertension (DASH) Eating Plan. (See Resources.)

- Engage in 40 minutes of aerobic physical activity at a moderate to vigorous intensity, at least 3 days a week.

- Referral to a registered dietitian/registered dietitian nutritionist can also be helpful.

Therapy Considerations

- People with a systolic blood pressure of 130 to 139 mmHg or a diastolic blood pressure of 80 to 89 mmHg may initially be treated with lifestyle therapy alone. Overweight people with higher blood pressure should receive both pharmacologic and lifestyle therapy at the time of diagnosis of hypertension.

- The primary goal of therapy is systolic blood pressure less than 140/90 mmHg. Lower blood pressure targets can be individualized, based upon shared decision making that addresses factors such as the level of CVD risk, presence of kidney disease, and burden of therapy.

- ACE inhibitors and angiotensin II receptor blockers (ARBs) are contraindicated in pregnancy.

Consider initial therapy with a thiazide, calcium channel blocker, ACE inhibitor, or an ARB. Multi-drug therapy (two or more agents at maximal doses) usually is required to achieve and maintain blood pressure targets. An ACE inhibitor or an ARB reduces progression of chronic kidney disease in people with albuminuria. Individualize further medication choices according to patient characteristics such as age, race, and response to therapy. Measure blood pressure at every health visit and adjust treatment as necessary.

Evidence for Statin Therapy

People with type 2 diabetes commonly have lipid patterns characterized by elevated triglyceride and reduced high-density lipoprotein cholesterol levels. Although their low-density lipoprotein (LDL) cholesterol values are generally not higher than those in non-diabetic individuals, they often have a greater number of smaller, denser, and more atherogenic LDL particles. Studies using the HMG-CoA reductase inhibitors (statins) have clearly shown that moderate to intensive statin therapy can reduce CVD events in people with diabetes.

Rather than targeting specific levels of LDL cholesterol, these studies have generally achieved 30 to 40 percent reductions from baseline LDL cholesterol levels. In people with diabetes over age 40 and with other CVD risk factors, moderate- to high-intensity statin therapy reduces CVD risk regardless of the baseline LDL cholesterol level.

Cholesterol Management

- Lifestyle modification to improve lipid profiles is indicated to reduce the risk of CVD in all people with diabetes. This involves actions to reduce intake of saturated fat, trans fat, and cholesterol; to increase intake of omega-3 fatty acids, viscous fiber, and plant stanols/sterols; to increase physical activity; and to reduce weight (if indicated).

- Statin therapy should be added to lifestyle therapy, regardless of baseline lipid levels, for people with diabetes who have overt CVD. Statin therapy should be considered in individuals with diabetes who are without overt CVD but are at substantial risk of developing CVD (e.g., over age 40).

- Risk of CVD is increased more in people with type 1 diabetes compared with type 2 diabetes, but it is not known if routine use of statins in people with type 1 diabetes under age 40 is useful for primary prevention of CVD.

- The strongest evidence for statin use is in people with diabetes who are 45 to 75 years old. Additional lipid-lowering medications have not been shown to reduce CVD risk in people with type 2 diabetes on statin therapy.

- Statins are contraindicated for women who are pregnant or considering pregnancy.

Statin therapy dosage should be carefully titrated according to individual responses to therapy and the occurrence of muscular and other side effects. Measurement of blood lipids may provide information on adherence to therapy. The small increase in the relative risk of developing diabetes with high dose statin therapy is outweighed by the major benefits of statin therapy in reducing CVD and mortality.

Multiple Risk Factor Reduction

In the Steno-2 Study, a target-driven, long-term, intensified intervention aimed at multiple risk factors in people with type 2 diabetes and microalbuminuria, the risk of cardiovascular and microvascular events was reduced by about 50 percent. This study demonstrated the value of comprehensively addressing CVD risk factors. Long-term follow-up of the participants found significant reductions in CVD deaths.

Anti-Platelet Therapy

Aspirin has been shown to be effective in reducing cardiovascular morbidity and mortality in high-risk people with diabetes and previous myocardial infarction or stroke (secondary prevention). Daily low-dose aspirin therapy (e.g., 75–81 mg) appears to have a modest effect at best on primary CVD prevention in patients with diabetes. In adults with 10-year coronary heart disease (CHD) risk lower than 10 percent (e.g., women under age 60 and men under age 50 without other CVD risk factors), the risk of bleeding may outweigh the atherosclerotic CVD benefits. Studies have not found a clear benefit of low-dose aspirin for primary prevention of atherosclerotic CVD in people without prior disease events.

- Use low-dose aspirin in adults with diabetes and a history of atherosclerotic CVD.

- In men over 50 and women over 60 with diabetes and other major atherosclerotic CVD risk factors, low-dose aspirin may be considered as a prevention strategy for cardiovascular events.

- For primary prevention of atherosclerotic CVD for people with diabetes, consider aspirin therapy in those who have a 10-year CHD risk of more than 10 percent.

Tobacco Use Cessation

Smoking more than doubles the risk for CVD in people with diabetes. While smokeless tobacco poses a lesser risk for CVD than cigarette smoking, all forms of tobacco should be discouraged. People who stop using tobacco greatly reduce their risk of premature death. Medications, counseling, telephone help lines, and smoking cessation programs increase a person's chances of success at stopping tobacco use. Additional effective therapies include nicotine replacement products (e.g., gum, inhaler, and patch).

Section 3.3

High Blood Pressure and Heart Disease

This section includes text excerpted from "High
Blood Pressure," National Heart, Lung, and Blood
Institute (NHLBI), September 10, 2015.

Description of High Blood Pressure

High blood pressure is a common disease in which blood flows
through blood vessels (arteries) at higher than normal pressures.

Measuring Blood Pressure

Blood pressure is the force of blood pushing against the walls of the
arteries as the heart pumps blood. High blood pressure, sometimes
called hypertension, happens when this force is too high. Healthcare
workers check blood pressure readings the same way for children,
teens, and adults. They use a gauge, stethoscope or electronic sensor,
and a blood pressure cuff. With this equipment, they measure:

- **Systolic Pressure:** blood pressure when the heart beats while
  pumping blood

- **Diastolic Pressure:** blood pressure when the heart is at rest
  between beats

Healthcare workers write blood pressure numbers with the systolic
number above the diastolic number. For example, 118/76 mmHg: people read "118 over 76" millimeters of mercury.

Normal Blood Pressure

Normal blood pressure for adults is defined as a systolic pressure
below 120 mmHg and a diastolic pressure below 80 mmHg. It is normal
for blood pressures to change when you sleep, wake up, or are excited
or nervous. When you are active, it is normal for your blood pressure to
increase. However, once the activity stops, your blood pressure returns
to your normal baseline range.

Blood pressure normally rises with age and body size. Newborn babies often have very low blood pressure numbers that are considered normal for babies, while older teens have numbers similar to adults.

Abnormal Blood Pressure

Abnormal increases in blood pressure are defined as having blood pressures higher than 120/80 mmHg. The following table outlines and defines high blood pressure severity levels.

Table 3.1. Stages of High Blood Pressure in Adults

Stages	Systolic (top number)		Diastolic (bottom number)
Prehypertension	120–139	OR	80–89
High blood pressure Stage 1	140–159	OR	90–99
High blood pressure Stage 2	160 or higher	OR	100 or higher

The ranges in the table are blood pressure guides for adults who do not have any short-term serious illnesses. **People with diabetes or chronic kidney disease should keep their blood pressure below 130/80 mmHg.**

Although blood pressure increases seen in prehypertension are less than those used to diagnose high blood pressure, prehypertension can progress to high blood pressure and should be taken seriously. Over time, consistently high blood pressure weakens and damages your blood vessels, which can lead to complications.

Types of High Blood Pressure

There are two main types of high blood pressure: primary and secondary high blood pressure.

1. Primary High Blood Pressure

Primary, or essential, high blood pressure is the most common type of high blood pressure. This type of high blood pressure tends to develop over years as a person ages.

2. Secondary High Blood Pressure

Secondary high blood pressure is caused by another medical condition or use of certain medicines. This type usually resolves after the cause is treated or removed.

Complications of High Blood Pressure

When blood pressure stays high over time, it can damage the body and cause complications. Some common complications and their signs and symptoms include:

- **Aneurysms:** When an abnormal bulge forms in the wall of an artery. Aneurysms develop and grow for years without causing signs or symptoms until they rupture, grow large enough to press on nearby body parts, or block blood flow. The signs and symptoms that develop depend on the location of the aneurysm.

- **Chronic Kidney Disease:** When blood vessels narrow in the kidneys, possibly causing kidney failure.

- **Cognitive Changes:** Research shows that over time, higher blood pressure numbers can lead to cognitive changes. Signs and symptoms include memory loss, difficulty finding words, and losing focus during conversations.

- **Eye Damage:** When blood vessels in the eyes burst or bleed. Signs and symptoms include vision changes or blindness.

- **Heart Attack:** When the flow of oxygen-rich blood to a section of heart muscle suddenly becomes blocked and the heart doesn't get oxygen. The most common warning symptoms of a heart attack are chest pain or discomfort, upper body discomfort, and shortness of breath.

- **Heart Failure:** When the heart can't pump enough blood to meet the body's needs. Common signs and symptoms of heart failure include shortness of breath or trouble breathing; feeling tired; and swelling in the ankles, feet, legs, abdomen, and veins in the neck.

- **Peripheral Artery Disease:** A disease in which plaque builds up in leg arteries and affects blood flow in the legs. When people have symptoms, the most common are pain, cramping, numbness, aching, or heaviness in the legs, feet, and buttocks after walking or climbing stairs.

- **Stroke:** When the flow of oxygen-rich blood to a portion of the brain is blocked. The symptoms of a stroke include sudden onset of weakness; paralysis or numbness of the face, arms, or legs; trouble speaking or understanding speech; and trouble seeing.

Section 3.4

High Cholesterol and Heart Disease

This section contains text excerpted from the following sources: Text under the heading "Cholesterol Facts" is excerpted from "Cholesterol Fact Sheet," Centers for Disease Control and Prevention (CDC), April 30, 2015; Text beginning with the heading "What is Cholesterol?" is excerpted from "High Blood Cholesterol," National Heart, Lung, and Blood Institute (NHLBI), March 30, 2016.

Cholesterol Facts

- Having high blood cholesterol puts you at risk of heart disease, the leading cause of death in the United States.

- People with high cholesterol have about **twice the risk** of heart disease as people with lower levels.

- Cholesterol is a waxy, fat-like substance. Your body needs some cholesterol, but it can build up on the walls of your arteries and lead to heart disease and stroke when you have too much in your blood.

- **71 million American adults (33.5%)** have high low-density lipoprotein (LDL), or "bad," cholesterol.

- Only **1 out of every 3** adults with high LDL cholesterol has the condition under control.

- **Less than half** of adults with high LDL cholesterol get treatment.

- Lowering your cholesterol can reduce your risk of having a heart attack, needing heart bypass surgery or angioplasty, and dying of heart disease.

- Exercising, eating a healthy diet, and not smoking will help you prevent high cholesterol and reduce your levels.

- High cholesterol has no symptoms, so many people don't know that their cholesterol is too high. Your doctor can do a simple blood test to check your levels. The National Cholesterol Education Program recommends that adults get their cholesterol checked every five years.

Table 3.2. Desirable Cholesterol Levels

Desirable Cholesterol Levels	
Total cholesterol	Less than 200 mg/dL
LDL ("bad" cholesterol)	Less than 100 mg/dL
HDL ("good" cholesterol)	60 mg/dL or higher
Triglycerides	Less than 150 mg/dL

What Is Cholesterol?

To understand high blood cholesterol, it helps to learn about cholesterol. Cholesterol is a waxy, fat-like substance that's found in all cells of the body.

Your body needs some cholesterol to make hormones, vitamin D, and substances that help you digest foods. Your body makes all the cholesterol it needs. However, cholesterol also is found in some of the foods you eat.

Cholesterol travels through your bloodstream in small packages called lipoproteins. These packages are made of fat (lipid) on the inside and proteins on the outside.

Two kinds of lipoproteins carry cholesterol throughout your body: low-density lipoproteins (LDL) and high-density lipoproteins (HDL). Having healthy levels of both types of lipoproteins is important.

LDL cholesterol sometimes is called "bad" cholesterol. A high LDL level leads to a buildup of cholesterol in your arteries. (Arteries are blood vessels that carry blood from your heart to your body.)

HDL cholesterol sometimes is called "good" cholesterol. This is because it carries cholesterol from other parts of your body back to your liver. Your liver removes the cholesterol from your body.

What Is High Blood Cholesterol?

High blood cholesterol is a condition in which you have too much cholesterol in your blood. By itself, the condition usually has no signs or symptoms. Thus, many people don't know that their cholesterol levels are too high.

People who have high blood cholesterol have a greater chance of getting coronary heart disease, also called coronary artery disease. (In this section, the term "heart disease" refers to coronary heart disease.)

The higher the level of LDL cholesterol in your blood, the GREATER your chance is of getting heart disease. The higher the level of HDL cholesterol in your blood, the LOWER your chance is of getting heart disease.

Coronary heart disease is a condition in which plaque builds up inside the coronary (heart) arteries. Plaque is made up of cholesterol, fat, calcium, and other substances found in the blood. When plaque builds up in the arteries, the condition is called atherosclerosis.

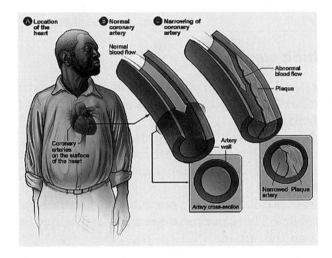

Figure 3.1. *Atherosclerosis*

(A) shows the location of the heart in the body. (B) shows a normal coronary artery with normal blood flow. The inset image shows a cross-section of a normal coronary artery. (C) shows a coronary artery narrowed by plaque. The buildup of plaque limits the flow of oxygen-rich blood through the artery. The inset image shows a cross-section of the plaque-narrowed artery.

Over time, plaque hardens and narrows your coronary arteries. This limits the flow of oxygen-rich blood to the heart.

Eventually, an area of plaque can rupture (break open). This causes a blood clot to form on the surface of the plaque. If the clot becomes large enough, it can mostly or completely block blood flow through a coronary artery.

If the flow of oxygen-rich blood to your heart muscle is reduced or blocked, angina or a heart attack may occur.

Angina is chest pain or discomfort. It may feel like pressure or squeezing in your chest. The pain also may occur in your shoulders, arms, neck, jaw, or back. Angina pain may even feel like indigestion.

A heart attack occurs if the flow of oxygen-rich blood to a section of heart muscle is cut off. If blood flow isn't restored quickly, the section of heart muscle begins to die.

Without quick treatment, a heart attack can lead to serious problems or death.

Plaque also can build up in other arteries in your body, such as the arteries that bring oxygen-rich blood to your brain and limbs. This can lead to problems such as carotid artery disease, stroke, and peripheral artery disease.

Outlook

Lowering your cholesterol may slow, reduce, or even stop the buildup of plaque in your arteries. It also may reduce the risk of plaque rupturing and causing dangerous blood clots.

Section 3.5

HIV and Heart Disease

This section includes text excerpted from "Cardiovascular Health," U.S. Department of Health and Human Services (HHS), March 19, 2016.

Good Heart Health Matters

Cardiovascular disease—or heart disease—is the leading cause of death in the United States for both men and women. Cardiovascular disease can include many different heart-related issues, including *heart attacks, strokes, coronary artery disease, congestive heart failure,* and *hypertension.* Each one of these diseases increases your risk of suffering a disabling health event, such as a major heart attack or stroke, and/or dying prematurely.

Evidence suggests that individuals with HIV have an increased chance of experiencing cardiovascular disease. A number of other factors are proven to increase your risk for cardiovascular disease:

- Alcohol use
- Age
- Depression
- Diabetes
- Diet that is high in saturated fats and sodium
- Family history of heart disease
- High blood cholesterol levels
- High blood pressure
- Obesity
- Other substance abuse
- Physical inactivity
- Tobacco use

HIV and Cardiovascular Disease

Since 1996, when *antiretroviral therapy* (ART) became available, people living with HIV have been living longer, healthier lives. However, as individuals with HIV age, they are more likely to be diagnosed with chronic illnesses. A growing body of evidence suggests cardiovascular disease in particular is a common occurrence in people over 40 living with HIV. Studies have shown that people living with HIV are 50-100% more likely to develop cardiovascular disease (including heart attack and stroke) than individuals without HIV.

A number of factors combine to put people with HIV at increased risk for cardiovascular disease.

- First, **HIV infection itself** increases your risk for cardiovascular disease. The virus causes chronic inflammation, which leads to plaque buildup in the arteries that can cause cardiovascular disease.

- Additionally, **some antiretroviral medications** used to treat HIV can increase your risk for heart disease by causing *insulin resistance*, and studies have shown that some kinds of HIV meds, including *protease inhibitors*, are associated with *hyperlipidemia*—high levels of fat in the blood, including choles-terol and triglycerides. If untreated, this increases the risk heart disease, as well as gall bladder disease, and pancreatitis.

- And finally, the rates of some **conventional risk factors for cardiovascular disease**, such as smoking, are also higher among people with HIV.

But the benefits of ART have been shown to greatly outweigh the risks, and researchers warn against stopping your HIV meds to pro-tect your heart. In fact, current research shows that stopping and starting HIV meds can make heart disease worse—while putting you in danger of more serious complications by allowing HIV to reproduce in your body.

Researchers are currently pursuing ways to address the problem of cardiovascular disease among people living with HIV. A current large-scale study with research sites throughout the United States called the Randomized Trial to Prevent Vascular Events in HIV, or REPRIEVE, is testing whether statin medications, which have been proven safe and effective in reducing cardiovascular disease risk in the general population, can also reduce that risk in people with HIV. And scientists say that newer antiretroviral drugs may be easier on your heart. Ask your healthcare provider what you can do to decrease your risk and to find the best HIV medications for you.

Prevention Is Still the Best Medicine

You can't control all of your risk factors for heart disease, but there is a lot you can do to reduce your risk:

- Quit smoking

- Maintain a healthy, low fat diet

- Exercise regularly

- See your healthcare provider regularly

- Get screened for cardiovascular risk factors

- Stay adherent to your HIV medication and keep your viral load low

Section 3.6

Metabolic Syndrome and Cardiovascular Disease

This section includes text excerpted from "Metabolic Syndrome," National Heart, Lung, and Blood Institute (NHLBI), November 6, 2015.

What Is Metabolic Syndrome?

Metabolic syndrome is the name for a group of risk factors that raises your risk for heart disease and other health problems, such as diabetes and stroke.

The term "metabolic" refers to the biochemical processes involved in the body's normal functioning. Risk factors are traits, conditions, or habits that increase your chance of developing a disease.

In this section, "heart disease" refers to coronary heart disease (CHD). CHD is a condition in which a waxy substance called plaque builds up inside the coronary (heart) arteries.

Plaque hardens and narrows the arteries, reducing blood flow to your heart muscle. This can lead to chest pain, a heart attack, heart damage, or even death.

Metabolic Risk Factors

The five conditions described below are metabolic risk factors. You can have any one of these risk factors by itself, but they tend to occur together. You must have at least three metabolic risk factors to be diagnosed with metabolic syndrome.

- **A large waistline.** This also is called abdominal obesity or "having an apple shape." Excess fat in the stomach area is a greater risk factor for heart disease than excess fat in other parts of the body, such as on the hips.

- **A high triglyceride level** (or you're on medicine to treat high triglycerides). Triglycerides are a type of fat found in the blood.

- **A low HDL cholesterol level** (or you're on medicine to treat low HDL cholesterol). HDL sometimes is called "good" cholesterol. This is because it helps remove cholesterol from your arteries. A low HDL cholesterol level raises your risk for heart disease.

- **High blood pressure** (or you're on medicine to treat high blood pressure). Blood pressure is the force of blood pushing against the walls of your arteries as your heart pumps blood. If this pressure rises and stays high over time, it can damage your heart and lead to plaque buildup.

- **High fasting blood sugar** (or you're on medicine to treat high blood sugar). Mildly high blood sugar may be an early sign of diabetes.

Who Is at Risk for Metabolic Syndrome?

People at greatest risk for metabolic syndrome have these underlying causes:

- Abdominal obesity (a large waistline)
- An inactive lifestyle
- Insulin resistance

Some people are at risk for metabolic syndrome because they take medicines that cause weight gain or changes in blood pressure, blood cholesterol, and blood sugar levels. These medicines most often are used to treat inflammation, allergies, HIV, and depression and other types of mental illness.

Populations Affected

Some racial and ethnic groups in the United States are at higher risk for metabolic syndrome than others. Mexican Americans have the highest rate of metabolic syndrome, followed by whites and blacks.

Other groups at increased risk for metabolic syndrome include:

- People who have a personal history of diabetes
- People who have a sibling or parent who has diabetes
- Women when compared with men
- Women who have a personal history of polycystic ovarian syndrome (a tendency to develop cysts on the ovaries)

Heart Disease Risk

Metabolic syndrome increases your risk for coronary heart disease. Other risk factors, besides metabolic syndrome, also increase your risk for heart disease. For example, a high LDL ("bad") cholesterol level and smoking are major risk factors for heart disease.

Even if you don't have metabolic syndrome, you should find out your short-term risk for heart disease. The National Cholesterol Education Program (NCEP) divides short-term heart disease risk into four categories. Your risk category depends on which risk factors you have and how many you have.

Your risk factors are used to calculate your 10-year risk of developing heart disease. The NCEP has an online calculator that you can use to estimate your 10-year risk of having a heart attack.

- **High risk:** You're in this category if you already have heart disease or diabetes, or if your 10-year risk score is more than 20 percent.

- **Moderately high risk:** You're in this category if you have two or more risk factors and your 10-year risk score is 10 percent to 20 percent.

- **Moderate risk:** You're in this category if you have two or more risk factors and your 10-year risk score is less than 10 percent.

- **Lower risk:** You're in this category if you have zero or one risk factor.

How Can Metabolic Syndrome Be Prevented?

Making heart-healthy lifestyle choices is the best way to prevent metabolic syndrome by:

- Being physically active

- Following a heart-healthy eating plan

- Knowing your weight, waist measurement, and body mass index

- Maintaining a healthy weight

Make sure to schedule routine doctor visits to keep track of your cholesterol, blood pressure, and blood sugar levels. Speak with your doctor about a blood test called a lipoprotein panel, which shows your levels of total cholesterol, LDL cholesterol, HDL cholesterol, and triglycerides.

Section 3.7

Sleep Apnea and Cardiovascular Disease

This section includes text excerpted from "Sleep Apnea,"
National Institute of Neurological Disorders and
Stroke (NINDS), October 21, 2015.

What Is Sleep Apnea?

Sleep apnea is a common sleep disorder characterized by brief interruptions of breathing during sleep. These episodes usually last 10 seconds or more and occur repeatedly throughout the night. People with sleep apnea will partially awaken as they struggle to breathe, but in the morning they will not be aware of the disturbances in their sleep. The most common type of sleep apnea is obstructive sleep apnea (OSA), caused by relaxation of soft tissue in the back of the throat that blocks the passage of air. Central sleep apnea (CSA) is caused by irregularities in the brain's normal signals to breathe. Most people with sleep apnea will have a combination of both types. The hallmark symptom of the disorder is excessive daytime sleepiness. Additional symptoms of sleep apnea include restless sleep, loud snoring (with periods of silence followed by gasps), falling asleep during the day, morning headaches, trouble concentrating, irritability, forgetfulness, mood or behavior changes, anxiety, and depression. Not everyone who has these symptoms will have sleep apnea, but it is recommended that people who are experiencing even a few of these symptoms visit their doctor for evaluation. Sleep apnea is more likely to occur in men than women, and in people who are overweight or obese.

Is There Any Treatment?

There are a variety of treatments for sleep apnea, depending on an individual's medical history and the severity of the disorder. Most treatment regimens begin with lifestyle changes, such as avoiding alcohol and medications that relax the central nervous system (for example, sedatives and muscle relaxants), losing weight, and quitting smoking. Some people are helped by special pillows or devices that keep them from sleeping on their backs, or oral appliances to keep the airway open during sleep. If these conservative methods are inadequate, doctors often recommend continuous positive airway pressure (CPAP), in which a face mask is attached to a tube and a machine that blows pressurized air into the mask and through the airway to keep it open. Also available are machines that offer variable positive airway pressure (VPAP) and automatic positive airway pressure (APAP). There are also surgical procedures that can be used to remove tissue and widen the airway. Some individuals may need a combination of therapies to successfully treat their sleep apnea.

What Is the Prognosis?

Untreated, sleep apnea can be life threatening. Excessive daytime sleepiness can cause people to fall asleep at inappropriate times, such as while driving. Sleep apnea also appears to put individuals at risk for stroke and transient ischemic attacks (TIAs, also known as "mini-strokes"), and is associated with coronary heart disease, heart failure, irregular heartbeat, heart attack, and high blood pressure. Although there is no cure for sleep apnea, recent studies show that successful treatment can reduce the risk of heart and blood pressure problems.

Section 3.8

Stress and Cardiovascular Disease

This section contains text excerpted from the following sources:
Text under the heading "Stress or Depression" is excerpted from
"Heart Disease in Women," National Heart, Lung, and Blood
Institute (NHLBI), April 21, 2014; Text beginning with the heading
"What is Broken Heart Syndrome" is excerpted from "Broken Heart
Syndrome," National Heart, Lung, and Blood Institute (NHLBI),
October 8, 2014.

Stress or Depression

Stress may play a role in causing CHD. Stress can trigger your arteries to narrow. This can raise your blood pressure and your risk for a heart attack.

Getting upset or angry also can trigger a heart attack. Stress also may indirectly raise your risk for CHD if it makes you more likely to smoke or overeat foods high in fat and sugar.

People who are depressed are two to three times more likely to develop CHD than people who are not. Depression is twice as common in women as in men.

What Is Broken Heart Syndrome

Broken heart syndrome is a condition in which extreme stress can lead to heart muscle failure. The failure is severe, but often short-term.

Most people who experience broken heart syndrome think they may be having a heart attack, a more common medical emergency caused by a blocked coronary (heart) artery. The two conditions have similar symptoms, including chest pain and shortness of breath. However, there's no evidence of blocked coronary arteries in broken heart syndrome, and most people have a full and quick recovery.

Broken Heart Syndrome versus Heart Attack

Symptoms of broken heart syndrome can look like those of a heart attack.

Most heart attacks are caused by blockages and blood clots forming in the coronary arteries, which supply the heart with blood. If these clots cut off the blood supply to the heart for a long enough period of time, heart muscle cells can die, leaving the heart with permanent damage. Heart attacks most often occur as a result of coronary heart disease (CHD), also called coronary artery disease.

Broken heart syndrome is quite different. Most people who experience broken heart syndrome have fairly normal coronary arteries, without severe blockages or clots. The heart cells are "stunned" by stress hormones but not killed. The "stunning" effects reverse quickly, often within just a few days or weeks. In most cases, there is no lasting damage to the heart.

Because symptoms are similar to a heart attack, it is important to seek help right away. You, and sometimes emergency care providers, may not be able to tell that you have broken heart syndrome until you have some tests.

All chest pain should be checked by a doctor. If you think you or someone else may be having heart attack symptoms or a heart attack, don't ignore it or feel embarrassed to call for help. Call 9–1–1 for emergency medical care. In the case of a heart attack, acting fast at the first sign of symptoms can save your life and limit damage to your heart.

Other Names for Broken Heart Syndrome

- Apical ballooning syndrome
- Stress cardiomyopathy
- Stress-induced cardiomyopathy
- Takotsubo cardiomyopathy
- Transient left ventricular apical ballooning syndrome

What Causes Broken Heart Syndrome?

The cause of broken heart syndrome isn't fully known. However, extreme emotional or physical stress is believed to play a role in causing the temporary disorder.

Although symptoms are similar to those of a heart attack, what is happening to the heart is quite different. Most heart attacks are caused by near or complete blockage of a coronary artery. In broken heart syndrome, the coronary arteries are not blocked, although blood flow may be reduced.

Potential Triggers

In most cases, broken heart syndrome occurs after an intense and upsetting emotional or physical event. Some potential triggers of broken heart syndrome are:

- **Emotional stressors**—extreme grief, fear, or anger, for example as a result of the unexpected death of a loved one, financial or legal trouble, intense fear, domestic abuse, confrontational argument, car accident, public speaking, or even a surprise party.
- **Physical stressors**—an asthma attack, serious illness or surgery, or exhausting physical effort.

Potential Causes

Researchers think that sudden stress releases hormones that overwhelm or "stun" the heart. (The term "stunned" is often used to indicate that the injury to the heart muscle is only temporary.) This can trigger changes in heart muscle cells or coronary blood vessels, or both. The heart becomes so weak that its left ventricle (which is the chamber that pumps blood from your heart to your body) bulges and cannot pump well, while the other parts of the heart work normally or with even more forceful contractions. As a result the heart is unable to pump properly.

Researchers are trying to identify the precise way in which the stress hormones affect the heart. Broken heart syndrome may result from a hormone surge, coronary artery spasm, or microvascular dysfunction.

Hormone Surge

Intense stress causes large amounts of the "fight or flight" hormones, such as adrenaline and noradrenaline, to be released into your bloodstream. The hormones are meant to help you cope with the stress. Researchers think that the sudden surge of hormones overwhelms and stuns the heart muscle, producing symptoms similar to those of a heart attack.

Coronary Artery Spasm

Some research suggests that the extreme stress causes a temporary, sudden narrowing of one of the coronary arteries as a result of a spasm. The spasm slows or stops blood flow through the artery and starves part of the heart of oxygen-rich blood.

Microvascular Dysfunction

Another theory that is gaining traction is that the very small coronary arteries (called microvascular arteries) do not function well due to low hormone levels occurring before or after menopause. The microvascular arteries fail to provide enough oxygen-rich blood to the heart muscle.

Who Is at Risk for Broken Heart Syndrome?

Broken heart syndrome affects women more often than men. Often, people who experience broken heart syndrome have previously been healthy. Research shows that the traditional risk factors for heart disease may not apply to broken heart syndrome.

People who might be at increased risk for broken heart syndrome include:

- Women who have gone through menopause, particularly women in their sixties and seventies

- People who often have no previous history of heart disease

- Asian and White populations

Although these are the characteristics for most cases of broken heart syndrome, the condition can occur in anyone.

What Are the Signs and Symptoms of Broken Heart Syndrome

All chest pain should be checked by a doctor. Because symptoms of broken heart syndrome are similar to those of a heart attack, it is important to seek help right away. Your doctor may not be able to diagnose broken heart syndrome until you have some tests.

Common Signs and Symptoms

The most common symptoms of broken heart syndrome are sudden, sharp chest pain and shortness of breath. Typically these symptoms begin just minutes to hours after experiencing a severe, and usually unexpected, stress.

Because the syndrome involves severe heart muscle weakness, some people also may experience signs and symptoms such as fainting, arrhythmias (fast or irregular heartbeats), cardiogenic shock (when the heart can't pump enough blood to meet the body's needs), low blood pressure, and heart failure.

Differences from a Heart Attack

Some of the signs and symptoms of broken heart syndrome differ from those of a heart attack. For example, in people who have broken heart syndrome:

- Symptoms (chest pain and shortness of breath) occur suddenly after having extreme emotional or physical stress.

- EKG (electrocardiogram) results don't look the same as the results for a person having a heart attack. (An EKG is a test that records the heart's electrical activity.)

- Blood tests show no signs or mild signs of heart damage.

- Tests show enlarged and unusual movement of the lower left heart chamber (the left ventricle).

- Tests show no signs of blockages in the coronary arteries.

- Recovery time is quick, usually within days or weeks (compared with the recovery time of a month or more for a heart attack).

Complications

Broken heart syndrome can be life threatening in some cases. It can lead to serious heart problems such as:

- Heart failure, a condition in which the heart can't pump enough blood to meet the body's needs

- Heart rhythm problems that cause the heart to beat much faster or slower than normal

- Heart valve problems

The good news is that most people who have broken heart syndrome make a full recovery within weeks. With medical care, even the most critically ill tend to make a quick and complete recovery.

How Is Broken Heart Syndrome Diagnosed?

Because the symptoms are similar, at first your doctor may not be able to tell whether you are experiencing broken heart syndrome or having a heart attack. Therefore, the doctor's immediate goals will be:

- To determine what's causing your symptoms

- To determine whether you're having or about to have a heart attack

Your doctor will diagnose broken heart syndrome based on your signs and symptoms, your medical and family histories, and the results from tests and procedures.

Specialists Involved

Your doctor may refer you to a cardiologist. A cardiologist is a doctor who specializes in diagnosing and treating heart diseases and conditions.

Physical Exam and Medical History

Your doctor will do a physical exam and ask you to describe your symptoms. He or she may ask questions such as when your symptoms began, where you are feeling pain or discomfort and what it feels like, and whether the pain is constant or varies.

To learn about your medical history, your doctor may ask about your overall health, risk factors for coronary heart disease (CHD) and other heart disease, and family history. Your doctor will ask whether you've recently experienced any major stresses.

Diagnostic Tests and Procedures

No single test can diagnose broken heart syndrome. The tests and procedures for broken heart syndrome are similar to those used to diagnose CHD or heart attack. The diagnosis is made based on the results of the following standards tests to rule out heart attack and imaging studies to help establish broken heart syndrome.

Standard Tests and Procedures

EKG (Electrocardiogram)

An EKG is a simple, painless test that detects and records the heart's electrical activity. The test shows how fast your heart is beating and whether its rhythm is steady or irregular. An EKG also records the strength and timing of electrical signals as they pass through each part of the heart.

The EKG may show abnormalities in your heartbeat, a sign of broken heart syndrome as well as heart damage due to CHD.

Blood Tests

Blood tests check the levels of certain substances in your blood, such as fats, cholesterol, sugar, and proteins. Blood tests help greatly in diagnosing broken heart syndrome, because certain enzymes (proteins in the blood) may be present in the blood to indicate the condition.

Imaging Procedures

Echocardiography

Echocardiography (echo) uses sound waves to create a moving picture of your heart. The test provides information about the size and shape of your heart and how well your heart chambers and valves are working. Echo also can show areas of heart muscle that aren't contracting well because of poor blood flow or previous injury.

The echo may show slowed blood flow in the left chamber of the heart.

Chest X-ray

A chest X-ray is a painless test that creates pictures of the structures in your chest, such as your heart, lungs, and blood vessels. Your doctor will need a chest X-ray to analyze whether your heart has the enlarged shape that is a sign of broken heart syndrome.

A chest X-ray can reveal signs of heart failure, as well as lung disorders and other causes of symptoms not related to broken heart syndrome.

Cardiac MRI

Cardiac magnetic resonance imaging (MRI) is a common test that uses radio waves, magnets, and a computer to make both still and moving pictures of your heart and major blood vessels. Doctors use cardiac MRI to get pictures of the beating heart and to look at its structure and function. These pictures can help them decide the best way to treat people who have heart problems.

Coronary Angiography and Cardiac Catheterization

Your doctor may recommend coronary angiography if other tests or factors suggest you have CHD. This test uses dye and special X-rays to look inside your coronary arteries.

To get the dye into your coronary arteries, your doctor will use a procedure called cardiac catheterization. A thin, flexible tube called a catheter is put into a blood vessel in your arm, groin (upper thigh), or neck. The tube is threaded into your coronary arteries, and the dye is released into your bloodstream.

Special X-rays are taken while the dye is flowing through your coronary arteries. The dye lets your doctor study the flow of blood through your heart and blood vessels.

Ventriculogram

Ventriculogram is another test that can be done during a cardiac catheterization that examines the left ventricle, which is the heart's main pumping chamber. During this test, a dye is injected into the inside of the heart and X-ray pictures are taken. The test can show the ventricle's size and how well it pumps blood. It also shows how well the blood flows through the aortic and mitral values.

How Is Broken Heart Syndrome Treated?

Even though broken heart syndrome may feel like a heart attack, it's a very different problem that needs a different type of treatment.

The good news is that broken heart syndrome is usually treatable, and most people make a full recovery. Most people who experience broken heart syndrome stay in the hospital for a few days to a week.

Initial treatment is aimed at improving blood flow to the heart, and may be similar to that for a heart attack until the diagnosis is clear. Further treatment can include medicines and lifestyle changes.

Medicines

Doctors may prescribe medicines to relieve fluid buildup, treat blood pressure problems, prevent blood clots, and manage stress hormones. Medicines are often discontinued once heart function has returned to normal.

Your doctor may prescribe the following medicines:

- **ACE inhibitors** (or angiotensin-converting enzyme inhibitors), to lower blood pressure and reduce strain on your heart

- **Beta blockers**, to slow your heart rate and lower your blood pressure to decrease your heart's workload

- **Diuretics** (water or fluid pills), to help reduce fluid buildup in your lungs and swelling in your feet and ankles

- **Anti-anxiety medicines**, to help manage stress hormones

Take all of your medicines as prescribed. If you have side effects or other problems related to your medicines, tell your doctor. He or she may be able to provide other options.

Treatment of Complications

Broken heart syndrome can be life threatening in some cases. Because the syndrome involves severe heart muscle weakness, patients can experience shock, heart failure, low blood pressure, and potentially life-threatening heart rhythm abnormalities.

The good news is that this condition improves very quickly, so with proper diagnosis and management, even the most critically ill tend to make a quick and complete recovery.

Lifestyle Changes

To stay healthy, it's important to find ways to reduce stress and cope with particularly upsetting situations. Learning how to manage stress, relax, and cope with problems can improve your emotional and physical health.

Having supportive people in your life with whom you can share your feelings or concerns can help relieve stress. Physical activity, medicine, and relaxation therapy also can help relieve stress. You may want to consider taking part in a stress management program.

Treatments Not Helpful for Broken Heart Syndrome

Several procedures used to treat a heart attack are not helpful in treating broken heart syndrome. These procedures—percutaneous coronary intervention (sometimes referred to as angioplasty), stent placement, and surgery—treat blocked arteries, which is not the cause of broken heart syndrome.

How Can Broken Heart Syndrome Be Prevented?

Researchers are still learning about broken heart syndrome, and no treatments have been shown to prevent it. For people who have experienced the condition, the risk of recurrence is low.

An emotionally upsetting or serious physical event can trigger broken heart syndrome. Learning how to manage stress, relax, and cope with problems can improve your emotional and physical health.

Having supportive people in your life with whom you can share your feelings or concerns can help relieve stress. Physical activity, medicine, and relaxation therapy also can help relieve stress. You may want to consider taking part in a stress management program.

Also, some of the ways people cope with stress—such as drinking, smoking, or overeating—aren't healthy. Learning to manage stress includes adopting healthy habits that will keep your stress levels low and make it easier to deal with stress when it does happen. A healthy lifestyle includes following a healthy diet, being physically active, maintaining a healthy weight, and quitting smoking.

Chapter 4

Aging and Cardiovascular Disease

Impact of Aging on Cardiovascular Disease

Age is the major risk factor for cardiovascular disease. Heart disease and stroke incidence rises steeply after age 65, accounting for more than 40 percent of all deaths among people age 65 to 74 and almost 60 percent at age 85 and above. People age 65 and older are much more likely than younger people to suffer a heart attack, to have a stroke, or to develop coronary heart disease and high blood pressure leading to heart failure. Cardiovascular disease is also a major cause of disability, limiting the activity and eroding the quality of life of millions of older people each year. The cost of these diseases to the Nation is in the billions of dollars.

To understand why aging is so closely linked to cardiovascular disease, and ultimately to understand the causes and develop cures for this group of diseases, it is essential to understand what is happening in the heart and arteries during normal aging—aging in the absence of disease. This understanding has moved forward dramatically in

This chapter contains text excerpted from the following sources: Text under the heading "Impact of Aging on Cardiovascular Disease" is excerpted from "Aging Hearts and Arteries: A Scientific Quest," National Institute on Aging (NIA), July 2014; Text under the heading "Changes to Your Heart with Age" is excerpted from "Heart Health," National Institute on Aging (NIA), May 4, 2016.

the past 30 years. The purpose of this chapter is to tell the story of this progress, describe some of the most important findings, and give a sense of what may lie ahead.

While we know a great deal about cardiovascular disease and its risk factors, new areas of research are beginning to shed further light on the link between aging and the development and course of the disease. For instance, scientists at the National Institute on Aging (NIA) are paying special attention to certain age-related changes that occur in the arteries and their influence on cardiac function. Many of these changes, once considered a normal part of aging, may put people at increased risk for cardiovascular disease.

This and other compelling research on the aging heart and blood vessels takes place at many different research centers. A great deal of the work is being done by researchers in the Laboratory of Cardiovascular Science at the NIA or by NIA-funded scientists at other institutions. Others have worked at or been funded by the National Heart, Lung, and Blood Institute (NHLBI). NIA and NHLBI are two of 27 research institutes and centers at the National Institutes of Health, and their work is complementary. NIA research focuses on the effects of aging on the heart, blood vessels, and other parts of the body, while NHLBI works to understand the diseases and risk factors that affect the heart and blood vessels.

Both perspectives are bringing us closer to the possibility that heart disease and stroke will someday be defeated. Research on the basic biology of the aging cardiovascular system nurtures hope that we as a Nation need not accept the high rates of death and disability and the enormous health care costs imposed by cardiovascular disease among older people in our society.

Changes to Your Heart with Age

Aging can cause changes in the heart and blood vessels. For example, as you get older, your heart can't beat as fast during physical activity or stress as when you were younger. However, the number of heart beats per minute (heart rate) at rest does not change as you age.

Many of the problems older people have with their heart and blood vessels are really caused by disease, not by aging. For example, an older heart can normally pump blood as strong as a younger heart; less ability to pump blood is caused by a disease. But, changes that happen with age may increase a person's risk of heart disease. The good news is there are things you can do to delay, lower, or possibly avoid or reverse your risk.

A common problem related to aging is "hardening of the arteries," called arteriosclerosis. This problem is why blood pressure goes up with age.

Age can cause other changes to the heart. For example:

- Blood vessels can become stiffer, and some parts of the heart wall will thicken to help with blood flow.

- Your valves (one-way, door-like parts that open and close to control the blood flow inside your heart) may become thicker and stiffer, causing leaks or problems with pumping blood out of the heart.

- The size of the sections of your heart may increase.

Other factors, such as thyroid disease or chemotherapy, may weaken the heart muscle. Things you can't control, like your family history, might also increase your risk of heart disease. But even so, leading a heart-healthy lifestyle might help you avoid or delay serious illness.

Chapter 5

Recent Research on Cardiovascular Disease

Chapter Contents

Section 5.1

When HDL Cholesterol Doesn't Protect against Heart Disease

This section includes text excerpted from "When HDL Cholesterol Doesn't Protect against Heart Disease," National Institutes of Health (NIH), March 22, 2016.

Cholesterol has many important functions. It's carried through the blood stream in several forms, including attached to low-density lipoproteins (LDL) and high-density lipoproteins (HDL). When there's too much cholesterol in your blood, the LDL-cholesterol can combine with other substances to form plaque that coats artery walls, causing them to narrow. This condition, called atherosclerosis, increases your risk for cardiovascular diseases such as heart attack and stroke.

HDL, in contrast, is thought to remove cholesterol from arteries and carry it to the liver for removal from the body. Higher levels of HDL have been associated with a lower risk of cardiovascular disease. However, pharmaceutical approaches to reduce heart disease risk by raising HDL levels have had disappointing results.

An international research team led by Dr. Daniel J. Rader at the University of Pennsylvania aimed to gain further insights into the relationship between HDL-cholesterol (HDL-C) and cardiovascular disease. They examined 328 people with very high HDL-C (average of 107 mg/dl) and 398 with low HDL-C (average of 30 mg/dl). The scientists sequenced nearly a thousand genes near genetic regions previously associated with plasma lipid levels. Their work was funded in part by NIH's National Center for Research Resources (NCRR) and National Center for Advancing Translational Sciences (NCATS). Results appeared on March 11, 2016 in *Science*.

In 5 people with high HDL-C, the researchers found a genetic variant within the gene *SCARB1*, which codes for the major HDL receptor on liver cells, scavenger receptor class BI (SR-BI). One of the individuals had 2 mutant copies of the variant. In mice, genetic manipulations of this gene had effects opposite from those expected if HDL-C were protective. Overexpression of the gene lowered HDL-C

60

levels but reduced atherosclerosis. Deletion raised HDL-C levels but increased atherosclerosis.

Genetic analyses of well over 300,000 people confirmed that the variant, called *SCARB1* P376L, was associated with elevated HDL-C levels. The researchers found that people with the variant had unusually high levels of large HDL-C particles in their blood.

To see whether *SCARB1* P376L was associated with heart disease, the team acquired data from nearly 50,000 people with coronary heart disease and about 88,000 controls. They found that those with the variant had a significantly higher risk of heart disease.

Experiments in cell cultures and mice revealed that the P376L SR-BI protein wasn't processed properly by the cell and often failed to reach the cell surface. As a result, liver cells became incapable of taking up HDL cholesterol from the blood.

"The work demonstrates that the protective effects of HDL are more dependent upon how it functions than merely how much of it is present," Rader says. "We still have a lot to learn about the relationship between HDL function and heart disease risk."

The team plans to study how other *SCARB1* mutations affect HDL levels and heart disease. Other genes, they suggest, may also have similar effects.

Section 5.2

Most Americans' Hearts Are Older than Their Age

This section includes text excerpted from "Most Americans' Hearts Are Older than Their Age," Centers for Disease Control and Prevention (CDC), September 1, 2015.

Your heart may be older than you are—and that's not good. According to a new CDC Vital Signs report, 3 out of 4 U.S. adults have a predicted heart age that is older than their actual age. This means they are at higher risk for heart attacks and stroke.

"Heart age" is the calculated age of a person's cardiovascular system based on his or her risk factor profile. The risks include high blood pressure, cigarette smoking, diabetes status, and body mass index as an indicator for obesity.

This is the first study to provide population-level estimates of heart age and to highlight disparities in heart age nationwide. The report shows that heart age varies by race/ethnicity, gender, region, and other sociodemographic characteristics.

CDC researchers used risk factor data collected from every U.S. state and information from the Framingham Heart Study to determine that nearly 69 million adults between the ages of 30 and 74 have a heart age older than their actual age. That's about the number of people living in the 130 largest U.S. cities combined.

"Too many U.S. adults have a heart age years older than their real age, increasing their risk of heart disease and stroke," said CDC Director Tom Frieden, M.D., M.P.H. "Everybody deserves to be young—or at least not old—at heart."

Key findings in the report include:

- Overall, the average heart age for adult men is 8 years older than their chronological age, compared to 5 years older for women.

- Although heart age exceeds chronological age for all race/ethnic groups, it is highest among African-American men and women (average of 11 years older for both).

- Among both U.S. men and women, excess heart age increases with age and decreases with greater education and household income.

- There are geographic differences in average heart age across states. Adults in the Southern U.S. typically have higher heart

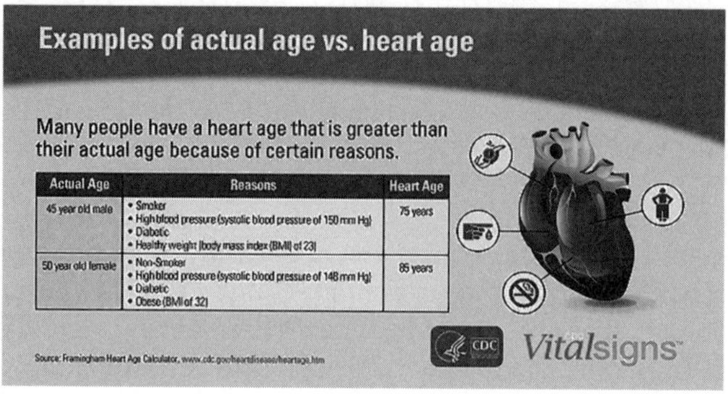

Figure 5.1. *Heart Age*

ages. For example, Mississippi, West Virginia, Kentucky, Louisiana, and Alabama have the highest percentage of adults with a heart age 5 years or more over their actual age, while Utah, Colorado, California, Hawaii, and Massachusetts have the lowest percentage.

Learn Your Heart Age

The heart age concept was created to more effectively communicate a person's risk of dying from heart attack or stroke—and to show what can be done to lower that risk. Despite the serious national problem of higher heart age, the report's findings can be used on both an individual and population level to boost heart health, particularly among groups that are most at risk of poor cardiovascular outcomes.

Healthcare providers can use cardiovascular risk assessment calculators to inform treatment decisions and work with patients on healthy habits. For example, a 53-year-old woman might find out through her doctor that her heart age is 68 because she smokes and has uncontrolled high blood pressure. Her doctor could then talk with her about finding a quit-smoking program that is right for her, and about lifestyle changes and medications that would put her in charge of her blood pressure.

U.S. adults can learn their own heart age and how to improve it. This could include quitting smoking or lowering blood pressure through eating a healthier diet, taking appropriate medication, or exercising more. State and local health departments can help by promoting healthier living spaces, such as tobacco-free areas, more access to healthy food options, and safe walking paths.

"Because so many U.S. adults don't understand their cardiovascular disease risk, they are missing out on early opportunities to prevent future heart attacks or strokes," said Barbara A. Bowman, Ph.D., director of CDC's Division for Heart Disease and Stroke Prevention. "About three in four heart attacks and strokes are due to risk factors that increase heart age, so it's important to continue focusing on efforts to improve heart health and increase access to early and affordable detection and treatment resources nationwide."

Section 5.3

Study Adds Evidence on Link between PTSD and Heart Disease

This section includes text excerpted from "Study Adds Evidence on Link between PTSD, Heart Disease," U.S. Department of Veterans Affairs (VA), March 31, 2015.

In a study of more than 8,000 Veterans living in Hawaii and the Pacific Islands, those with posttraumatic stress disorder (PTSD) had a nearly 50 percent greater risk of developing heart failure over about a seven-year follow-up period, compared with their non-PTSD peers.

The study adds to a growing body of evidence linking PTSD and heart disease. The research to date—including these latest findings—doesn't show a clear cause-and-effect relationship. But most experts believe PTSD, like other forms of chronic stress or anxiety, can damage the heart over time.

"There are many theories as to how exactly PTSD contributes to heart disease," says Dr. Alyssa Mansfield, one of the study authors. "Overall, the evidence to date seems to point in the direction of a causal relationship."

Mansfield was senior author on the study while with the Pacific Islands Division of the National Center for PTSD of the Department of Veterans Affairs (VA). She is now with the VA Pacific Islands Healthcare System and also an assistant adjunct professor of epidemiology at the University of Hawaii.

Study Tracked More than 8,000 Veterans

The study tracked 8,248 Veterans who had been outpatients in the VA Pacific Islands system. The researchers followed them an average of just over seven years. Those with a PTSD diagnosis were 47 percent more likely to develop heart failure during the follow-up period. The researchers controlled for differences between the groups in health and demographic factors.

Out of the total study group, about 21 percent were diagnosed with PTSD. Of the total 371 cases of heart failure during the study, 287 occurred among those with PTSD, whereas only 84 cases occurred among the group without PTSD.

Combat service, whether or not it led to a full-blown PTSD diagnosis, was itself a strong predictor of heart failure. Those Veterans with combat experience were about five times more likely to develop heart failure during the study period, compared with those who had not seen combat. Other predictors of heart failure were advanced age, diabetes, high blood pressure, and overweight or obesity.

Evidence of Nexus between Mental Health and Physical Health

The authors of the study say they didn't have access to a full range of data that would have provided further clues as to the PTSD-heart disease link. For example, they were not able to distinguish in the data between those who had served in the Gulf during 1990 and 1991, and those who served more recently in Iraq or Afghanistan. Nor were they able to analyze whether racial or ethnic identity plays a role one way or the other, as that information was not complete for most Veterans in study.

Nonetheless, the authors point out that the work is the "first large-scale longitudinal study to report an association between PTSD and incident heart failure in an outpatient sample of U.S. Veterans."

Heart failure, in which the heart grows weaker and can't pump enough blood to adequately supply the body's needs, affects about 5 million Americans in all, with some 500,000 new cases each year. People with the condition feel tired with physical activity, as the muscles aren't getting enough blood.

The new results, says Mansfield, provide further potent evidence of the nexus between mental and physical health. The practical upshot of the findings, she says, is that Veterans with PTSD should realize that by treating their PTSD, they may also be helping to prevent heart disease down the road.

By the same token, the authors point out that VA and other health-care systems may need to step up efforts to prevent and treat heart failure among those with PTSD.

Section 5.4

Air Pollution May Be "Hard" on the Body's Blood Vessels

This section includes text excerpted from "Air Pollution May Be "Hard" on the Body's Blood Vessels," U.S. Environmental Protection Agency (EPA), February 11, 2014.

Can air pollution affect your heart? The short answer is—yes. It can trigger heart attacks, stroke and cause other cardiovascular health problems. The long answer is that while we know that air pollution impacts the heart, additional research is needed to learn more about how this happens and what pollutants or mixtures are responsible.

An unprecedented 10-year study funded by EPA and the National Institutes of Health, called the Multi-Ethnic Study of Atherosclerosis and Air Pollution (MESA Air), is providing new information about the impacts of fine particle pollution on the arteries—the blood vessels that supply blood to the heart and other parts of the body. Fine particles are microscopic bits of matter that are emitted mostly from the burning of fossil fuel. They have been found to be bad for the heart, at high levels.

MESA Air is expanding our knowledge of a condition that can set you up for a heart attack—atherosclerosis. You may have heard of the term "hardening of the arteries." Well, that refers to atherosclerosis when there is a buildup of fats, cholesterol, and calcium in and on the artery walls, most commonly known as plaque. The buildup of plaques can result in a blood clot, which can block the flow of blood and trigger a heart attack. While atherosclerosis is often considered a heart problem, it can affect arteries anywhere in your body; in the brain, it may lead to strokes.

The MESA Air study is finding evidence of associations between long-term fine particle pollution and the progression of atherosclerosis. Another important observation from the MESA Air study shows that long-term exposure to fine particle pollution limited the ability of arteries to widen when the body needs more blood flow to the heart, say, when running up a flight of stairs.

These are among the many discoveries coming out of the MESA Air study that are providing new insights into how air pollution can contribute to atherosclerosis and lead to heart attacks and strokes.

Those with heart disease who may be exposed to high levels of air pollutants can take action to protect their heart. A good first step is to be aware of high air pollution days.

Section 5.5

Seafood Consumption Can Reduce Risk of Heart Disease

This section includes text excerpted from "Consumers Missing out on Seafood Benefits," United States Department of Agriculture (USDA), August 2015.

Consumers Missing out on Seafood Benefits

Seafood, which is defined as both fish and shellfish, is a nutrient-rich protein food, and its consumption has been associated with reduced risk of heart disease. But while most U.S. consumers eat some seafood, the amounts are inadequate to meet federal dietary guidelines, according to a study conducted by Agricultural Research Service scientists.

Seafood contains healthful natural compounds known as omega-3 fatty acids. Two omega-3s—EPA (eicosapentaenoic acid) and DHA (docosahexaenoic acid)—are abundantly available in oily fish such as salmon, mackerel, herring, sardines, anchovies, trout, and tuna. The *2010 Dietary Guidelines for Americans*, or DGAs, recommend eating two servings of seafood weekly, or about 8 ounces, to get at least 1,750 milligrams of EPA and DHA weekly.

The study, led by ARS nutritionist Lisa Jahns, was conducted with colleagues at the Grand Forks Human Nutrition Research Center in Grand Forks, North Dakota. The study was based on an evaluation of food-intake data collected from a representative sampling of the U.S. population. That data is collected during the national survey known as

"What We Eat in America/NHANES." Because little has been known about how well Americans meet the guidelines for eating seafood, the authors wanted to group people's seafood consumption by sex, age, income, education, and race-ethnicity.

Overall, about 80 to 90 percent of U.S. consumers did not meet their seafood recommendations. The researchers also found that the proportions of seafood consumption varied by sex, income, and education level but not by race-ethnicity. Groups associated with eating less (or no) seafood were women, people aged 19 to 30, and people of lower income and education levels. "Much work remains to move U.S. consumers toward eating seafood at current recommended levels," says Jahns. The scientists published their findings in December 2014 in the research journal Nutrients.

Also at the Grand Forks center, lead author and nutritionist Susan Raatz and colleagues reviewed published studies that explored fish consumption's link to reduced heart-disease risk. They found consistent evidence supporting reduced risk of heart disease due particularly to eating oily fish, which is high in EPA and DHA. In the published study, the authors concluded that getting the message of the benefits of fish consumption to consumers is key, and they suggested a public health education program on the health benefits of eating fish. The study was published in March 2013 in Nutrients.

Recently, USDA's interactive website for helping consumers use the federal dietary guidelines—ChooseMyPlate.gov—launched a board on Pinterest that highlights healthful seafood recipes from a variety of sources.

USDA-ARS provides the science-based food nutrition databases that support the interactive consumer-nutrition resources found at ChooseMyPlate.gov. A 5-ounce serving of cooked farmed Atlantic salmon provides about 290 calories and more than 1,800 mg of omega-3s. A 4.5-ounce serving of cooked, farmed rainbow trout provides 214 calories and about 1,115 mg of omega-3s.

Section 5.6

Relationship between Added Sugars and Risk of Cardiovascular Disease

This section includes text excerpted from "What Is the Relationship between Added Sugars and Risk of Cardiovascular Disease (2015 DGAC)?" U.S. Department of Agriculture (USDA), February 19, 2015.

Moderate evidence from prospective cohort studies indicates that higher intake of added sugars, especially in the form of sugar-sweetened beverages, is consistently associated with increased risk of hypertension, stroke and coronary heart disease (CHD) in adults. Observational and intervention studies indicate a consistent relationship between higher added sugars intake and higher blood pressure and serum triglycerides.

Key Findings

- NEL systematic review (SR) included 23 articles that examined the relationship between added sugars and risk of cardiovascular disease (CVD) or CVD risk factors such as high blood lipids and blood pressure. This literature included 11 intervention studies and 12 prospective cohort studies.

- The majority of intervention and observational studies provide some evidence among adults in support of an association between higher intake of added sugars, especially in the form of sugar-sweetened beverages (SSB), and higher risk of CVD or increased CVD risk factors:

  - More consistent associations were seen between added sugars and elevated serum triglycerides, blood pressure and increased risk of hypertension, stroke, or coronary heart disease (CHD)

  - Evidence for associations between added sugars and dyslipidemia [i.e., low high-density lipoproteins (HDL), high low-density lipoproteins (LDL), and high total cholesterol (TC)] was not as consistent, especially among intervention studies.

69

- The body of evidence examined in this SR had a number of limitations. For example, the intervention studies had extensive heterogeneity in terms of the types and forms of sugars used (i.e., fructose, glucose, sucrose, sugar-sweetened beverages (SSBs), sweetened milk) and the type of control and isocaloric condition used. In addition, most intervention studies had a short duration of the intervention and a small sample size. Most of the observational studies assessed dietary intake only at baseline, and did not take assessments during follow-up. Residual confounding by other dietary and lifestyle factors in observational analyses could not be completely ruled out.

Chapter 6

Research Regarding Genetics and Heart Disease

Chapter Contents

Section 6.1

Researchers Discover Underlying Genetics, Marker for Stroke and Cardiovascular Disease

This section includes text excerpted from "Researchers Discover Underlying Genetics, Marker for Stroke, Cardiovascular Disease," National Institutes of Health (NIH), March 20, 2014.

Scientists studying the genomes of nearly 5,000 people have pinpointed a genetic variant tied to an increased risk for stroke, and have also uncovered new details about an important metabolic pathway that plays a major role in several common diseases. Together, their findings may provide new clues to underlying genetic and biochemical influences in the development of stroke and cardiovascular disease, and may also help lead to new treatment strategies.

"Our findings have the potential to identify new targets in the prevention and treatment of stroke, cardiovascular disease and many other common diseases," said Stephen R. Williams, Ph.D., a postdoctoral fellow at the University of Virginia Cardiovascular Research Center and the University of Virginia Center for Public Health Genomics, Charlottesville.

Dr. Williams, Michele Sale, Ph.D., associate professor of medicine, Brad Worrall, M.D., professor of neurology and public health sciences, all at the University of Virginia, and their team reported their findings March 20, 2014 in PLoS Genetics. The investigators were supported by the National Human Genome Research Institute (NHGRI) Genomics and Randomized Trials Network (GARNET) program.

Stroke is the fourth leading cause of death and a major cause of adult disability in this country, yet its underlying genetics have been difficult to understand. Numerous genetic and environmental factors can contribute to a person having a stroke. "Our goals were to break down the risk factors for stroke," Dr. Williams said.

The researchers focused on one particular biochemical pathway called the folate one-carbon metabolism (FOCM) pathway. They knew that abnormally high blood levels of the amino acid homocysteine are associated with an increased risk of common diseases such as stroke, cardiovascular disease and dementia. Homocysteine is a breakdown product of methionine, which is part of the FOCM pathway. The same pathway can affect many important cellular processes, including the methylation of proteins, DNA and RNA. DNA methylation is a mechanism that cells use to control which genes are turned on and off, and when.

But clinical trials of homocysteine-lowering therapies have not prevented disease, and the genetics underlying high homocysteine levels—and methionine metabolism gone awry—are not well defined.

Dr. Williams and his colleagues conducted genome-wide association studies of participants from two large long-term projects: the Vitamin Intervention for Stroke Prevention (VISP), a trial looking at ways to prevent a second ischemic stroke, and the Framingham Heart Study (FHS), which has followed the cardiovascular health and disease in a general population for decades. They also measured methionine metabolism—the ability to convert methionine to homocysteine—in both groups. In all, they studied 2,100 VISP participants and 2,710 FHS subjects.

In a genome-wide association study, researchers scan the genome to identify specific genomic variants associated with a disease. In this case, the scientists were trying to identify variants associated with a trait—the ability to metabolize methionine into homocysteine.

Investigators identified variants in five genes in the FOCM pathway that were associated with differences in a person's ability to convert methionine to homocysteine. They found that among the five genes, one—the ALDH1L1 gene—was also strongly associated with stroke in the Framingham study. When the gene is not working properly, it has been associated with a breakdown in a normal cellular process called programmed cell death, and cancer cell survival.

They also made important discoveries about the methionine-homocysteine process. "GNMT produces a protein that converts methionine to homocysteine. Of the five genes that we identified, it was the one most significantly associated with this process," Dr. Williams said. "The analyses suggest that differences in GNMT are the major drivers behind the differences in methionine metabolism in humans."

"It's striking that the genes are in the same pathway, so we know that the genomic variants affecting that pathway contribute to the variability in disease and risk that we're seeing," he said. "We may have found how genetic information controls the regulation of GNMT."

The group determined that the five genes accounted for 6 percent of the difference in individuals' ability to process methionine into homocysteine among those in the VISP trial. The genes also accounted for 13 percent of the difference in those participants in the FHS, a remarkable result given the complex nature of methionine metabolism and its impact on cerebrovascular risk. In many complex diseases, genomic variants often account for less than 5 percent of such differences.

"This is a great example of the kinds of successful research efforts coming out of the GARNET program," said program director Ebony Madden, Ph.D. "GARNET scientists aim to identify variants that affect treatment response by doing association studies in randomized trials. These results show that variants in genes are associated with the differences in homocysteine levels in individuals."

The association of the ALDH1L1 gene variant with stroke is just one example of how the findings may potentially lead to new prevention efforts, and help develop new targets for treating stroke and heart disease, Dr. Williams said.

"As genome sequencing becomes more widespread, clinicians may be able to determine if a person's risk for abnormally high levels of homocysteine is elevated," he said. "Changes could be made to an individual's diet because of a greater risk for stroke and cardiovascular disease."

The investigators plan to study the other four genes in the pathway to try to better understand their potential roles in stroke and cardiovascular disease risk.

Section 6.2

Link between Congenital Heart Disease and Neurodevelopment Issues in Children

This section includes text excerpted from "Link between Congenital Heart Disease and Neurodevelopment Issues in Children," National Heart, Lung, and Blood Institute (NHLBI), December 3, 2015.

Scientists have confirmed the role of a set of gene mutations in the development of congenital heart disease and simultaneously discovered a link between them and some neurodevelopmental abnormalities in children. These abnormalities include cognitive, motor, social, and language impairments.

"The risk of developing neurodevelopmental disabilities is so high when these particular gene mutations are present that we might consider testing for them in all patients with congenital heart disease," said Jonathan R. Kaltman, M.D., a study investigator and program administrator of the National Heart, Lung, and Blood Institute's (NHLBI) Bench to Bassinet Program, which funded the study. Dr. Kaltman noted that the findings from the study would have to be replicated and refined before a clinical test could be available. NHLBI is part of the National Institutes of Health.

Congenital heart disease—in which there are structural defects in the heart—is the most common type of birth defect in the United States, and one of the leading causes of infant death. Nearly 40,000 children are born with congenital heart disease each year, and experts estimate that approximately 1 to 2 million adults and 800,000 children in the United States currently live with the disease.

"Surgery is often performed early in life to repair heart defects," said Dr. Kaltman. "However, we have found that once children reach school age, many exhibit various attention deficits, including attention deficit hyperactivity disorder, and other neurobehavioral problems."

In their study, published Dec. 4 in the journal Science, investigators from the Bench to Bassinet Program's Pediatric Cardiac Genomics Consortium used a technique called exome sequencing to genetically evaluate 1,220 family trios—composed of a child with congenital heart disease and the mother and father. Through this technique, which examines only the protein-coding regions of DNA, they found that children with moderate-to-severe congenital heart disease had a substantial number of "de novo" gene mutations. De novo mutations occur within egg, sperm, and fertilized cells, but are not part of the genetic makeup of the mother or father.

"This finding was especially high in patients who had congenital heart disease and another structural birth defect and/or a neurodevelopmental abnormality," said senior investigator Christine Seidman, M.D., of Brigham and Women's Hospital, Howard Hughes Medical Institute, and Harvard Medical School, Boston. "When the consortium examined the specific genes involved, many of them were highly expressed in both the developing heart and brain, suggesting that a single mutation can contribute to both congenital heart disease and neurodevelopmental abnormalities."

Dr. Seidman noted that the findings have implications for basic research and clinical medicine. "Through further analyses of these mutated genes, we expect to uncover new pathways that are critical for the development of the heart, brain, and other organs—information that will contribute basic insights into the causes of many human congenital malformations," she said.

75

Dr. Seidman added that if the relationship between the de novo mutations and neurodevelopmental abnormalities in children continues to hold, clinical genetic tests could be created for newborns with moderate-to-severe congenital heart abnormalities. The patients found to carry the gene mutations could then be targeted for greater surveillance and early interventions that might address and limit developmental delays and improve their outcomes.

Section 6.3

Risk Factors Identified at Diagnosis Help Predict Outcomes for Children with Rare Heart Condition

This section includes text excerpted from "Risk Factors Identified at Diagnosis Help Predict Outcomes for Children with Rare Heart Condition," National Heart, Lung, and Blood Institute (NHLBI), October 24, 2013.

A long-term study of children with a potentially life-threatening heart condition called hypertrophic cardiomyopathy (HCM) found that the risk of death or need for immediate heart transplantation was greatest for those who developed certain subtypes of this disease as infants with congestive heart failure and for children who also had inborn errors of metabolism, a group of rare genetic disorders in which one or more of the body's key metabolic processes are disrupted. These findings present an immediate opportunity to improve outcomes for affected children.

The findings were published online September 3 in The Lancet to coincide with a presentation at the European Society of Cardiology Congress 2013 meeting in Amsterdam.

"Predicting the clinical outcome for children with hypertrophic cardiomyopathy, or HCM, is challenging because of the complexity and diversity of causes and symptoms," said Steven E. Lipshultz, M.D., director of the Batchelor Children's Research Institute from the University of Miami Leonard Miller School of Medicine and principal investigator of the study. "Although children with HCM comprise the smallest proportion of children with cardiomyopathy listed for heart transplantation, selected patient groups may benefit from early listing for heart transplantation given the malignant course and high death rates shown in certain subgroups."

Hypertrophic cardiomyopathy, a type of pediatric cardiomyopathy (diseases of the heart muscle) with varied causes and outcomes, is characterized by increased thickness (hypertrophy) of the heart wall. HCM is rare, with less than one out of 100,000 children (ages birth to 18 years) diagnosed annually in the United States. The condition is more frequently diagnosed in infants (under the age of one year), with 2-3 out of every 100,000 identified each year.

Despite all that modern medicine has to offer, too many infants and children with HCM still die unexpectedly or prematurely. To better understand how diagnostic factors and patient characteristics predict the risk of death or the need for immediate heart transplantation in this rare condition, researchers from the University of Miami Miller School of Medicine, along with colleagues from other institutions, spent 19 years amassing data on more than 1,000 affected children at 98 pediatric cardiology centers in the United States and Canada through the National Heart, Lung, and Blood Institute (NHLBI)-funded Pediatric Cardiomyopathy Registry.

They found that children with HCM caused by inborn errors of metabolism had the lowest rate of transplant-free survival within two years after diagnosis (43 percent). At two years after diagnosis, the rate of transplant-free survival was 55 percent for children with a mixed version of the disease that included thickening of the heart walls and enlargement and weakening of the heart and 62 percent for those with a restrictive form of the disease characterized by both a thickening and hardening of the heart walls. Children diagnosed after age one with hypertrophic cardiomyopathy of unknown cause had the most favorable outcome, a 97 percent rate of transplant-free survival.

Infants and children who had two or more of the following risk factors at HCM diagnosis (depending on the cause of HCM)—lower weight or body size, female gender, diagnosis during infancy, congestive heart failure, and abnormal heart function—had an increased risk of poor outcomes (death or need for immediate heart transplantation).

"Progress has been slow in properly diagnosing and finding treatments for this heart disease that took the life of my two young sons at age 11 months and 9 months," said Lisa Yue, founding executive director of the Children's Cardiomyopathy Foundation. "When my second son was diagnosed with hypertrophic cardiomyopathy in 2000, very few children had this condition and there was not an understanding that his symptoms were life-threatening and required immediate evaluation for heart transplantation. These new population-based findings will allow families to work with medical professionals to make more informed treatment decisions."

The study's findings are expected to assist clinicians in identifying which children are likely to have the worst outcomes (death or need for heart transplantation) within two years of diagnosis thereby enabling medical teams, genetic counselors, and family planners to jointly and quickly determine the best treatment approach.

"This study is a good example of public-private collaboration to address one of the most serious and complex heart conditions that affects children," said Gail Pearson, M.D., Sc.D., a pediatric cardiologist and director of the Adult and Pediatric Cardiac Research Program in the NHLBI's Division of Cardiovascular Sciences. "Where we don't have good treatment options, such as with hypertrophic cardiomyopathy, determining risk level takes on more importance. The long-term follow-up made possible through the Pediatric Cardiomyopathy Registry has improved our ability to determine which children are at the highest risk for needing a heart transplant and for dying from this condition and thus need more intensive monitoring or earlier listing for transplantation."

Section 6.4

Researchers Find Gene Variant Linked to Aortic Valve Disease

This section includes text excerpted from "Researchers Find Gene Variant Linked to Aortic Valve Disease," National Heart, Lung, and Blood Institute (NHLBI), February 6, 2013.

A newly identified genetic variant doubles the risk of calcium buildup in the heart's aortic valve. Calcium buildup is the most common cause of aortic stenosis, a narrowing of the aortic valve that can lead to heart failure, stroke, and sudden cardiac death.

An international genomics team called CHARGE (Cohorts for Heart and Aging Research in Genomic Epidemiology) found the variant in the gene for lipoprotein(a), a cholesterol-rich particle that circulates in the blood. CHARGE oversees genomic studies of five large study populations in the United States and Europe, including the Framingham Heart Study (FHS), which is a part of the National Heart, Lung, and Blood Institute (NHLBI) at the National Institutes of Health.

"No medications tested to date have shown an ability to prevent or even slow progression of aortic stenosis, and treatments are limited beyond the major step of replacing the aortic valve," said study co-author Christopher O'Donnell, M.D., M.P.H., senior director for genome research at the NHLBI and associate director of the FHS. "By identifying for the first time a common genetic link to aortic stenosis, we might be able to open up new therapeutic options."

The CHARGE researchers conducted a genome-wide analysis of 2.5 million known genetic variants in a group of nearly 7,000 white participants. The analysis identified a variant in the lipoprotein(a), or Lp(a), gene that was highly correlated with calcification of the aortic valve, as measured by computed tomography (CT) scanning. Follow-up analysis in more than 6,000 additional participants, including Hispanics, African-Americans, and Chinese-Americans, confirmed this correlation. The variant was present in about 7 percent of the study population and the people who carry it generally had higher amounts of Lp(a) circulating in their blood. The function of Lp(a) is unknown, but it is associated with an elevated risk of heart disease.

Another independent analysis carried out by CHARGE followed participants in Sweden and Denmark, and found that people with the Lp(a) variant had higher risks of clinical heart valve disease and of needing valve replacement surgery.

"What makes these findings provocative is that we linked the genetic variant with a physiological change in lipoprotein levels, disease precursor in the form of calcium buildup, and fully diagnosed aortic valve disease, across multiple ethnicities," O'Donnell said. "The study suggests a causal relation between Lp(a) and aortic valve disease, but further work will be needed to see whether medications that lower Lp(a) levels can lower the risk or slow the development of valve disease."

In addition to the FHS, this work included data from the NHLBI's Multi-Ethnic Study of Atherosclerosis, the Age Gene/Environment Susceptibility Study, the Heinz Nixdorf Recall Study, the Malmo Diet and Cancer Study, and the Copenhagen City Heart Study.

Chapter 7

Warning Signs of Cardiovascular Emergencies

Chapter Contents

Section 7.1

Signs and Symptoms of a Heart Attack

This section contains text excerpted from the following sources: Text under the heading "About Heart Attack" is excerpted from "Know the Signs and Symptoms of a Heart Attack," Centers for Disease Control and Prevention (CDC), November 30, 2015; Text beginning with the heading "Heart Attack Signs and Symptoms" is excerpted from "Heart Attack Signs and Symptoms," Centers for Disease Control and Prevention (CDC), August 5, 2015.

About Heart Attack

- A heart attack happens when the **blood supply** to the heart is **cut off**. Cells in the heart muscle that do not receive enough oxygen-carrying blood begin to die. The more time that passes without treatment to restore blood flow, the greater the damage to the heart.

- Every year about **735,000** Americans have a heart attack. Of these, **525,000** are a first heart attack and **210,000** happen in people who have already had a heart attack.

- About **15%** of people who have a heart attack will die from it.

- **Almost half** of sudden cardiac deaths happen outside a hospital.

- Having high blood pressure or high blood cholesterol, smoking, having had a previous heart attack or stroke, or having diabetes can increase your chance of developing heart disease and having a heart attack.

- It is important to recognize the signs of a heart attack and to **act immediately** by **calling 911**. A person's chance of surviving a heart attack increases if emergency treatment is administered as soon as possible.

Heart Attack Signs and Symptoms

The five major symptoms of a heart attack are

1. Pain or discomfort in the jaw, neck, or back.

2. Feeling weak, light-headed, or faint.

3. Chest pain or discomfort.

4. Pain or discomfort in arms or shoulder.

5. Shortness of breath.

Other symptoms of a heart attack could include unusual or unexplained tiredness and nausea or vomiting. Women are more likely to have these other symptoms.

Call 9-1-1

If you notice the symptoms of a heart attack in yourself or someone else, call 9-1-1 immediately. The sooner you get to an emergency room, the sooner you can receive treatment to prevent total blockage and heart muscle damage or reduce the amount of damage. At the hospital, healthcare professionals can run tests to determine whether a heart attack is occurring and decide the best treatment.

In some cases, a heart attack requires cardiopulmonary resuscitation (CPR) or electrical shock (defibrillation). Bystanders trained to use CPR or a defibrillator may be able to help until emergency medical personnel arrive.

Remember, the chances of surviving a heart attack are greater the sooner emergency treatment begins.

Section 7.2

Warning Signs of a Stroke

This section contains text excerpted from the following sources: Text beginning with the heading "Stroke Signs and Symptoms" is excerpted from "Stroke Signs and Symptoms," Centers for Disease Control and Prevention (CDC), April 30, 2015; Text beginning with the heading "Why It's Important to Act Fast" is excerpted from "Stroke: Warning Signs of Stroke," National Institutes of Health (NIH), February 2013.

Stroke Signs and Symptoms

During a stroke, every minute counts! Fast treatment can reduce the brain damage that stroke can cause.

By knowing the signs and symptoms of stroke, you can be prepared to take quick action and perhaps save a life—maybe even your own.

Signs of Stroke in Men and Women

- Sudden **numbness** or weakness in the face, arm, or leg, especially on one side of the body.

- Sudden **confusion**, trouble speaking, or difficulty understanding speech.

- Sudden **trouble seeing** in one or both eyes.

- Sudden **trouble walking**, dizziness, loss of balance, or lack of coordination.

- Sudden **severe headache** with no known cause.

Call 9-1-1 immediately if you or someone else has any of these symptoms.

Acting F.A.S.T. Is Key for Stroke

Acting F.A.S.T. can help stroke patients get the treatments they desperately need. The most effective stroke treatments are only available if the stroke is recognized and diagnosed within 3 hours of the first symptoms. Stroke patients may not be eligible for the most effective treatments if they don't arrive at the hospital in time.

If you think someone may be having a stroke, act F.A.S.T. and do the following simple test:

F—Face: Ask the person to smile. Does one side of the face droop?

A—Arms: Ask the person to raise both arms. Does one arm drift downward?

S—Speech: Ask the person to repeat a simple phrase. Is their speech slurred or strange?

T—Time: If you observe any of these signs, call 9-1-1 immediately.

Note the time when any symptoms first appear. Some treatments for stroke only work if given in the first 3 hours after symptoms appear. Do not drive to the hospital or let someone else drive you. Call an ambulance so that medical personnel can begin life-saving treatment on the way to the emergency room.

Treating a Transient Ischemic Attack

If your symptoms go away after a few minutes, you may have had a transient ischemic attack (TIA). Although brief, a TIA is a sign of a serious condition that will not go away without medical help. Tell your healthcare team about your symptoms right away.

Unfortunately, because TIAs clear up, many people ignore them. Don't be one of those people. Paying attention to a TIA can save your life.

Why It's Important to Act Fast

Stroke is a medical emergency. Every minute counts when someone is having a stroke. The longer blood flow is cut off to the brain, the greater the damage. Immediate treatment can save people's lives and enhance their chances for successful recovery.

Ischemic strokes, the most common type of strokes, can be treated with a drug called t-PA that dissolves blood clots obstructing blood flow to the brain. The window of opportunity to start treating stroke patients is three hours, but to be evaluated and receive treatment, patients need to get to the hospital within 60 minutes.

What Should You Do?

Don't wait for the symptoms of stroke to improve or worsen. If you believe you are having a stroke, call 911 immediately. Making the decision to call for medical help can make the difference in avoiding a lifelong disability and in greatly improving your chances for recovery.

If you observe someone having a stroke—if he or she suddenly loses the ability to speak, or move an arm or leg on one side, or experiences facial paralysis on one side—call 911 immediately.

Chapter 8

What to Do in a Cardiac Emergency?

Chapter Contents

Section 8.1

Heart Attack and Sudden Cardiac Arrest: How Are They Different?

"Heart Attack and Sudden Cardiac Arrest: How Are They Different?"
© 2016 Omnigraphics. Reviewed June 2016.

Although the terms "heart attack" and "sudden cardiac arrest" are often confused with one another, there are important differences between these two emergency medical conditions. Sudden cardiac arrest occurs when the heart stops beating unexpectedly. Without immediate treatment, a person who experiences this abrupt loss of heart function will lose consciousness, stop breathing, and die in a matter of minutes. A heart attack, on the other hand, occurs when a blockage in a coronary artery prevents blood from circulating through part of the heart muscle. The heart usually continues beating during a heart attack, although it can lead to cardiac arrest if the disruption to the blood supply affects a large enough area of the heart.

Heart Attack Symptoms and Causes

The heart muscle is nourished by oxygen-rich blood that flows through the coronary arteries. When a coronary artery becomes blocked, the part of the heart that is fed by that artery is deprived of oxygen. If the blockage is not treated quickly, the heart muscle suffers damage and begins to die. This process is known as a heart attack. Most people experience physical symptoms during a heart attack. The symptoms may come on suddenly and be very intense, or they may appear gradually over several hours, days, or even weeks and be fairly mild. Although the symptoms vary greatly from person to person, some of the most common ones include:

- Pain or tightness in the center of the chest that may spread to the neck, back, arms, or abdomen
- Shortness of breath, even when resting
- Wheezing or coughing

- Dizziness, light-headedness, or weakness

- Nausea

- Anxiety

- Sweating

- Palpitations (rapid, strong, or irregular heartbeats)

Heart attacks are generally caused by the buildup of fatty deposits or plaques in the coronary arteries. Over time, the arteries narrow and harden, creating a condition known as atherosclerosis. If a plaque ruptures and creates a blood clot, the artery may become blocked and cause a heart attack. There are a number of factors that increase a person's risk of developing cardiovascular disease and having a heart attack, including the following:

- Smoking

- Obesity

- High blood pressure

- Unhealthy eating habits

- Lack of exercise

- Diabetes

- Family history of cardiovascular disease

- Exposure to high levels of air pollution

- Exposure to high levels of stress or anxiety

Cardiac Arrest Symptoms and Causes

Sudden cardiac arrest occurs when an electrical malfunction in the heart disrupts its rhythmic pumping action. The heart stops beating, which means that the brain, lungs, and other organs no longer receive the oxygen-rich blood they require to function. Within a matter of seconds, a person who experiences cardiac arrest will lose consciousness, stop breathing, and have no pulse. Although these are the main symptoms of sudden cardiac arrest, some people may experience early warning signs that are similar to the symptoms of a heart attack, such as chest pain, shortness of breath, dizziness, weakness, nausea, or palpitations.

Like heart attacks, sudden cardiac arrest is often related to cardiovascular disease. But sudden cardiac arrest can have many other causes, as well, including both cardiac and non-cardiac conditions. Some potential causes include:

- Arrhythmias (abnormal heart rhythms) such as ventricular fibrillation or ventricular tachycardia

- Other cardiac abnormalities, such as cardiomyopathy, myocarditis, congestive heart failure, or long QT syndrome

- Pacemaker failure

- Respiratory arrest

- Dramatic drop in blood pressure

- Trauma, choking, drowning, or electrocution

- Hypothermia

- Drug overdose or excessive alcohol consumption

- Poisoning

- Severe allergic reaction (anaphylaxis)

The Link between Heart Attack and Cardiac Arrest

Despite the differences between heart attack and sudden cardiac arrest, the two conditions are linked. Heart attack is one of the more common causes of cardiac arrest, which may occur after the heart attack or during the recovery process. Although most heart attacks do not lead to cardiac arrest, having a heart attack does increase a person's risk for sudden cardiac arrest.

In addition, both heart conditions are life-threatening emergency medical situations. If a person experiences chest pain or other symptoms of a heart attack, experts recommend calling for emergency medical services immediately. Calling 9-1-1 is also the first step for responders in cases of cardiac arrest, where a person is unresponsive and has no pulse. Since sudden cardiac arrest can lead to death within minutes, however, responders should also use an automated external defibrillator (AED) if one is available and perform cardiopulmonary resuscitation (CPR) until professional help arrives. Cardiac arrest is often reversible with immediate treatment, and performing CPR significantly increases the victim's chances of survival.

References

1. Cashin-Garbutt, April. "Heart Attack and Cardiac Arrest Difference," News Medical, December 6, 2013.

2. "Heart Attack or Sudden Cardiac Arrest: How Are They Different?" American Heart Association, July 2015.

Section 8.2

What to Do during a Heart Attack?

This section includes text excerpted from "Heart Attack," National Heart, Lung, and Blood Institute (NHLBI), November 6, 2015.

How Is a Heart Attack Treated?

Early treatment for a heart attack can prevent or limit damage to the heart muscle. Acting fast, **by calling 9–1–1** at the first symptoms of a heart attack, can save your life. Medical personnel can begin diagnosis and treatment even before you get to the hospital.

Immediate Treatment

Certain treatments usually are started right away if a heart attack is suspected, even before the diagnosis is confirmed. These include:

- Aspirin to prevent further blood clotting

- Nitroglycerin to reduce your heart's workload and improve blood flow through the coronary arteries

- Oxygen therapy

- Treatment for chest pain

Once the diagnosis of a heart attack is confirmed or strongly suspected, doctors start treatments promptly to try to restore blood flow through the blood vessels supplying the heart. The two main treatments are clot-busting medicines and percutaneous coronary intervention, also known as coronary angioplasty, a procedure used to open blocked coronary arteries.

Clot-Busting Medicines

Thrombolytic medicines, also called clot busters, are used to dissolve blood clots that are blocking the coronary arteries. To work best, these medicines must be given within several hours of the start of heart attack symptoms. Ideally, the medicine should be given as soon as possible.

Percutaneous Coronary Intervention

Percutaneous coronary intervention is a nonsurgical procedure that opens blocked or narrowed coronary arteries. A thin, flexible tube (catheter) with a balloon or other device on the end is threaded through a blood vessel, usually in the groin (upper thigh), to the narrowed or blocked coronary artery. Once in place, the balloon located at the tip of the catheter is inflated to compress the plaque and related clot against the wall of the artery. This restores blood flow through the artery. During the procedure, the doctor may put a small mesh tube called a stent in the artery. The stent helps to keep the blood vessel open to prevent blockages in the artery in the months or years after the procedure.

Section 8.3

Symptoms and Emergency Treatment of Cardiac Arrest

This section includes text excerpted from "Sudden Cardiac Arrest," National Heart, Lung, and Blood Institute (NHLBI), October 29, 2015.

What Are the Signs and Symptoms of Sudden Cardiac Arrest?

Usually, the first sign of sudden cardiac arrest (SCA) is loss of consciousness (fainting). At the same time, no heartbeat (or pulse) can be felt.

Some people may have a racing heartbeat or feel dizzy or light-headed just before they faint. Within an hour before SCA, some people have chest pain, shortness of breath, nausea (feeling sick to the stomach), or vomiting.

How Is Sudden Cardiac Arrest Treated?

Emergency Treatment

Sudden cardiac arrest (SCA) is an emergency. A person having SCA needs to be treated with a defibrillator right away. This device sends an electric shock to the heart. The electric shock can restore a normal rhythm to a heart that's stopped beating.

To work well, defibrillation must be done within minutes of SCA. With every minute that passes, the chances of surviving SCA drop rapidly.

Police, emergency medical technicians, and other first responders usually are trained and equipped to use a defibrillator. Call 9–1–1 right away if someone has signs or symptoms of SCA. The sooner you call for help, the sooner lifesaving treatment can begin.

Automated External Defibrillators

Automated external defibrillators (AEDs) are special defibrillators that untrained bystanders can use. These portable devices often are found in public places, such as shopping malls, golf courses, businesses, airports, airplanes, casinos, convention centers, hotels, sports venues, and schools.

AEDs are programmed to give an electric shock if they detect a dangerous arrhythmia, such as ventricular fibrillation. This prevents giving a shock to someone who may have fainted but isn't having SCA.

You should give cardiopulmonary resuscitation (CPR) to a person having SCA until defibrillation can be done.

People who are at risk for SCA may want to consider having an AED at home. When considering a home-use AED, talk with your doctor. He or she can help you decide whether having an AED in your home will benefit you.

Treatment in a Hospital

If you survive SCA, you'll likely be admitted to a hospital for ongoing care and treatment. In the hospital, your medical team will closely watch your heart. They may give you medicines to try to reduce the risk of another SCA.

While in the hospital, your medical team will try to find out what caused your SCA. If you're diagnosed with coronary heart disease, you may have percutaneous coronary intervention, also known as coronary angioplasty, or coronary artery bypass grafting. These procedures help restore blood flow through narrowed or blocked coronary arteries.

Often, people who have SCA get a device called an implantable cardioverter defibrillator (ICD). This small device is surgically placed under the skin in your chest or abdomen. An ICD uses electric pulses or shocks to help control dangerous arrhythmias.

Section 8.4

What to Do during a Stroke?

This section includes text excerpted from "Stroke," National Heart, Lung, and Blood Institute (NHLBI), October 28, 2015.

How Is a Stroke Treated?

Treatment for a stroke depends on whether it is ischemic or hemorrhagic. Treatment for a transient ischemic attack (TIA) depends on its cause, how much time has passed since symptoms began, and whether you have other medical conditions.

Strokes and TIAs are medical emergencies. If you have stroke symptoms, call 9–1–1 right away. Do not drive to the hospital or let someone else drive you. Call an ambulance so that medical personnel can begin lifesaving treatment on the way to the emergency room. During a stroke, every minute counts.

Once you receive immediate treatment, your doctor will try to treat your stroke risk factors and prevent complications by recommending heart-healthy lifestyle changes.

Treating an Ischemic Stroke or Transient Ischemic Attack

An ischemic stroke or TIA occurs if an artery that supplies oxygen-rich blood to the brain becomes blocked. Often, blood clots cause the blockages that lead to ischemic strokes and TIAs. Treatment for an ischemic stroke or TIA may include medicines and medical procedures.

Medicines

If you have a stroke caused by a blood clot, you may be given a clot-dissolving, or clot-busting, medication called tissue plasminogen activator (tPA). A doctor will inject tPA into a vein in your arm. This type of medication must be given within 4 hours of symptom onset. Ideally, it should be given as soon as possible. The sooner treatment begins, the better your chances of recovery. Thus, it's important to know the signs and symptoms of a stroke and to call 9–1–1 right away for emergency care.

If you can't have tPA for medical reasons, your doctor may give you antiplatelet medicine that helps stop platelets from clumping together to form blood clots or anticoagulant medicine (blood thinner) that keeps existing blood clots from getting larger. Two common medicines are aspirin and clopidogrel.

Medical Procedures

If you have carotid artery disease, your doctor may recommend a carotid endarterectomy or carotid artery angioplasty. Both procedures open blocked carotid arteries.

Researchers are testing other treatments for ischemic stroke, such as intra-arterial thrombolysis and mechanical clot removal in cerebral ischemia (MERCI).

In intra-arterial thrombolysis, a long flexible tube called a catheter is put into your groin (upper thigh) and threaded to the tiny arteries of the brain. Your doctor can deliver medicine through this catheter to break up a blood clot in the brain.

MERCI is a device that can remove blood clots from an artery. During the procedure, a catheter is threaded through a carotid artery to the affected artery in the brain. The device is then used to pull the blood clot out through the catheter.

Treating a Hemorrhagic Stroke

A hemorrhagic stroke occurs if an artery in the brain leaks blood or ruptures. The first steps in treating a hemorrhagic stroke are to find the cause of bleeding in the brain and then control it. Unlike ischemic strokes, hemorrhagic strokes aren't treated with antiplatelet medicines and blood thinners because these medicines can make bleeding worse.

If you're taking antiplatelet medicines or blood thinners and have a hemorrhagic stroke, you'll be taken off the medicine. If high blood pressure is the cause of bleeding in the brain, your doctor may prescribe medicines to lower your blood pressure. This can help prevent further bleeding.

Surgery also may be needed to treat a hemorrhagic stroke. The types of surgery used include aneurysm clipping, coil embolization, and arteriovenous malformation (AVM) repair.

Aneurysm Clipping and Coil Embolization

If an aneurysm (a balloon-like bulge in an artery) is the cause of a stroke, your doctor may recommend aneurysm clipping or coil embolization.

Aneurysm clipping is done to block off the aneurysm from the blood vessels in the brain. This surgery helps prevent further leaking of blood from the aneurysm. It also can help prevent the aneurysm from bursting again. During the procedure, a surgeon will make an incision (cut) in the brain and place a tiny clamp at the base of the aneurysm. You'll be given medicine to make you sleep during the surgery. After the surgery, you'll need to stay in the hospital's intensive care unit for a few days.

Coil embolization is a less complex procedure for treating an aneurysm. The surgeon will insert a tube called a catheter into an artery in the groin. He or she will thread the tube to the site of the aneurysm. Then, a tiny coil will be pushed through the tube and into the aneurysm. The coil will cause a blood clot to form, which will block blood flow through the aneurysm and prevent it from bursting again. Coil embolization is done in a hospital. You'll be given medicine to make you sleep during the surgery.

Arteriovenous Malformation Repair

If an AVM is the cause of a stroke, your doctor may recommend an AVM repair. (An AVM is a tangle of faulty arteries and veins that can rupture within the brain.) AVM repair helps prevent further bleeding in the brain.

Doctors use several methods to repair AVMs. These methods include:

- Injecting a substance into the blood vessels of the AVM to block blood flow

- Surgery to remove the AVM

- Using radiation to shrink the blood vessels of the AVM

Chapter 9

Cardiopulmonary Resuscitation (CPR)

About CPR

CPR (or **cardiopulmonary resuscitation**) is a combination of chest compressions and rescue breathing (mouth-to-mouth resuscitation). If someone isn't circulating blood or breathing adequately, CPR can restore circulation of oxygen-rich blood to the brain. Without oxygen, permanent brain damage or death can happen in less than 8 minutes.

CPR might be necessary in many different emergencies, including accidents, near-drowning, suffocation, poisoning, smoke inhalation, electrocution injuries, and suspected sudden infant death syndrome (SIDS).

Reading about CPR and learning when it's needed will give you a basic understanding of the concept and procedure, but it's strongly recommended that you learn the details of how to perform CPR by taking a course. If CPR is needed, using the correct technique will give someone the best chance of survival.

CPR is most successful when started as quickly as possible, but you must first determine if it's necessary. It should only be performed when a person isn't breathing or circulating blood adequately.

Text in this chapter is excerpted from "CPR," ©1995–2016. The Nemours Foundation/KidsHealth®. Reprinted with permission.

First, determine that it's safe to approach the person in trouble. For instance, if someone was injured in an accident on a busy highway, you'd have to be extremely careful about ongoing traffic as you try to help. Or if someone touched an exposed wire and was electrocuted, you'd have to be certain that he or she is no longer in contact with electricity before offering assistance to prevent becoming electrocuted yourself. (For instance, turn off the source of electricity, such as a light switch or a circuit breaker.)

Once you know that you can safely approach someone who needs help, quickly evaluate whether the person is responsive. Look for things such as eye opening, sounds from the mouth, chest movement, or other signs of life such as movement of the arms and legs.

In infants and younger kids, rubbing the chest (over the breastbone) can help determine if there is any level of responsiveness. In older kids and adults, this also can be done by gently tapping the shoulders and asking if they're all right.

Whenever CPR is needed, remember to call for emergency medical assistance. Current CPR courses teach you that if you are alone with an unresponsive infant or child, you should perform CPR for about 2 minutes before calling for help.

Three Parts of CPR

The three basic parts of CPR are easily remembered as "CAB": **C** for compressions, **A** for airway, and **B** for breathing.

1. **C is for compressions**. Chest compressions can help improve the flow of blood to the heart, brain, and other organs. CPR begins with 30 chest compressions, followed by two rescue breaths. This cycle is immediately repeated and continued until the child recovers or help arrives. It is not necessary to check for signs of circulation to perform this technique. According to the American Heart Association (AHA), rescuers doing compressions should "push hard, fast, and in the center of the chest." A CPR course will teach you how to perform chest compressions in infants, kids, and adults, and how to coordinate the compressions with rescue breathing.

2. **A is for airway.** After 30 compressions have been completed, the victim's airway must be open for breathing to be restored. The airway may be blocked by the tongue when someone loses consciousness or may be obstructed by food or another foreign object. In a CPR course, participants learn how to open the

airway and position the person so the airway is ready for rescue breathing. The course will include what to do to clear the airway if you believe an infant or child has choked and the airway is blocked.

3. **B is for breathing**. Rescue breathing is begun after 30 compressions have been completed and the airway is open. Someone performing rescue breathing essentially breathes for the victim by forcing air into the lungs. This procedure includes breathing into the victim's mouth at correct intervals and checking for signs of life.

A CPR course will review correct techniques and procedures for rescuers to position themselves to give mouth-to-mouth resuscitation to infants, kids, and adults.

Taking a CPR Course

Nearby hospitals and your local chapters of the AHA and the American Red Cross are good resources for finding a CPR course in your area.

Qualified instructors may use videos, printed materials, and demonstrations on mannequins representing infants, kids, and adults to teach proper techniques for performing CPR.

The AHA offers many levels of CPR courses. A basic course that includes CPR lasts several hours and takes place within one session. It covers adult, child, and infant CPR and choking. Participants practice the techniques on mannequins and can ask questions and get individualized instruction.

Because CPR is a skill that must be practiced, it's wise to repeat the course at least every 2 years to maintain your skills. Doing so also allows you to learn about any new advances or discoveries in CPR techniques.

Remember, taking a CPR course could help you save your child's—or someone else's—life someday.

Chapter 10

Automated External Defibrillators

What Is an Automated External Defibrillator?

An automated external defibrillator (AED) is a portable device that checks the heart rhythm and can send an electric shock to the heart to try to restore a normal rhythm. AEDs are used to treat sudden cardiac arrest (SCA).

SCA is a condition in which the heart suddenly and unexpectedly stops beating. When this happens, blood stops flowing to the brain and other vital organs.

SCA usually causes death if it's not treated within minutes. In fact, each minute of SCA leads to a 10 percent reduction in survival. Using an AED on a person who is having SCA may save the person's life.

Overview

To understand how AEDs work, it helps to understand how the heart works.

The heart has an internal electrical system that controls the rate and rhythm of the heartbeat. With each heartbeat, an electrical signal spreads from the top of the heart to the bottom. As the signal travels,

---

This chapter includes text excerpted from "Automated External Defibrillator," National Heart, Lung, and Blood Institute (NHLBI), December 2, 2011. Reviewed June 2016.

it causes the heart to contract and pump blood. The process repeats with each new heartbeat.

Problems with the electrical system can cause abnormal heart rhythms called arrhythmias. During an arrhythmia, the heart can beat too fast, too slow, or with an irregular rhythm. Some arrhythmias can cause the heart to stop pumping blood to the body. These arrhythmias cause SCA.

Outlook

Ninety-five percent of people who have SCA die from it—most within minutes. Rapid treatment of SCA with an AED can be lifesaving.

When Should an Automated External Defibrillator Be Used?

Using an automated external defibrillator (AED) on a person who is having sudden cardiac arrest (SCA) may save the person's life.

The most common cause of SCA is an arrhythmia called ventricular fibrillation (v-fib). In v-fib, the ventricles (the heart's lower chambers) don't beat normally. Instead, they quiver very rapidly and irregularly.

Another arrhythmia that can lead to SCA is ventricular tachycardia. This is a fast, regular beating of the ventricles that may last for a few seconds or much longer.

In people who have either of these arrhythmias, an electric shock from an AED can restore the heart's normal rhythm (if done within minutes of the onset of SCA).

What Are the Signs of Sudden Cardiac Arrest?

If someone is having SCA, you may see him or her suddenly collapse and lose consciousness. Or, you may find the person unconscious and unable to respond when you call or shake him or her.

The person may not be breathing, or he or she may have an abnormal breathing pattern. If you check, you usually can't find a pulse. The person's skin also may become dark or blue from lack of oxygen. Also, the person may not move, or his or her movements may look like a seizure (spasms).

An AED can check the person's heart rhythm and determine whether an electric shock is needed to try to restore a normal rhythm.

How Does an Automated External Defibrillator Work?

Automated external defibrillators (AEDs) are lightweight, battery-operated, portable devices that are easy to use. Sticky pads with sensors (called electrodes) are attached to the chest of the person who is having sudden cardiac arrest (SCA).

The electrodes send information about the person's heart rhythm to a computer in the AED. The computer analyzes the heart rhythm to find out whether an electric shock is needed. If a shock is needed, the AED uses voice prompts to tell you when to give the shock, and the electrodes deliver it.

Using an AED to shock the heart within minutes of the start of SCA may restore a normal heart rhythm. Every minute counts. Each minute of SCA leads to a 10 percent reduction in survival.

Training To Use an Automated External Defibrillator

Learning how to use an AED and taking a CPR (cardiopulmonary resuscitation) course are helpful. However, if trained personnel aren't available, untrained people also can use an AED to help save someone's life.

Some people are afraid to use an AED to help save someone's life. They're worried that something might go wrong and that they might be sued. However, Good Samaritan laws in each State and the Federal Cardiac Arrest Survival Act (CASA) provide some protection for untrained bystanders who respond to emergencies.

Facility owners who are thinking about buying an AED should provide initial and ongoing training to likely rescuers (usually people who work in the facility). Also, it's important to properly maintain an AED and notify local emergency officials of its location.

How to Use an Automated External Defibrillator

Before using an automated external defibrillator (AED) on someone who you think is having sudden cardiac arrest (SCA), check him or her.

If you see a person suddenly collapse and pass out, or if you find a person already unconscious, confirm that the person can't respond. Shout at and shake the person to make sure he or she isn't sleeping.

Never shake an infant or young child. Instead, you can pinch the child to try to wake him or her up.

Call 9–1–1 or have someone else call 9–1–1. If two rescuers are present, one can provide CPR (cardiopulmonary resuscitation) while the other calls 9–1–1 and gets the AED.

Check the person's breathing and pulse. If breathing and pulse are absent or irregular, prepare to use the AED as soon as possible. (SCA causes death if it's not treated within minutes.)

If no one knows how long the person has been unconscious, or if an AED isn't readily available, do 2 minutes of CPR. Then use the AED (if you have one) to check the person.

After you use the AED, or if you don't have an AED, give CPR until emergency medical help arrives or until the person begins to move. Try to limit pauses in CPR.

After 2 minutes of CPR, you can use the AED again to check the person's heart rhythm and give another shock, if needed. If a shock isn't needed, continue CPR.

Using an Automated External Defibrillator

AEDs are user-friendly devices that untrained bystanders can use to save the life of someone having SCA.

Before using an AED, check for puddles or water near the person who is unconscious. Move him or her to a dry area, and stay away from wetness when delivering shocks (water conducts electricity).

Turn on the AED's power. The device will give you step-by-step instructions. You'll hear voice prompts and see prompts on a screen.

Expose the person's chest. If the person's chest is wet, dry it. AEDs have sticky pads with sensors called electrodes. Apply the pads to the person's chest as pictured on the AED's instructions.

Place one pad on the right center of the person's chest above the nipple. Place the other pad slightly below the other nipple and to the left of the ribcage.

Make sure the sticky pads have good connection with the skin. If the connection isn't good, the machine may repeat the phrase "check electrodes."

If the person has a lot of chest hair, you may have to trim it. (AEDs usually come with a kit that includes scissors and/or a razor.) If the person is wearing a medication patch that's in the way, remove it and clean the medicine from the skin before applying the sticky pads.

Remove metal necklaces and underwire bras. The metal may conduct electricity and cause burns. You can cut the center of the bra and pull it away from the skin.

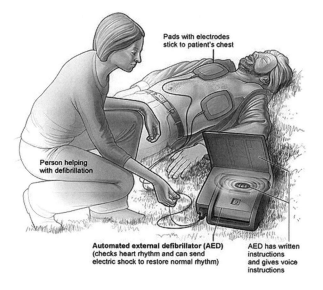

Figure 10.1. *Using an Automated External Defibrillator*

The image shows a typical setup using an automated external defibrillator (AED). The AED has step-by-step instructions and voice prompts that enable an untrained bystander to correctly use the machine.

Check the person for implanted medical devices, such as a pacemaker or implantable cardioverter defibrillator. (The outline of these devices is visible under the skin on the chest or abdomen, and the person may be wearing a medical alert bracelet.) Also check for body piercings.

Move the defibrillator pads at least 1 inch away from implanted devices or piercings so the electric current can flow freely between the pads.

Check that the wires from the electrodes are connected to the AED. Make sure no one is touching the person, and then press the AED's "analyze" button. Stay clear while the machine checks the person's heart rhythm.

If a shock is needed, the AED will let you know when to deliver it. Stand clear of the person and make sure others are clear before you push the AED's "shock" button.

Start or resume CPR until emergency medical help arrives or until the person begins to move. Stay with the person until medical help arrives, and report all of the information you know about what has happened.

What Are the Risks of Using an Automated External Defibrillator?

Automated external defibrillators (AEDs) are safe to use. There are no reports of AEDs harming bystanders or users. Also, there are no reports of AEDs delivering inappropriate shocks.

If someone is having sudden cardiac arrest, using an AED and giving CPR (cardiopulmonary resuscitation) can improve the person's chance of survival.

Part Two

Heart Disorders

Chapter 11

Problems with the Heart's Blood Supply

Chapter Contents

Section 11.1

Coronary Heart Disease

This section includes text excerpted from "Coronary Heart
Disease," National Heart, Lung, and Blood Institute
(NHLBI), October 23, 2015.

What Is Coronary Heart Disease?

Coronary heart disease (CHD) is a disease in which a waxy substance called plaque builds up inside the coronary arteries. These
arteries supply oxygen-rich blood to your heart muscle.

When plaque builds up in the arteries, the condition is called atherosclerosis. The buildup of plaque occurs over many years.

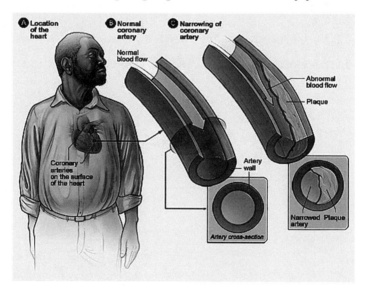

Figure 11.1. *Atherosclerosis*

*(A) shows the location of the heart in the body. (B) shows a normal coronary artery
with normal blood flow. The inset image shows a cross-section of a normal coronary
artery. (C) shows a coronary artery narrowed by plaque. The buildup of plaque limits
the flow of oxygen-rich blood through the artery. The inset image shows a cross-section of the plaque-narrowed artery.*

Over time, plaque can harden or rupture (break open). Hardened plaque narrows the coronary arteries and reduces the flow of oxygen-rich blood to the heart.

If the plaque ruptures, a blood clot can form on its surface. A large blood clot can mostly or completely block blood flow through a coronary artery. Over time, ruptured plaque also hardens and narrows the coronary arteries.

Other Names for Coronary Heart Disease

- Atherosclerosis

- Heart disease

- Ischemic heart disease

- Narrowing of the arteries

- Coronary artery disease

- Hardening of the arteries

What Causes Coronary Heart Disease?

Research suggests that coronary heart disease (CHD) starts when certain factors damage the inner layers of the coronary arteries. These factors include:

- Smoking

- High levels of certain fats and cholesterol in the blood

- High blood pressure

- High levels of sugar in the blood due to insulin resistance or diabetes

- Blood vessel inflammation

Plaque might begin to build up where the arteries are damaged. The buildup of plaque in the coronary arteries may start in childhood.

Over time, plaque can harden or rupture (break open). Hardened plaque narrows the coronary arteries and reduces the flow of oxygen-rich blood to the heart. This can cause angina (chest pain or discomfort).

If the plaque ruptures, blood cell fragments called platelets stick to the site of the injury. They may clump together to form blood clots.

Blood clots can further narrow the coronary arteries and worsen angina. If a clot becomes large enough, it can mostly or completely block a coronary artery and cause a heart attack.

Who Is at Risk for Coronary Heart Disease?

In the United States, coronary heart disease (CHD) is a leading cause of death for both men and women. Each year, about 370,000 Americans die from coronary heart disease.

Certain traits, conditions, or habits may raise your risk for CHD. The more risk factors you have, the more likely you are to develop the disease.

You can control many risk factors, which may help prevent or delay CHD.

Major Risk Factors

- Unhealthy blood cholesterol levels
- High blood pressure
- Smoking
- Insulin resistance
- Diabetes
- Overweight or obesity
- Metabolic syndrome
- Lack of physical activity
- Unhealthy diet
- Older age
- A family history of early coronary heart disease

Although older age and a family history of early heart disease are risk factors, it doesn't mean that you'll develop CHD if you have one or both. Controlling other risk factors often can lessen genetic influences and help prevent CHD, even in older adults.

Emerging Risk Factors

Researchers continue to study other possible risk factors for CHD.

High levels of a protein called C-reactive protein (CRP) in the blood may raise the risk of CHD and heart attack. High levels of CRP are a sign of inflammation in the body.

Inflammation is the body's response to injury or infection. Damage to the arteries' inner walls may trigger inflammation and help plaque grow.

Research is under way to find out whether reducing inflammation and lowering CRP levels also can reduce the risk of CHD and heart attack.

High levels of triglycerides in the blood also may raise the risk of CHD, especially in women. Triglycerides are a type of fat.

Other Risks Related to Coronary Heart Disease

Other conditions and factors also may contribute to CHD, including:

- Sleep apnea

- Stress

- Alcohol

- Preeclampsia

What Are the Signs and Symptoms of Coronary Heart Disease?

A common symptom of coronary heart disease (CHD) is angina. Angina is chest pain or discomfort that occurs if an area of your heart muscle doesn't get enough oxygen-rich blood.

Angina may feel like pressure or squeezing in your chest. You also may feel it in your shoulders, arms, neck, jaw, or back. Angina pain may even feel like indigestion. The pain tends to get worse with activity and go away with rest. Emotional stress also can trigger the pain.

Another common symptom of CHD is shortness of breath. This symptom occurs if CHD causes heart failure. When you have heart failure, your heart can't pump enough blood to meet your body's needs. Fluid builds up in your lungs, making it hard to breathe.

The severity of these symptoms varies. They may get more severe as the buildup of plaque continues to narrow the coronary arteries.

Signs and Symptoms of Heart Problems Related to Coronary Heart Disease

Some people who have CHD have no signs or symptoms—a condition called silent CHD. The disease might not be diagnosed until a person has signs or symptoms of a heart attack, heart failure, or an arrhythmia (an irregular heartbeat).

How Is Coronary Heart Disease Diagnosed?

Your doctor will diagnose coronary heart disease (CHD) based on your medical and family histories, your risk factors for CHD, a physical exam, and the results from tests and procedures.

No single test can diagnose CHD. If your doctor thinks you have CHD, he or she may recommend one or more of the following tests.

- EKG (Electrocardiogram)
- Stress testing
- Echocardiography
- Chest X-ray
- Blood tests
- Coronary angiography and cardiac catheterization

How Is Coronary Heart Disease Treated?

Treatments for coronary heart disease include heart-healthy lifestyle changes, medicines, medical procedures and surgery, and cardiac rehabilitation. Treatment goals may include:

- Lowering the risk of blood clots forming (blood clots can cause a heart attack)
- Preventing complications of coronary heart disease
- Reducing risk factors in an effort to slow, stop, or reverse the buildup of plaque
- Relieving symptoms
- Widening or bypassing clogged arteries

Heart-Healthy Lifestyle Changes

Your doctor may recommend heart-healthy lifestyle changes if you have coronary heart disease. Heart-healthy lifestyle changes include:

- Heart-healthy eating
- Maintaining a healthy weight
- Managing stress
- Physical activity
- Quitting smoking

Section 11.2

Coronary Microvascular Disease

This section includes text excerpted from "Coronary Heart
Disease," National Heart, Lung, and Blood Institute
(NHLBI), October 27, 2015.

What Is Coronary Microvascular Disease?

Coronary microvascular disease (MVD) is heart disease that affects
the tiny coronary (heart) arteries. In coronary MVD, the walls of the
heart's tiny arteries are damaged or diseased.

Coronary MVD is different from traditional coronary heart disease
(CHD), also called coronary artery disease. In CHD, a waxy substance
called plaque builds up in the large coronary arteries.

Plaque narrows the heart's large arteries and reduces the flow of
oxygen-rich blood to your heart muscle. The buildup of plaque also
makes it more likely that blood clots will form in your arteries. Blood
clots can mostly or completely block blood flow through a coronary
artery.

In coronary MVD, however, the heart's tiny arteries are affected.
Plaque doesn't create blockages in these vessels as it does in the heart's
large arteries.

Other Names for Coronary Microvascular Disease

• Cardiac syndrome X

• Nonobstructive coronary heart disease

What Causes Coronary Microvascular Disease?

The same risk factors that cause atherosclerosis may cause coronary
microvascular disease. Atherosclerosis is a disease in which plaque
builds up inside the arteries.

Risk factors for atherosclerosis include:

• Diabetes

- Family history of early heart disease

- High blood pressure

- Insulin resistance

- Lack of physical activity

- Older age

- Overweight and obesity

- Unhealthy blood cholesterol levels

- Unhealthy diet

In women, coronary microvascular disease also may be linked to low estrogen levels occurring before or after menopause. Also, the disease may be linked to anemia or conditions that affect blood clotting. Anemia is thought to slow the growth of cells needed to repair damaged blood vessels.

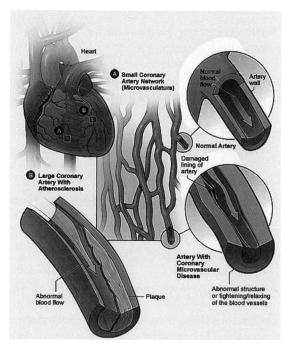

Figure 11.2. *Coronary Microvascular Disease*

(A) shows the small coronary artery network (microvasculature), containing a normal artery and an artery with coronary MVD. (B) shows a large coronary artery with plaque buildup.

Who Is at Risk for Coronary Microvascular Disease?

Coronary microvascular disease can affect both men and women. However, women may be at risk for coronary microvascular disease if they have lower than normal levels of estrogen at any point in their adult lives. (This refers to the estrogen that the ovaries produce, not the estrogen used in hormone therapy.) Low estrogen levels before menopause can raise younger women's risk for the disease. Causes of low estrogen levels in younger women can be mental stress or a problem with the function of the ovaries.

The causes of coronary microvascular disease and atherosclerosis are also considered risk factors for the disease.

What Are the Signs and Symptoms of Coronary Microvascular Disease?

The signs and symptoms of coronary microvascular disease (MVD) often differ from the signs and symptoms of traditional coronary heart disease (CHD).

Many women with coronary MVD have angina. Angina is chest pain or discomfort that occurs when your heart muscle doesn't get enough oxygen-rich blood.

Angina may feel like pressure or squeezing in your chest. You also may feel it in your shoulders, arms, neck, jaw, or back. Angina pain may even feel like indigestion.

Angina also is a common symptom of CHD. However, the angina that occurs in coronary MVD may differ from the typical angina that occurs in CHD. In coronary MVD, the chest pain usually lasts longer than 10 minutes, and it can last longer than 30 minutes. Typical angina is more common in women older than 65.

Other signs and symptoms of coronary MVD are shortness of breath, sleep problems, fatigue (tiredness), and lack of energy.

Coronary MVD symptoms often are first noticed during routine daily activities (such as shopping, cooking, cleaning, and going to work) and times of mental stress. It's less likely that women will notice these symptoms during physical activity (such as jogging or walking fast).

This differs from CHD, in which symptoms often first appear while a person is being physically active—such as while jogging, walking on a treadmill, or going up stairs.

How Is Coronary Microvascular Disease Diagnosed?

Your doctor will diagnose coronary microvascular disease (MVD) based on your medical history, a physical exam, and test results. He or she will check to see whether you have any risk factors for heart disease.

For example, your doctor may measure your weight and height to check for overweight or obesity. He or she also may recommend tests for high blood cholesterol, metabolic syndrome, and diabetes.

Your doctor may ask you to describe any chest pain, including when it started and how it changed during physical activity or periods of stress. He or she also may ask about other symptoms, such as fatigue (tiredness), lack of energy, and shortness of breath. Women may be asked about their menopausal status.

Diagnostic Tests

The risk factors for coronary MVD and traditional coronary heart disease (CHD) often are the same. Thus, your doctor may recommend tests for CHD, such as:

- Coronary angiography

- Stress testing

- Cardiac MRI (magnetic resonance imaging) stress test

Unfortunately, standard tests for CHD aren't designed to detect coronary MVD. These tests look for blockages in the large coronary arteries. Coronary MVD affects the tiny coronary arteries.

If test results show that you don't have CHD, your doctor might still diagnose you with coronary MVD. This could happen if signs are present that not enough oxygen is reaching your heart's tiny arteries.

Coronary MVD symptoms often first occur during routine daily tasks. Thus, your doctor may ask you to fill out a questionnaire called the Duke Activity Status Index (DASI). The questionnaire will ask you how well you're able to do daily activities, such as shopping, cooking, and going to work.

The DASI results will help your doctor decide which kind of stress test you should have. The results also give your doctor information about how well blood is flowing through your coronary arteries.

Your doctor also may recommend blood tests, including a test for anemia. Anemia is thought to slow the growth of cells needed to repair damaged blood vessels.

Research is ongoing for better ways to detect and diagnose coronary MVD. Currently, researchers have not agreed on the best way to diagnose the disease.

How Is Coronary Microvascular Disease Treated?

Relieving pain is one of the main goals of treating coronary microvascular disease (MVD). Treatments also are used to control risk factors and other symptoms. Treatments may include medicines, such as:

- ACE inhibitors and beta blockers to lower blood pressure and decrease the heart's workload

- Aspirin to help prevent blood clots or control inflammation

- Nitroglycerin to relax blood vessels, improve blood flow to the heart muscle, and treat chest pain

- Statin medicines to control or lower your blood cholesterol.

Take all medicines regularly, as your doctor prescribes. Don't change the amount of your medicine or skip a dose unless your doctor tells you to.

If you're diagnosed with coronary MVD and also have anemia, you may benefit from treatment for that condition. Anemia is thought to slow the growth of cells needed to repair damaged blood vessels.

If you're diagnosed with and treated for coronary MVD, you should get ongoing care from your doctor. Research is under way to find the best treatments for coronary MVD.

How Can Coronary Microvascular Disease Be Prevented?

No specific studies have been done on how to prevent coronary microvascular disease.

Researchers don't yet know how or in what way preventing coronary microvascular disease differs from preventing coronary heart disease. Coronary microvascular disease affects the tiny coronary arteries; coronary heart disease affects the large coronary arteries.

Taking action to control risk factors for heart disease can help prevent or delay coronary heart disease. You can't control some risk factors, such as older age and family history of heart disease. However, you can take steps to prevent or control other risk factors, such as high blood pressure, overweight and obesity, high blood cholesterol, diabetes, and smoking.

Heart-healthy lifestyle changes and ongoing medical care can help you lower your risk for heart disease.

Heart-Healthy Lifestyle Changes

Your doctor may recommend heart-healthy lifestyle changes if you have coronary microvascular disease. Heart-healthy lifestyle changes include:

- Heart-healthy eating
- Maintaining a healthy weight
- Managing stress
- Physical activity
- Quitting smoking

Chapter 12

Angina

What Is Angina?

Angina is chest pain or discomfort that occurs if an area of your heart muscle doesn't get enough oxygen-rich blood.

Angina may feel like pressure or squeezing in your chest. The pain also can occur in your shoulders, arms, neck, jaw, or back. Angina pain may even feel like indigestion.

Angina isn't a disease; it's a symptom of an underlying heart problem. Angina usually is a symptom of coronary heart disease (CHD).

CHD is the most common type of heart disease in adults. It occurs if a waxy substance called plaque builds up on the inner walls of your coronary arteries. These arteries carry oxygen-rich blood to your heart.

Types of Angina

The major types of angina are stable, unstable, variant (Prinzmetal's), and microvascular. Knowing how the types differ is important. This is because they have different symptoms and require different treatments.

Stable Angina

Stable angina is the most common type of angina. It occurs when the heart is working harder than usual. Stable angina has a regular

---

This chapter includes text excerpted from "Angina," National Heart, Lung, and Blood Institute (NHLBI), June 1, 2011. Reviewed June 2016.

pattern. ("Pattern" refers to how often the angina occurs, how severe it is, and what factors trigger it.)

If you have stable angina, you can learn its pattern and predict when the pain will occur. The pain usually goes away a few minutes after you rest or take your angina medicine.

Stable angina isn't a heart attack, but it suggests that a heart attack is more likely to happen in the future.

Unstable Angina

Unstable angina doesn't follow a pattern. It may occur more often and be more severe than stable angina. Unstable angina also can occur with or without physical exertion, and rest or medicine may not relieve the pain.

Unstable angina is very dangerous and requires emergency treatment. This type of angina is a sign that a heart attack may happen soon.

Variant (Prinzmetal's) Angina

Variant angina is rare. A spasm in a coronary artery causes this type of angina. Variant angina usually occurs while you're at rest, and the pain can be severe. It usually happens between midnight and early morning. Medicine can relieve this type of angina.

Microvascular Angina

Microvascular angina can be more severe and last longer than other types of angina. Medicine may not relieve this type of angina.

Overview

Experts believe that nearly 7 million people in the United States suffer from angina. The condition occurs equally among men and women. Angina can be a sign of CHD, even if initial tests don't point to the disease. However, not all chest pain or discomfort is a sign of CHD.

Other conditions also can cause chest pain, such as:

- Pulmonary embolism (a blockage in a lung artery)

- A lung infection

- Aortic dissection (tearing of a major artery)

- Aortic stenosis (narrowing of the heart's aortic valve)

- Hypertrophic cardiomyopathy (Heart muscle disease)
- Pericarditis (inflammation in the tissues that surround the heart)
- A panic attack

All chest pain should be checked by a doctor.

Other Names for Angina

- Acute coronary syndrome
- Angina pectoris
- Chest pain
- Coronary artery spasms
- Microvascular angina
- Prinzmetal's angina
- Stable or common angina
- Unstable angina
- Variant angina

What Causes Angina?

Immediate Causes

Many factors can trigger angina pain, depending on the type of angina you have.

Stable Angina

Physical exertion is the most common trigger of stable angina. Severely narrowed arteries may allow enough blood to reach the heart when the demand for oxygen is low, such as when you're sitting.

However, with physical exertion—like walking up a hill or climbing stairs—the heart works harder and needs more oxygen.

Other triggers of stable angina include:

- Emotional stress
- Exposure to very hot or cold temperatures
- Heavy meals
- Smoking

Unstable Angina

Blood clots that partially or totally block an artery cause unstable angina.

If plaque in an artery ruptures, blood clots may form. This creates a blockage. A clot may grow large enough to completely block the artery and cause a heart attack.

Blood clots may form, partially dissolve, and later form again. Angina can occur each time a clot blocks an artery.

Variant Angina

A spasm in a coronary artery causes variant angina. The spasm causes the walls of the artery to tighten and narrow. Blood flow to the heart slows or stops. Variant angina can occur in people who have CHD and in those who don't.

The coronary arteries can spasm as a result of:

• Exposure to cold

• Emotional stress

• Medicines that tighten or narrow blood vessels

• Smoking

• Cocaine use

Microvascular Angina

This type of angina may be a symptom of coronary microvascular disease (MVD). Coronary MVD is heart disease that affects the heart's smallest coronary arteries.

Reduced blood flow in the small coronary arteries may cause microvascular angina. Plaque in the arteries, artery spasms, or damaged or diseased artery walls can reduce blood flow through the small coronary arteries.

Who Is at Risk for Angina?

Angina is a symptom of an underlying heart problem. It's usually a symptom of coronary heart disease (CHD), but it also can be a symptom of coronary microvascular disease (MVD). So, if you're at risk for CHD or coronary MVD, you're also at risk for angina.

The major risk factors for CHD and coronary MVD include:

• Unhealthy cholesterol levels.

- High blood pressure.

- Smoking.

- Insulin resistance or diabetes.

- Overweight or obesity.

- Metabolic syndrome.

- Lack of physical activity.

- Unhealthy diet.

- Older age. (The risk increases for men after 45 years of age and for women after 55 years of age.)

- Family history of early heart disease.

People sometimes think that because men have more heart attacks than women, men also suffer from angina more often. In fact, overall, angina occurs equally among men and women.

Microvascular angina, however, occurs more often in women. About 70 percent of the cases of microvascular angina occur in women around the time of menopause.

Unstable angina occurs more often in older adults. Variant angina is rare; it accounts for only about 2 out of 100 cases of angina. People who have variant angina often are younger than those who have other forms of angina.

What Are the Signs and Symptoms of Angina?

Pain and discomfort are the main symptoms of angina. Angina often is described as pressure, squeezing, burning, or tightness in the chest. The pain or discomfort usually starts behind the breastbone.

Pain from angina also can occur in the arms, shoulders, neck, jaw, throat, or back. The pain may feel like indigestion. Some people say that angina pain is hard to describe or that they can't tell exactly where the pain is coming from.

Signs and symptoms such as nausea (feeling sick to your stomach), fatigue (tiredness), shortness of breath, sweating, light-headedness, and weakness also may occur.

Women are more likely to feel discomfort in the neck, jaw, throat, abdomen, or back. Shortness of breath is more common in older people and those who have diabetes. Weakness, dizziness, and confusion can mask the signs and symptoms of angina in elderly people.

Symptoms also vary based on the type of angina you have.

Because angina has so many possible symptoms and causes, all chest pain should be checked by a doctor. Chest pain that lasts longer than a few minutes and isn't relieved by rest or angina medicine may be a sign of a heart attack. Call 9–1–1 right away.

Stable Angina

The pain or discomfort:

- Occurs when the heart must work harder, usually during physical exertion
- Doesn't come as a surprise, and episodes of pain tend to be alike
- Usually lasts a short time (5 minutes or less)
- Is relieved by rest or medicine
- May feel like gas or indigestion
- May feel like chest pain that spreads to the arms, back, or other areas

Unstable Angina

The pain or discomfort:

- Often occurs at rest, while sleeping at night, or with little physical exertion
- Comes as a surprise
- Is more severe and lasts longer than stable angina (as long as 30 minutes)
- Usually isn't relieved by rest or medicine
- May get worse over time
- May mean that a heart attack will happen soon

Variant Angina

The pain or discomfort:

- Usually occurs at rest and during the night or early morning hours
- Tends to be severe
- Is relieved by medicine

Microvascular Angina

The pain or discomfort:

- May be more severe and last longer than other types of angina pain

- May occur with shortness of breath, sleep problems, fatigue, and lack of energy

- Often is first noticed during routine daily activities and times of mental stress

Diagnostic Tests and Procedures

If your doctor thinks that you have unstable angina or that your angina is related to a serious heart condition, he or she may recommend one or more tests.

- EKG (Electrocardiogram)

- Stress testing

- Chest X-ray

- Coronary angiography and cardiac catheterization

- Computed tomography angiography

- Blood tests

How Is Angina Treated?

Treatments for angina include lifestyle changes, medicines, medical procedures, cardiac rehabilitation (rehab), and other therapies. The main goals of treatment are to:

- Reduce pain and discomfort and how often it occurs

- Prevent or lower your risk for heart attack and death by treating your underlying heart condition

Lifestyle changes and medicines may be the only treatments needed if your symptoms are mild and aren't getting worse. If lifestyle changes and medicines don't control angina, you may need medical procedures or cardiac rehab.

Unstable angina is an emergency condition that requires treatment in a hospital.

Lifestyle Changes

Making lifestyle changes can help prevent episodes of angina. You can:

- Slow down or take rest breaks if physical exertion triggers angina.

- Avoid large meals and rich foods that leave you feeling stuffed if heavy meals trigger angina.

- Try to avoid situations that make you upset or stressed if emotional stress triggers angina. Learn ways to handle stress that can't be avoided.

Medicines

Nitrates are the medicines most commonly used to treat angina. They relax and widen blood vessels. This allows more blood to flow to the heart, while reducing the heart's workload.

Nitroglycerin is the most commonly used nitrate for angina. Nitroglycerin that dissolves under your tongue or between your cheek and gum is used to relieve angina episodes.

Nitroglycerin pills and skin patches are used to prevent angina episodes. However, pills and skin patches act too slowly to relieve pain during an angina attack.

Other medicines also are used to treat angina, such as beta blockers, calcium channel blockers, ACE inhibitors, oral antiplatelet medicines, or anticoagulants (blood thinners). These medicines can help:

- Lower blood pressure and cholesterol levels

- Slow the heart rate

- Relax blood vessels

- Reduce strain on the heart

- Prevent blood clots from forming

People who have stable angina may be advised to get annual flu shots.

Medical Procedures

If lifestyle changes and medicines don't control angina, you may need a medical procedure to treat the underlying heart disease. Both angioplasty and coronary artery bypass grafting (CABG) are commonly used to treat heart disease.

You will work with your doctor to decide which treatment is better for you.

Cardiac Rehabilitation

Your doctor may recommend cardiac rehab for angina or after angioplasty, CABG, or a heart attack. Cardiac rehab is a medically supervised program that can help improve the health and well-being of people who have heart problems.

Rehab has two parts:

1. **Exercise training.** This part helps you learn how to exercise safely, strengthen your muscles, and improve your stamina. Your exercise plan will be based on your personal abilities, needs, and interests.

2. **Education, counseling, and training.** This part of rehab helps you understand your heart condition and find ways to reduce your risk for future heart problems. The rehab team will help you learn how to adjust to a new lifestyle and deal with your fears about the future.

Enhanced External Counterpulsation Therapy

Enhanced external counterpulsation (EECP) therapy is helpful for some people who have angina. Large cuffs, similar to blood pressure cuffs, are put on your legs. The cuffs are inflated and deflated in sync with your heartbeat.

EECP therapy improves the flow of oxygen-rich blood to your heart muscle and helps relieve angina. You typically get 35 1-hour treatments over 7 weeks.

How Can Angina Be Prevented?

You can prevent or lower your risk for angina and heart disease by making lifestyle changes and treating related conditions.

Making Lifestyle Changes

Healthy lifestyle choices can help prevent or delay angina and heart disease. To adopt a healthy lifestyle, you can:

- Quit smoking and avoid secondhand smoke
- Avoid angina triggers

- Follow a healthy diet

- Be physically active

- Maintain a healthy weight

- Learn ways to handle stress and relax

- Take your medicines as your doctor prescribes

Treating Related Conditions

You also can help prevent or delay angina and heart disease by treating related conditions, such as high blood cholesterol, high blood pressure, diabetes, and overweight or obesity.

If you have one or more of these conditions, talk with your doctor about how to control them. Follow your treatment plan and take all of your medicines as your doctor prescribes.

Chapter 13

Heart Attack
(Myocardial Infarction)

What Is a Heart Attack?

A heart attack happens when the flow of oxygen-rich blood to a section of heart muscle suddenly becomes blocked and the heart can't get oxygen. If blood flow isn't restored quickly, the section of heart muscle begins to die.

Heart attack treatment works best when it's given right after symptoms occur. If you think you or someone else is having a heart attack, even if you're not sure, **call 9–1–1 right away.**

Don't Wait—Get Help Quickly

Acting fast at the first sign of heart attack symptoms can save your life and limit damage to your heart. Treatment works best when it's given right after symptoms occur.

Many people aren't sure what's wrong when they are having symptoms of a heart attack.

Not all heart attacks begin with the sudden, crushing chest pain that often is shown on TV or in the movies, or other common symptoms such as chest discomfort. The symptoms of a heart attack can vary from person to person. Some people can have few symptoms and are

---

This chapter includes text excerpted from "Heart Attack," National Heart, Lung, and Blood Institute (NHLBI), November 6, 2015.

surprised to learn they've had a heart attack. If you've already had a heart attack, your symptoms may not be the same for another one.

Quick Action Can Save Your Life: Call 9–1–1

If you think you or someone else may be having heart attack symptoms or a heart attack, don't ignore it or feel embarrassed to call for help. **Call 9–1–1 for emergency medical care**. Acting fast can save your life.Do not drive to the hospital or let someone else drive you. Call an ambulance so that medical personnel can begin life-saving treatment on the way to the emergency room. Take a nitroglycerin pill if your doctor has prescribed this type of treatment.

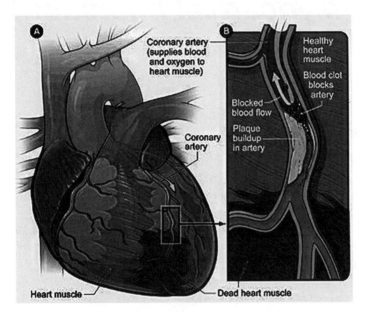

Figure 13.1. *Heart with Muscle Damage and a Blocked Artery*

(A) is an overview of a heart and coronary artery showing damage (dead heart muscle) caused by a heart attack. (B) is a cross-section of the coronary artery with plaque buildup and a blood clot.

Other Names for a Heart Attack

- Myocardial infarction (MI)

- Acute myocardial infarction (AMI)

- Acute coronary syndrome

- Coronary thrombosis
- Coronary occlusion

What Causes a Heart Attack?

Coronary Heart Disease

A heart attack happens if the flow of oxygen-rich blood to a section of heart muscle suddenly becomes blocked and the heart can't get oxygen. Most heart attacks occur as a result of coronary heart disease (CHD).

CHD is a condition in which a waxy substance called plaque builds up inside of the coronary arteries. These arteries supply oxygen-rich blood to your heart.

When plaque builds up in the arteries, the condition is called atherosclerosis. The buildup of plaque occurs over many years.

Eventually, an area of plaque can rupture (break open) inside of an artery. This causes a blood clot to form on the plaque's surface. If the clot becomes large enough, it can mostly or completely block blood flow through a coronary artery.

If the blockage isn't treated quickly, the portion of heart muscle fed by the artery begins to die. Healthy heart tissue is replaced with scar tissue. This heart damage may not be obvious, or it may cause severe or long-lasting problems.

Coronary Artery Spasm

A less common cause of heart attack is a severe spasm (tightening) of a coronary artery. The spasm cuts off blood flow through the artery. Spasms can occur in coronary arteries that aren't affected by atherosclerosis.

What causes a coronary artery to spasm isn't always clear. A spasm may be related to:

- Taking certain drugs, such as cocaine
- Emotional stress or pain
- Exposure to extreme cold
- Cigarette smoking

Who Is at Risk for a Heart Attack?

Certain risk factors make it more likely that you'll develop coronary heart disease (CHD) and have a heart attack. You can control many of these risk factors.

Risk Factors You Can Control

The major risk factors for a heart attack that you can control include:

- Smoking

- High blood pressure

- High blood cholesterol

- Overweight and obesity

- An unhealthy diet (for example, a diet high in saturated fat, trans fat, cholesterol, and sodium)

- Lack of routine physical activity

- High blood sugar due to insulin resistance or diabetes

Some of these risk factors—such as obesity, high blood pressure, and high blood sugar—tend to occur together. When they do, it's called metabolic syndrome.

In general, a person who has metabolic syndrome is twice as likely to develop heart disease and five times as likely to develop diabetes as someone who doesn't have metabolic syndrome.

Risk Factors You Can't Control

Risk factors that you can't control include:

- Age

- Family history of early heart disease

- Preeclampsia

What Are the Symptoms of a Heart Attack?

Not all heart attacks begin with the sudden, crushing chest pain that often is shown on TV or in the movies. In one study, for example, one-third of the patients who had heart attacks had no chest pain. These patients were more likely to be older, female, or diabetic.

The symptoms of a heart attack can vary from person to person. Some people can have few symptoms and are surprised to learn they've had a heart attack. If you've already had a heart attack, your symptoms may not be the same for another one. It is important for you to know the most common symptoms of a heart attack and also remember these facts:

- Heart attacks can start slowly and cause only mild pain or discomfort. Symptoms can be mild or more intense and sudden. Symptoms also may come and go over several hours.

- People who have high blood sugar (diabetes) may have no symptoms or very mild ones.

- The most common symptom, in both men and women, is chest pain or discomfort.

- Women are somewhat more likely to have shortness of breath, nausea and vomiting, unusual tiredness (sometimes for days), and pain in the back, shoulders, and jaw.

Some people don't have symptoms at all. Heart attacks that occur without any symptoms or with very mild symptoms are called silent heart attacks.

Most Common Symptoms

The most common warning symptoms of a heart attack for both men and women are:

- Chest pain or discomfort

- Upper body discomfort

- Shortness of breath

The symptoms of angina can be similar to the symptoms of a heart attack. Angina is chest pain that occurs in people who have coronary heart disease, usually when they're active. Angina pain usually lasts for only a few minutes and goes away with rest.

Chest pain or discomfort that doesn't go away or changes from its usual pattern (for example, occurs more often or while you're resting) can be a sign of a heart attack.

All chest pain should be checked by a doctor.

Other Common Signs and Symptoms

Pay attention to these other possible symptoms of a heart attack:

- Breaking out in a cold sweat

- Feeling unusually tired for no reason, sometimes for days (especially if you are a woman)

- Nausea (feeling sick to the stomach) and vomiting

- Light-headedness or sudden dizziness

- Any sudden, new symptoms or a change in the pattern of symptoms you already have (for example, if your symptoms become stronger or last longer than usual)

Not everyone having a heart attack has typical symptoms. If you've already had a heart attack, your symptoms may not be the same for another one. However, some people may have a pattern of symptoms that recur.

The more signs and symptoms you have, the more likely it is that you're having a heart attack.

Quick Action Can Save Your Life: Call 9–1–1

The signs and symptoms of a heart attack can develop suddenly. However, they also can develop slowly—sometimes within hours, days, or weeks of a heart attack.

Any time you think you might be having heart attack symptoms or a heart attack, don't ignore it or feel embarrassed to call for help. Call 9–1–1 for emergency medical care, even if you are not sure whether you're having a heart attack. Here's why:

- Acting fast can save your life.

- An ambulance is the best and safest way to get to the hospital. Emergency medical services (EMS) personnel can check how you are doing and start life-saving medicines and other treatments right away. People who arrive by ambulance often receive faster treatment at the hospital.

- The 9–1–1 operator or EMS technician can give you advice. You might be told to crush or chew an aspirin if you're not allergic, unless there is a medical reason for you not to take one. Aspirin taken during a heart attack can limit the damage to your heart and save your life.

How Is a Heart Attack Diagnosed?

Your doctor will diagnose a heart attack based on your signs and symptoms, your medical and family histories, and test results.

Diagnostic Tests

- EKG (Electrocardiogram)

- Blood Tests
- Coronary Angiography

How Is a Heart Attack Treated?

Early treatment for a heart attack can prevent or limit damage to the heart muscle. Acting fast, **by calling 9–1–1** at the first symptoms of a heart attack, can save your life. Medical personnel can begin diagnosis and treatment even before you get to the hospital.

Immediate Treatment

Certain treatments usually are started right away if a heart attack is suspected, even before the diagnosis is confirmed. These include:

- Aspirin to prevent further blood clotting
- Nitroglycerin to reduce your heart's workload and improve blood flow through the coronary arteries
- Oxygen therapy
- Treatment for chest pain

Once the diagnosis of a heart attack is confirmed or strongly suspected, doctors start treatments promptly to try to restore blood flow through the blood vessels supplying the heart. The two main treatments are clot-busting medicines and percutaneous coronary intervention, also known as coronary angioplasty, a procedure used to open blocked coronary arteries.

Clot-Busting Medicines

Thrombolytic medicines, also called clot busters, are used to dissolve blood clots that are blocking the coronary arteries. To work best, these medicines must be given within several hours of the start of heart attack symptoms. Ideally, the medicine should be given as soon as possible.

Percutaneous Coronary Intervention

Percutaneous coronary intervention is a nonsurgical procedure that opens blocked or narrowed coronary arteries. A thin, flexible tube (catheter) with a balloon or other device on the end is threaded through a blood vessel, usually in the groin (upper thigh), to the narrowed or blocked coronary artery. Once in place, the balloon located at the tip of the catheter is inflated to compress the plaque and related clot against the wall of the artery. This restores blood flow through the artery. During the procedure, the doctor may put a small mesh tube called a stent in the artery. The stent helps to keep the blood vessel open to prevent blockages in the artery in the months or years after the procedure.

Other Treatments for Heart Attack

Other treatments for heart attack include:

- Medicines
- Medical procedures
- Heart-healthy lifestyle changes
- Cardiac rehabilitation

Medicines

Your doctor may prescribe one or more of the following medicines.

- **ACE inhibitors.** ACE inhibitors lower blood pressure and reduce strain on your heart. They also help slow down further weakening of the heart muscle.

- **Anticlotting medicines.** Anticlotting medicines stop platelets from clumping together and forming unwanted blood clots. Examples of anticlotting medicines include aspirin and clopidogrel.

- **Anticoagulants.** Anticoagulants, or blood thinners, prevent blood clots from forming in your arteries. These medicines also keep existing clots from getting larger.

- **Beta blockers.** Beta blockers decrease your heart's workload. These medicines also are used to relieve chest pain and discomfort and to help prevent another heart attack. Beta blockers also are used to treat arrhythmias (irregular heartbeats).

- **Statin medicines.** Statins control or lower your blood cholesterol. By lowering your blood cholesterol level, you can decrease your chance of having another heart attack or stroke.

You also may be given medicines to relieve pain and anxiety, and treat arrhythmias. Take all medicines regularly, as your doctor prescribes. Don't change the amount of your medicine or skip a dose unless your doctor tells you to.

Medical Procedures

Coronary artery bypass grafting also may be used to treat a heart attack. During coronary artery bypass grafting, a surgeon removes a healthy artery or vein from your body. The artery or vein is then connected, or grafted, to bypass the blocked section of the coronary artery. The grafted artery or vein bypasses (that is, goes around) the blocked portion of the coronary artery. This provides a new route for blood to flow to the heart muscle.

Heart-Healthy Lifestyle Changes

Treatment for a heart attack usually includes making heart-healthy lifestyle changes. Your doctor also may recommend:

- Heart-healthy eating
- Maintaining a healthy weight
- Managing stress
- Physical activity
- Quitting smoking

Taking these steps can lower your chances of having another heart attack.

Cardiac Rehabilitation

Your doctor may recommend cardiac rehabilitation (cardiac rehab) to help you recover from a heart attack and to help prevent another heart attack. Nearly everyone who has had a heart attack can benefit from rehab. Cardiac rehab is a medically supervised program that may help improve the health and well-being of people who have heart problems.

Rehab has two parts:

1. **Education, counseling, and training.** This part of rehab helps you understand your heart condition and find ways to reduce your risk for future heart problems. The rehab team will help you learn how to cope with the stress of adjusting to a new lifestyle and how to deal with your fears about the future.

2. **Exercise training.** This part helps you learn how to exercise safely, strengthen your muscles, and improve your stamina. Your exercise plan will be based on your personal abilities, needs, and interests.

How Can a Heart Attack Be Prevented?

Lowering your risk factors for coronary heart disease can help you prevent a heart attack. Even if you already have coronary heart disease, you still can take steps to lower your risk for a heart attack. These steps involve following a heart-healthy lifestyle and getting ongoing medical care.

Risk of a Repeat Heart Attack

Once you've had a heart attack, you're at higher risk for another one. Knowing the difference between angina and a heart attack is important. Angina is chest pain that occurs in people who have CHD.

The pain from angina usually occurs after physical exertion and goes away in a few minutes when you rest or take medicine as directed.

The pain from a heart attack usually is more severe than the pain from angina. Heart attack pain doesn't go away when you rest or take medicine.

If you don't know whether your chest pain is angina or a heart attack, call 9–1–1.

The symptoms of a second heart attack may not be the same as those of a first heart attack. Don't take a chance if you're in doubt. Always call 9–1–1 right away if you or someone else has heart attack symptoms.

Unfortunately, most heart attack victims wait 2 hours or more after their symptoms start before they seek medical help. This delay can result in lasting heart damage or death.

Chapter 14

Sudden Cardiac Arrest

What Is Sudden Cardiac Arrest?

Sudden cardiac arrest (SCA) is a condition in which the heart suddenly and unexpectedly stops beating. If this happens, blood stops flowing to the brain and other vital organs.

SCA usually causes death if it's not treated within minutes.

What Causes Sudden Cardiac Arrest?

Ventricular fibrillation (v-fib) causes most sudden cardiac arrests (SCAs). V-fib is a type of arrhythmia.

During v-fib, the ventricles (the heart's lower chambers) don't beat normally. Instead, they quiver very rapidly and irregularly. When this happens, the heart pumps little or no blood to the body. V-fib is fatal if not treated within a few minutes.

Other problems with the heart's electrical system also can cause SCA. For example, SCA can occur if the rate of the heart's electrical signals becomes very slow and stops. SCA also can occur if the heart muscle doesn't respond to the heart's electrical signals.

Certain diseases and conditions can cause the electrical problems that lead to SCA. Examples include coronary heart disease (CHD), also called coronary artery disease; severe physical stress; certain inherited disorders; and structural changes in the heart.

This chapter includes text excerpted from "Sudden Cardiac Arrest," National Heart, Lung, and Blood Institute (NHLBI), October 29, 2015.

Several research studies are under way to try to find the exact causes of SCA and how to prevent them.

Coronary Heart Disease

CHD is a disease in which a waxy substance called plaque builds up in the coronary arteries. These arteries supply oxygen-rich blood to your heart muscle.

Plaque narrows the arteries and reduces blood flow to your heart muscle. Eventually, an area of plaque can rupture (break open). This may cause a blood clot to form on the plaque's surface.

A blood clot can partly or fully block the flow of oxygen-rich blood to the portion of heart muscle fed by the artery. This causes a heart attack.

During a heart attack, some heart muscle cells die and are replaced with scar tissue. The scar tissue damages the heart's electrical system. As a result, electrical signals may spread abnormally throughout the heart. These changes to the heart increase the risk of dangerous arrhythmias and SCA.

CHD seems to cause most cases of SCA in adults. Many of these adults, however, have no signs or symptoms of CHD before having SCA.

Physical Stress

Certain types of physical stress can cause your heart's electrical system to fail. Examples include:

- Intense physical activity. The hormone adrenaline is released during intense physical activity. This hormone can trigger SCA in people who have heart problems.

- Very low blood levels of potassium or magnesium. These minerals play an important role in your heart's electrical signaling.

- Major blood loss.

- Severe lack of oxygen.

Inherited Disorders

A tendency to have arrhythmias runs in some families. This tendency is inherited, which means it's passed from parents to children through the genes. Members of these families may be at higher risk for SCA.

An example of an inherited disorder that makes you more likely to have arrhythmias is long QT syndrome (LQTS). LQTS is a disorder of the heart's electrical activity. Problems with tiny pores on the surface of heart muscle cells cause the disorder. LQTS can cause sudden, uncontrollable, dangerous heart rhythms.

People who inherit structural heart problems also may be at higher risk for SCA. These types of problems often are the cause of SCA in children.

Structural Changes in the Heart

Changes in the heart's normal size or structure may affect its electrical system. Examples of such changes include an enlarged heart due to high blood pressure or advanced heart disease. Heart infections also may cause structural changes in the heart.

Who Is at Risk for Sudden Cardiac Arrest?

The risk of sudden cardiac arrest (SCA) increases:

• With age

• If you are a man. Men are more likely than women to have SCA.

• Some studies show that blacks—particularly those with underlying conditions such as diabetes, high blood pressure, heart failure, and chronic kidney disease or certain cardiac findings on tests such as an electrocardiogram—have a higher risk for SCA.

Major Risk Factor

The major risk factor for SCA is coronary heart disease. Most people who have SCA have some degree of coronary heart disease; however, many people may not know that they have coronary heart disease until SCA occurs. Usually their coronary heart disease is "silent"—that is, it has no signs or symptoms. Because of this, doctors and nurses have not detected it.

Many people who have SCA also have silent, or undiagnosed, heart attacks before sudden cardiac arrest happens. These people have no clear signs of heart attack, and they don't even realize that they've had one.

Other Risk Factors

Other risk factors for SCA include:

• A personal history of arrhythmias

- A personal or family history of SCA or inherited disorders that make you prone to arrhythmias
- Drug or alcohol abuse
- Heart attack
- Heart failure

What Are the Signs and Symptoms of Sudden Cardiac Arrest?

Usually, the first sign of sudden cardiac arrest (SCA) is loss of consciousness (fainting). At the same time, no heartbeat (or pulse) can be felt.

Some people may have a racing heartbeat or feel dizzy or light-headed just before they faint. Within an hour before SCA, some people have chest pain, shortness of breath, nausea (feeling sick to the stomach), or vomiting.

How Is Sudden Cardiac Arrest Diagnosed?

Sudden cardiac arrest (SCA) happens without warning and requires emergency treatment. Doctors rarely diagnose SCA with medical tests as it's happening. Instead, SCA often is diagnosed after it happens. Doctors do this by ruling out other causes of a person's sudden collapse.

Diagnostic Tests and Procedures

Doctors use several tests to help detect the factors that put people at risk for SCA.

- EKG (Electrocardiogram)
- Echocardiography
- MUGA Test or Cardiac MRI
- Cardiac Catheterization
- Electrophysiology Study
- Blood Tests

How Is Sudden Cardiac Arrest Treated?

Emergency Treatment

Sudden cardiac arrest (SCA) is an emergency. A person having SCA needs to be treated with a defibrillator right away. This device sends an electric shock to the heart. The electric shock can restore a normal rhythm to a heart that's stopped beating.

To work well, defibrillation must be done within minutes of SCA. With every minute that passes, the chances of surviving SCA drop rapidly.

Police, emergency medical technicians, and other first responders usually are trained and equipped to use a defibrillator. Call 9–1–1 right away if someone has signs or symptoms of SCA. The sooner you call for help, the sooner lifesaving treatment can begin.

Automated External Defibrillators

Automated external defibrillators (AEDs) are special defibrillators that untrained bystanders can use. These portable devices often are found in public places, such as shopping malls, golf courses, businesses, airports, airplanes, casinos, convention centers, hotels, sports venues, and schools.

AEDs are programmed to give an electric shock if they detect a dangerous arrhythmia, such as ventricular fibrillation. This prevents giving a shock to someone who may have fainted but isn't having SCA.

You should give cardiopulmonary resuscitation (CPR) to a person having SCA until defibrillation can be done.

People who are at risk for SCA may want to consider having an AED at home. When considering a home-use AED, talk with your doctor. He or she can help you decide whether having an AED in your home will benefit you.

Treatment in a Hospital

If you survive SCA, you'll likely be admitted to a hospital for ongoing care and treatment. In the hospital, your medical team will closely watch your heart. They may give you medicines to try to reduce the risk of another SCA.

While in the hospital, your medical team will try to find out what caused your SCA. If you're diagnosed with coronary heart disease, you may have percutaneous coronary intervention, also known as coronary angioplasty, or coronary artery bypass grafting. These procedures help restore blood flow through narrowed or blocked coronary arteries.

Often, people who have SCA get a device called an implantable cardioverter defibrillator (ICD). This small device is surgically placed under the skin in your chest or abdomen. An ICD uses electric pulses or shocks to help control dangerous arrhythmias.

How Can Death due to Sudden Cardiac Arrest Be Prevented?

Ways to prevent death due to sudden cardiac arrest (SCA) differ depending on whether:

- You've already had SCA
- You've never had SCA but are at high risk for the condition
- You've never had SCA and have no known risk factors for the condition

For People Who Have Survived Sudden Cardiac Arrest

If you've already had SCA, you're at high risk of having it again. Research shows that an implantable cardioverter defibrillator (ICD) reduces the chances of dying from a second SCA. An ICD is surgically placed under the skin in your chest or abdomen. The device has wires with electrodes on the ends that connect to your heart's chambers. The ICD monitors your heartbeat.

If the ICD detects a dangerous heart rhythm, it gives an electric shock to restore the heart's normal rhythm. Your doctor may give you medicine to limit irregular heartbeats that can trigger the ICD.

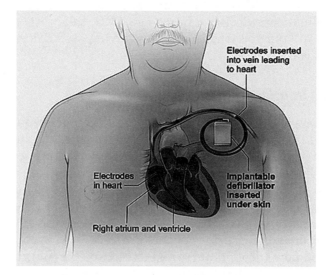

Figure 14.1. *Implantable Cardioverter Defibrillator*

The illustration shows the location of an implantable cardioverter defibrillator in the upper chest. The electrodes are inserted into the heart through a vein.

An ICD isn't the same as a pacemaker. The devices are similar, but they have some differences. Pacemakers give off low-energy electrical pulses. They're often used to treat less dangerous heart rhythms, such as those that occur in the upper chambers of the heart. Most new ICDs work as both pacemakers and ICDs.

For People at High Risk for a First Sudden Cardiac Arrest

If you have severe coronary heart disease (CHD), you're at increased risk for SCA. This is especially true if you've recently had a heart attack.

Your doctor may prescribe a type of medicine called a beta blocker to help lower your risk for SCA. Your doctor also may discuss beginning statin treatment if you have an elevated risk for developing heart disease or having a stroke. Doctors usually prescribe statins for people who have:

- Diabetes

- Heart disease or had a prior stroke

- High LDL cholesterol levels

Your doctor also may prescribe other medications to:

- Decrease your chance of having a heart attack or dying suddenly.

- Lower blood pressure.

- Prevent blood clots, which can lead to heart attack or stroke.

- Prevent or delay the need for a procedure or surgery, such as angioplasty or coronary artery bypass grafting.

- Reduce your heart's workload and relieve coronary heart disease symptoms.

Take all medicines regularly, as your doctor prescribes. Don't change the amount of your medicine or skip a dose unless your doctor tells you to. You should still follow a heart-healthy lifestyle, even if you take medicines to treat your coronary heart disease.

Other treatments for coronary heart disease—such as percutaneous coronary intervention, also known as coronary angioplasty, or coronary artery bypass grafting—also may lower your risk for SCA. Your doctor also may recommend an ICD if you're at high risk for SCA.

For People Who Have No Known Risk Factors for Sudden Cardiac Arrest

CHD seems to be the cause of most SCAs in adults. CHD also is a major risk factor for angina (chest pain or discomfort) and heart attack, and it contributes to other heart problems.

Following a healthy lifestyle can help you lower your risk for CHD, SCA, and other heart problems. A heart-healthy lifestyle includes:

- Heart-healthy eating
- Maintaining a healthy weight
- Managing stress
- Physical activity
- Quitting smoking

Chapter 15

Cardiogenic Shock

What Is Cardiogenic Shock?

Cardiogenic shock is a condition in which a suddenly weakened heart isn't able to pump enough blood to meet the body's needs. The condition is a medical emergency and is fatal if not treated right away.

The most common cause of cardiogenic shock is damage to the heart muscle from a severe heart attack. However, not everyone who has a heart attack has cardiogenic shock. In fact, on average, only about 7 percent of people who have heart attacks develop the condition.

If cardiogenic shock does occur, it's very dangerous. When people die from heart attacks in hospitals, cardiogenic shock is the most common cause of death.

What Is Shock?

The medical term "shock" refers to a state in which not enough blood and oxygen reach important organs in the body, such as the brain and kidneys. Shock causes very low blood pressure and may be life threatening.

Shock can have many causes. Cardiogenic shock is only one type of shock. Other types of shock include hypovolemic shock and vasodilatory shock.

Hypovolemic shock is a condition in which the heart can't pump enough blood to the body because of severe blood loss.

This chapter includes text excerpted from "Cardiogenic Shock," National Heart, Lung, and Blood Institute (NHLBI), July 1, 2011. Reviewed June 2016.

In vasodilatory shock, the blood vessels suddenly relax. When the blood vessels are too relaxed, blood pressure drops and blood flow becomes very low. Without enough blood pressure, blood and oxygen don't reach the body's organs.

A bacterial infection in the bloodstream, a severe allergic reaction, or damage to the nervous system (brain and nerves) may cause vasodilatory shock.

When a person is in shock (from any cause), not enough blood and oxygen are reaching the body's organs. If shock lasts more than a few minutes, the lack of oxygen starts to damage the body's organs. If shock isn't treated quickly, it can cause permanent organ damage or death.

Some of the signs and symptoms of shock include:

- Confusion or lack of alertness

- Loss of consciousness

- A sudden and ongoing rapid heartbeat

- Sweating

- Pale skin

- A weak pulse

- Rapid breathing

- Decreased or no urine output

- Cool hands and feet

If you think that you or someone else is in shock, call 9–1–1 right away for emergency treatment. Prompt medical care can save your life and prevent or limit damage to your body's organs.

What Causes Cardiogenic Shock?

Immediate Causes

Cardiogenic shock occurs if the heart suddenly can't pump enough oxygen-rich blood to the body. The most common cause of cardiogenic shock is damage to the heart muscle from a severe heart attack.

This damage prevents the heart's main pumping chamber, the left ventricle, from working well. As a result, the heart can't pump enough oxygen-rich blood to the rest of the body.

In about 3 percent of cardiogenic shock cases, the heart's lower right chamber, the right ventricle, doesn't work well. This means the heart can't properly pump blood to the lungs, where it picks up oxygen to bring back to the heart and the rest of the body.

Without enough oxygen-rich blood reaching the body's major organs, many problems can occur. For example:

- Cardiogenic shock can cause death if the flow of oxygen-rich blood to the organs isn't restored quickly. This is why emergency medical treatment is required.

- If organs don't get enough oxygen-rich blood, they won't work well. Cells in the organs die, and the organs may never work well again.

- As some organs stop working, they may cause problems with other bodily functions. This, in turn, can worsen shock. For example:

  - If the kidneys aren't working well, the levels of important chemicals in the body change. This may cause the heart and other muscles to become even weaker, limiting blood flow even more.

  - If the liver isn't working well, the body stops making proteins that help the blood clot. This can lead to more bleeding if the shock is due to blood loss.

How well the brain, kidneys, and other organs recover will depend on how long a person is in shock. The less time a person is in shock, the less damage will occur to the organs. This is another reason why emergency treatment is so important.

Underlying Causes

The underlying causes of cardiogenic shock are conditions that weaken the heart and prevent it from pumping enough oxygen-rich blood to the body.

Heart Attack

Most heart attacks occur as a result of coronary heart disease (CHD). CHD is a condition in which a waxy substance called plaque narrows or blocks the coronary (heart) arteries.

Plaque reduces blood flow to your heart muscle. It also makes it more likely that blood clots will form in your arteries. Blood clots can partially or completely block blood flow.

Conditions Caused by Heart Attack

Heart attacks can cause some serious heart conditions that can lead to cardiogenic shock. One example is ventricular septal rupture. This condition occurs if the wall that separates the ventricles (the heart's two lower chambers) breaks down.

The breakdown happens because cells in the wall have died due to a heart attack. Without the wall to separate them, the ventricles can't pump properly.

Heart attacks also can cause papillary muscle infarction or rupture. This condition occurs if the muscles that help anchor the heart valves stop working or break because a heart attack cuts off their blood supply. If this happens, blood doesn't flow correctly between the heart's chambers. This prevents the heart from pumping properly.

Other Heart Conditions

Serious heart conditions that may occur with or without a heart attack can cause cardiogenic shock. Examples include:

Myocarditis. This is inflammation of the heart muscle.

Endocarditis. This is an infection of the inner lining of the heart chambers and valves.

Life-threatening arrhythmias. These are problems with the rate or rhythm of the heartbeat.

Pericardial tamponade. This is too much fluid or blood around the heart. The fluid squeezes the heart muscle so it can't pump properly.

Pulmonary Embolism

Pulmonary embolism (PE) is a sudden blockage in a lung artery. This condition usually is caused by a blood clot that travels to the lung from a vein in the leg. PE can damage your heart and other organs in your body.

Who Is at Risk for Cardiogenic Shock?

The most common risk factor for cardiogenic shock is having a heart attack. If you've had a heart attack, the following factors can further increase your risk for cardiogenic shock:

- Older age

- A history of heart attacks or heart failure

- Coronary heart disease that affects all of the heart's major blood vessels

- High blood pressure

- Diabetes

Women who have heart attacks are at higher risk for cardiogenic shock than men who have heart attacks.

What Are the Signs and Symptoms of Cardiogenic Shock?

A lack of oxygen-rich blood reaching the brain, kidneys, skin, and other parts of the body causes the signs and symptoms of cardiogenic shock.

Some of the typical signs and symptoms of shock usually include at least two or more of the following:

- Confusion or lack of alertness

- Loss of consciousness

- A sudden and ongoing rapid heartbeat

- Sweating

- Pale skin

- A weak pulse

- Rapid breathing

- Decreased or no urine output

- Cool hands and feet

Any of these alone is unlikely to be a sign or symptom of shock.

If you or someone else is having these signs and symptoms, call 9–1–1 right away for emergency treatment. Prompt medical care can save your life and prevent or limit organ damage.

How Is Cardiogenic Shock Diagnosed?

The first step in diagnosing cardiogenic shock is to identify that a person is in shock. At that point, emergency treatment should begin.

Once emergency treatment starts, doctors can look for the specific cause of the shock. If the reason for the shock is that the heart isn't pumping strongly enough, then the diagnosis is cardiogenic shock.

Tests and Procedures To Diagnose Shock and Its Underlying Causes

- Blood Pressure Test
- EKG (Electrocardiogram)
- Echocardiography
- Chest X-Ray
- Cardiac Enzyme Test
- Coronary Angiography
- Pulmonary Artery Catheterization
- Blood Tests

How Is Cardiogenic Shock Treated?

Cardiogenic shock is life threatening and requires emergency medical treatment. The condition usually is diagnosed after a person has been admitted to a hospital for a heart attack. If the person isn't already in a hospital, emergency treatment can start as soon as medical personnel arrive.

The first goal of emergency treatment for cardiogenic shock is to improve the flow of blood and oxygen to the body's organs.

Sometimes both the shock and its cause are treated at the same time. For example, doctors may quickly open a blocked blood vessel that's damaging the heart. Often, this can get the patient out of shock with little or no additional treatment.

Emergency Life Support

Emergency life support treatment is needed for any type of shock. This treatment helps get oxygen-rich blood flowing to the brain, kidneys, and other organs.

Restoring blood flow to the organs keeps the patient alive and may prevent long-term damage to the organs. Emergency life support treatment includes:

- Giving the patient extra oxygen to breathe so that more oxygen reaches the lungs, the heart, and the rest of the body.

- Providing breathing support if needed. A ventilator might be used to protect the airway and provide the patient with extra oxygen. A ventilator is a machine that supports breathing.

- Giving the patient fluids, including blood and blood products, through a needle inserted in a vein (when the shock is due to blood loss). This can help get more blood to major organs and the rest of the body. This treatment usually isn't used for cardiogenic shock because the heart can't pump the blood that's already in the body. Also, too much fluid is in the lungs, making it hard to breathe.

Medicines

During and after emergency life support treatment, doctors will try to find out what's causing the shock. If the reason for the shock is that the heart isn't pumping strongly enough, then the diagnosis is cardiogenic shock.

Treatment for cardiogenic shock will depend on its cause. Doctors may prescribe medicines to:

- Prevent blood clots from forming

- Increase the force with which the heart muscle contracts

- Treat a heart attack

Medical Devices

Medical devices can help the heart pump and improve blood flow. Devices used to treat cardiogenic shock may include:

- An intra-aortic balloon pump. This device is placed in the aorta, the main blood vessel that carries blood from the heart to the body. A balloon at the tip of the device is inflated and deflated in a rhythm that matches the heart's pumping rhythm. This allows the weakened heart muscle to pump as much blood as it can, which helps get more blood to vital organs, such as the brain and kidneys.

- A left ventricular assist device (LVAD). This device is a battery-operated pump that takes over part of the heart's pumping action. An LVAD helps the heart pump blood to the body. This device may be used if damage to the left ventricle, the heart's main pumping chamber, is causing shock.

Medical Procedures and Surgery

Sometimes medicines and medical devices aren't enough to treat cardiogenic shock.

Medical procedures and surgery can restore blood flow to the heart and the rest of the body, repair heart damage, and help keep a patient alive while he or she recovers from shock.

Surgery also can improve the chances of long-term survival. Surgery done within 6 hours of the onset of shock symptoms has the greatest chance of improving survival.

The types of procedures and surgery used to treat underlying causes of cardiogenic shock include:

- **Percutaneous coronary intervention (PCI) and stents.** PCI, also known as coronary angioplasty, is a procedure used to open narrowed or blocked coronary (heart) arteries and treat an ongoing heart attack. A stent is a small mesh tube that's placed in a coronary artery during PCI to help keep it open.

- **Coronary artery bypass grafting.** For this surgery, arteries or veins from other parts of the body are used to bypass (that is, go around) narrowed coronary arteries. This creates a new passage for oxygen-rich blood to reach the heart.

- **Surgery to repair damaged heart valves.**

- **Surgery to repair a break in the wall that separates the heart's chambers.** This break is called a septal rupture.

- **Heart transplant.** This type of surgery rarely is done during an emergency situation like cardiogenic shock because of other available options. Also, doctors need to do very careful testing to make sure a patient will benefit from a heart transplant and to find a matching heart from a donor. Still, in some cases, doctors may recommend a transplant if they feel it's the best way to improve a patient's chances of long-term survival.

How Can Cardiogenic Shock Be Prevented?

The best way to prevent cardiogenic shock is to lower your risk for coronary heart disease (CHD) and heart attack.

If you already have CHD, it's important to get ongoing treatment from a doctor who has experience treating heart problems.

If you have a heart attack, you should get treatment right away to try to prevent cardiogenic shock and other possible complications.

- Act in time. Know the warning signs of a heart attack so you can act fast to get treatment. Many heart attack victims wait 2 hours or more after their symptoms begin before they seek medical help. Delays in treatment increase the risk of complications and death.

- If you think you're having a heart attack, call 9–1–1 for help. Don't drive yourself or have friends or family drive you to the hospital. Call an ambulance so that medical personnel can begin life-saving treatment on the way to the emergency room.

Chapter 16

Cardiomyopathy

What Is Cardiomyopathy?

Cardiomyopathy refers to diseases of the heart muscle. These diseases have many causes, signs and symptoms, and treatments.

In cardiomyopathy, the heart muscle becomes enlarged, thick, or rigid. In rare cases, the muscle tissue in the heart is replaced with scar tissue.

As cardiomyopathy worsens, the heart becomes weaker. It's less able to pump blood through the body and maintain a normal electrical rhythm. This can lead to heart failure or irregular heartbeats called arrhythmias. In turn, heart failure can cause fluid to build up in the lungs, ankles, feet, legs, or abdomen.

The weakening of the heart also can cause other complications, such as heart valve problems.

Types of Cardiomyopathy

The types of cardiomyopathy include:

• Hypertrophic cardiomyopathy

• Dilated cardiomyopathy

• Restrictive cardiomyopathy

This chapter includes text excerpted from "Cardiomyopathy," National Heart, Lung, and Blood Institute (NHLBI), October 23, 2015.

- Arrhythmogenic right ventricular cardiomyopathy
- Unclassified cardiomyopathy

Hypertrophic Cardiomyopathy

Hypertrophic cardiomyopathy is very common and can affect people of any age. Hypertrophic cardiomyopathy affects men and women equally, and about 1 out of every 500 people has the disease.

Hypertrophic cardiomyopathy happens when the heart muscle enlarges and thickens without an obvious cause. Usually the ventricles, the lower chambers of the heart, and septum (the wall that separates the left and right side of the heart) thicken. The thickened areas create narrowing or blockages in the ventricles, making it harder for the heart to pump blood. Hypertrophic cardiomyopathy also can cause stiffness of the ventricles, changes in the mitral valve, and cellular changes in the heart tissue.

Dilated Cardiomyopathy

Dilated cardiomyopathy develops when the ventricles enlarge and weaken. The condition usually starts in the left ventricle and over time can affect the right ventricle. The weakened chambers of the heart don't pump effectively, causing the heart muscle to work harder. Over time, the heart loses the ability to pump blood effectively. Dilated cardiomyopathy can lead to heart failure, heart valve disease, irregular heart rate, and blood clots in the heart.

Restrictive Cardiomyopathy

Restrictive cardiomyopathy develops when the ventricles become stiff and rigid but the walls of the heart do not thicken. As a result, the ventricles do not relax and don't fill with the normal blood volume. As the disease progresses, the ventricles do not pump as well and the heart muscle weakens. Over time, restrictive cardiomyopathy can lead to heart failure and problems with the heart valves.

Arrhythmogenic Right Ventricular Dysplasia

Arrhythmogenic right ventricular dysplasia is a rare type of cardiomyopathy that occurs when the muscle tissue in the right ventricle is replaced with fatty or fibrous tissue. This can lead to disruptions in the heart's electrical signals and causes arrhythmias. Arrhythmogenic right ventricular dysplasia usually affects teens or young adults and can cause sudden cardiac arrest in young athletes.

Unclassified Cardiomyopathy

Other types of cardiomyopathy are grouped into this category and can include:

- Left ventricular noncompaction happens when the left ventricle has trabeculations, projections of muscle inside the ventricle.
- Takotsubo cardiomyopathy, or broken heart syndrome, happens when extreme stress leads to heart muscle failure. Though rare, this condition is more common in post-menopausal women.

Other Names for Cardiomyopathy

Other Names for Dilated Cardiomyopathy

- Alcoholic cardiomyopathy. This term is used when overuse of alcohol causes the disease.
- Congestive cardiomyopathy.
- Diabetic cardiomyopathy.
- Familial dilated cardiomyopathy.
- Idiopathic cardiomyopathy.
- Ischemic cardiomyopathy. This term is used when coronary heart disease (also called coronary artery disease) or heart attack causes the disease.
- Peripartum cardiomyopathy. This term is used when the disease develops in a woman shortly before or after she gives birth.
- Primary cardiomyopathy.

Other Names for Hypertrophic Cardiomyopathy

- Asymmetric septal hypertrophy
- Familial hypertrophic cardiomyopathy
- Hypertrophic nonobstructive cardiomyopathy
- Hypertrophic obstructive cardiomyopathy
- Idiopathic hypertrophic subaortic stenosis

Other Names for Restrictive Cardiomyopathy

- Idiopathic restrictive cardiomyopathy
- Infiltrative cardiomyopathy

Other Names for Arrhythmogenic Right Ventricular Dysplasia

- Arrhythmogenic right ventricular cardiomyopathy
- Right ventricular cardiomyopathy
- Right ventricular dysplasia

What Causes Cardiomyopathy?

Cardiomyopathy can be acquired or inherited. "Acquired" means you aren't born with the disease, but you develop it due to another disease, condition, or factor.

"Inherited" means your parents passed the gene for the disease on to you. Researchers continue to look for the genetic links to cardiomyopathy and to explore how these links cause or contribute to the various types of the disease.

Many times, the cause of cardiomyopathy isn't known. This often is the case when the disease occurs in children.

Hypertrophic Cardiomyopathy

Hypertrophic cardiomyopathy usually is inherited. It's caused by a mutation or change in some of the genes in heart muscle proteins. Hypertrophic cardiomyopathy also can develop over time because of high blood pressure, aging, or other diseases, such as diabetes or thyroid disease. Sometimes the cause of the disease isn't known.

Dilated Cardiomyopathy

The cause of dilated cardiomyopathy often isn't known. About one-third of the people who have dilated cardiomyopathy inherit it from their parents.

Certain diseases, conditions, and substances also can cause the disease, such as:

- Alcohol, especially if you also have a poor diet
- Certain toxins, such as poisons and heavy metals

- Complications during the last months of pregnancy

- Coronary heart disease, heart attack, high blood pressure, diabetes, thyroid disease, viral hepatitis, and HIV

- Illegal drugs, such as cocaine and amphetamines, and some medicines used to treat cancer

- Infections, especially viral infections that inflame the heart muscle

Restrictive Cardiomyopathy

Certain diseases, conditions, and factors can cause restrictive cardiomyopathy, including:

- **Amyloidosis:** A disease in which abnormal proteins build up in the body's organs, including the heart

- Connective tissue disorders

- **Hemochromatosis:** A disease in which too much iron builds up in the body. The extra iron is toxic to the body and can damage the organs, including the heart.

- **Sarcoidosis:** A disease that causes inflammation and can affect various organs in the body. Researchers believe that an abnormal immune response may cause sarcoidosis. This abnormal response causes tiny lumps of cells to form in the body's organs, including the heart.

- Some cancer treatments, such as radiation and chemotherapy

Arrhythmogenic Right Ventricular Dysplasia

Researchers think that arrhythmogenic right ventricular dysplasia is an inherited disease.

Who Is at Risk for Cardiomyopathy?

People of all ages and races can have cardiomyopathy. However, certain types of the disease are more common in certain groups.

Dilated cardiomyopathy is more common in African Americans than Whites. This type of the disease also is more common in men than women.

Teens and young adults are more likely than older people to have arrhythmogenic right ventricular dysplasia, although it's rare in both groups.

Major Risk Factors

Certain diseases, conditions, or factors can raise your risk for cardiomyopathy. Major risk factors include:

- A family history of cardiomyopathy, heart failure, or sudden cardiac arrest (SCA)

- A disease or condition that can lead to cardiomyopathy, such as coronary heart disease, heart attack, or a viral infection that inflames the heart muscle

- Diabetes or other metabolic diseases, or severe obesity

- Diseases that can damage the heart, such as hemochromatosis, sarcoidosis, or amyloidosis

- Long-term alcoholism

- Long-term high blood pressure

Some people who have cardiomyopathy never have signs or symptoms. Thus, it's important to identify people who may be at high risk for the disease. This can help prevent future problems, such as serious arrhythmias (irregular heartbeats) or SCA.

What Are the Signs and Symptoms of Cardiomyopathy?

Some people who have cardiomyopathy never have signs or symptoms. Others don't have signs or symptoms in the early stages of the disease.

As cardiomyopathy worsens and the heart weakens, signs and symptoms of heart failure usually occur. These signs and symptoms include:

- Shortness of breath or trouble breathing, especially with physical exertion

- Fatigue (tiredness)

- Swelling in the ankles, feet, legs, abdomen, and veins in the neck

Other signs and symptoms may include dizziness; light-headedness; fainting during physical activity; arrhythmias (irregular heartbeats); chest pain, especially after physical exertion or heavy meals; and heart murmurs. (Heart murmurs are extra or unusual sounds heard during a heartbeat.)

How Is Cardiomyopathy Diagnosed?

Your doctor will diagnose cardiomyopathy based on your medical and family histories, a physical exam, and the results from tests and procedures.

Medical and Family Histories

Your doctor will want to learn about your medical history. He or she will want to know what signs and symptoms you have and how long you've had them.

Your doctor also will want to know whether anyone in your family has had cardiomyopathy, heart failure, or sudden cardiac arrest.

Physical Exam

Your doctor will use a stethoscope to listen to your heart and lungs for sounds that may suggest cardiomyopathy. These sounds may even suggest a certain type of the disease.

For example, the loudness, timing, and location of a heart murmur may suggest obstructive hypertrophic cardiomyopathy. A "crackling" sound in the lungs may be a sign of heart failure. (Heart failure often develops in the later stages of cardiomyopathy.)

Physical signs also help your doctor diagnose cardiomyopathy. Swelling of the ankles, feet, legs, abdomen, or veins in your neck suggests fluid buildup, a sign of heart failure.

Your doctor may notice signs and symptoms of cardiomyopathy during a routine exam. For example, he or she may hear a heart murmur, or you may have abnormal test results.

Diagnostic Tests

Your doctor may recommend one or more of the following tests to diagnose cardiomyopathy.

- Blood Tests
- Chest X-Ray
- EKG (Electrocardiogram)
- Holter and Event Monitors
- Echocardiography
- Stress Test

Diagnostic Procedures

You may have one or more medical procedures to confirm a diagnosis or to prepare for surgery (if surgery is planned). These procedures may include cardiac catheterization, coronary angiography, or myocardial biopsy.

- Cardiac Catheterization
- Coronary Angiography
- Myocardial Biopsy

Genetic Testing

Some types of cardiomyopathy run in families. Thus, your doctor may suggest genetic testing to look for the disease in your parents, brothers and sisters, or other family members.

Genetic testing can show how the disease runs in families. It also can find out the chances of parents passing the genes for the disease on to their children.

Genetic testing also may be useful if your doctor thinks you have cardiomyopathy, but you don't yet have signs or symptoms. If the test shows you have the disease, your doctor can start treatment early, when it may work best.

How Is Cardiomyopathy Treated?

People who have cardiomyopathy but no signs or symptoms may not need treatment. Sometimes, dilated cardiomyopathy that comes on suddenly may go away on its own. For other people who have cardiomyopathy, treatment is needed. Treatment depends on the type of cardiomyopathy you have, the severity of your symptoms and complications, and your age and overall health. Treatments may include:

- Heart-healthy lifestyle changes
- Medicines
- Nonsurgical procedure
- Surgery and implanted devices

The main goals of treating cardiomyopathy include:

- Controlling signs and symptoms so that you can live as normally as possible

- Managing any conditions that cause or contribute to the disease
- Reducing complications and the risk of sudden cardiac arrest
- Stopping the disease from getting worse

Heart-Healthy Lifestyle Changes

Your doctor may suggest lifestyle changes to manage a condition that's causing your cardiomyopathy including:

- Heart-healthy eating
- Maintaining a healthy weight
- Managing stress
- Physical activity
- Quitting smoking

Medicines

Many medicines are used to treat cardiomyopathy. Your doctor may prescribe medicines to:

- **Balance electrolytes in your body.** Electrolytes are minerals that help maintain fluid levels and acid-base balance in the body. They also help muscle and nerve tissues work properly. Abnormal electrolyte levels may be a sign of dehydration (lack of fluid in your body), heart failure, high blood pressure, or other disorders. Aldosterone blockers are an example of a medicine used to balance electrolytes.

- **Keep your heart beating with a normal rhythm.** These medicines, called antiarrhythmics, help prevent arrhythmias.

- **Lower your blood pressure.** ACE inhibitors, angiotensin II receptor blockers, beta blockers, and calcium channel blockers are examples of medicines that lower blood pressure.

- **Prevent blood clots from forming.** Anticoagulants, or blood thinners, are an example of a medicine that prevents blood clots. Blood thinners often are used to prevent blood clots from forming in people who have dilated cardiomyopathy.

- **Reduce inflammation.** Corticosteroids are an example of a medicine used to reduce inflammation.

- **Remove excess sodium from your body.** Diuretics, or water pills, are an example of medicines that help remove excess sodium from the body, which reduces the amount of fluid in your blood.

- **Slow your heart rate.** Beta blockers, calcium channel blockers, and digoxin are examples of medicines that slow the heart rate. Beta blockers and calcium channel blockers also are used to lower blood pressure.

Take all medicines regularly, as your doctor prescribes. Don't change the amount of your medicine or skip a dose unless your doctor tells you to.

Surgery and Implanted Devices

Doctors use several types of surgery to treat cardiomyopathy, including septal myectomy, surgically implanted devices, and heart transplant.

Septal Myectomy

Septal myectomy is open-heart surgery and is used to treat people who have hypertrophic cardiomyopathy and severe symptoms. This surgery generally is used for younger patients and for people whose medicines aren't working well.

A surgeon removes part of the thickened septum that's bulging into the left ventricle. This improves blood flow through the heart and out to the body. The removed tissue doesn't grow back. If needed, the surgeon also can repair or replace the mitral valve at the same time. Septal myectomy often is successful and allows you to return to a normal life with no symptoms.

Surgically Implanted Devices

Surgeons can place several types of devices in the heart to improve function and symptoms, including:

- **Cardiac resynchronization therapy (CRT) device.** A CRT device coordinates contractions between the heart's left and right ventricles.

- **Implantable cardioverter defibrillator (ICD).** An ICD helps control life-threatening arrhythmias that may lead to sudden cardiac arrest. This small device is implanted in the chest or abdomen and connected to the heart with wires. If an ICD senses a dangerous change in heart rhythm, it will send an electric shock to the heart to restore a normal heartbeat.

- **Left ventricular assist device (LVAD).** This device helps the heart pump blood to the body. An LVAD can be used as a long-term therapy or as a short-term treatment for people who are waiting for a heart transplant.

- **Pacemaker.** This small device is placed under the skin of your chest or abdomen to help control arrhythmias. The device uses electrical pulses to prompt the heart to beat at a normal rate.

Heart Transplant

For this surgery, a surgeon replaces a person's diseased heart with a healthy heart from a deceased donor. A heart transplant is a last resort treatment for people who have end-stage heart failure. "End-stage" means the condition has become so severe that all treatments, other than heart transplant, have failed.

Nonsurgical Procedure

Doctors may use a nonsurgical procedure called alcohol septal ablation to treat cardiomyopathy. During this procedure, the doctor injects ethanol (a type of alcohol) through a tube into the small artery that supplies blood to the thickened area of heart muscle. The alcohol kills cells, and the thickened tissue shrinks to a more normal size. This procedure allows blood to flow freely through the ventricle, which improves symptoms.

How Can Cardiomyopathy Be Prevented?

You can't prevent inherited types of cardiomyopathy. However, you can take steps to lower your risk for diseases or conditions that may lead to or complicate cardiomyopathy. Examples include coronary heart disease, high blood pressure, and heart attack.

Your doctor may advise you to make heart-healthy lifestyle changes, such as:

- Avoiding the use of alcohol and illegal drugs

- Getting enough sleep and rest

- Heart-healthy eating

- Physical activity

- Quitting smoking

- Managing stress

Your cardiomyopathy may be due to an underlying disease or condition. If you treat that condition early enough, you may be able to prevent cardiomyopathy complications. For example, to control high blood pressure, high blood cholesterol, and diabetes:

- Follow your doctor's advice about lifestyle changes.

- Get regular checkups with your doctor.

- Take all of your medicines as your doctor prescribes.

Chapter 17

Heart Failure

What Is Heart Failure?

Heart failure is a condition in which the heart can't pump enough blood to meet the body's needs. In some cases, the heart can't fill with enough blood. In other cases, the heart can't pump blood to the rest of the body with enough force. Some people have both problems.

The term "heart failure" doesn't mean that your heart has stopped or is about to stop working. However, heart failure is a serious condition that requires medical care.

Other Names for Heart Failure

- Congestive heart failure.

- Left-side heart failure. This is when the heart can't pump enough oxygen-rich blood to the body.

- Right-side heart failure. This is when the heart can't fill with enough blood.

- Cor pulmonale. This term refers to right-side heart failure caused by high blood pressure in the pulmonary arteries and right ventricle (lower right heart chamber).

This chapter includes text excerpted from "Heart Failure," National Heart, Lung, and Blood Institute (NHLBI), November 6, 2015.

What Causes Heart Failure?

Conditions that damage or overwork the heart muscle can cause heart failure. Over time, the heart weakens. It isn't able to fill with and/or pump blood as well as it should. As the heart weakens, certain proteins and substances might be released into the blood. These substances have a toxic effect on the heart and blood flow, and they worsen heart failure.

Causes of heart failure include:

- Coronary heart disease
- Diabetes
- High blood pressure
- Other heart conditions or diseases
- Other factors

Coronary Heart Disease

Coronary heart disease is a condition in which a waxy substance called plaque builds up inside the coronary arteries. These arteries supply oxygen-rich blood to your heart muscle.

Plaque narrows the arteries and reduces blood flow to your heart muscle. The buildup of plaque also makes it more likely that blood clots will form in your arteries. Blood clots can partially or completely block blood flow. Coronary heart disease can lead to chest pain or discomfort called angina, a heart attack, and heart damage.

Diabetes

Diabetes is a disease in which the body's blood glucose (sugar) level is too high. The body normally breaks down food into glucose and then carries it to cells throughout the body. The cells use a hormone called insulin to turn the glucose into energy.

In diabetes, the body doesn't make enough insulin or doesn't use its insulin properly. Over time, high blood sugar levels can damage and weaken the heart muscle and the blood vessels around the heart, leading to heart failure.

High Blood Pressure

Blood pressure is the force of blood pushing against the walls of the arteries. If this pressure rises and stays high over time, it can weaken your heart and lead to plaque buildup.

Blood pressure is considered high if it stays at or above 140/90 mmHg over time. (The mmHg is millimeters of mercury—the units used to measure blood pressure.) If you have diabetes or chronic kidney disease, high blood pressure is defined as 130/80 mmHg or higher.

Other Heart Conditions or Diseases

Other conditions and diseases also can lead to heart failure, such as:

- **Arrhythmia.** Happens when a problem occurs with the rate or rhythm of the heartbeat.

- **Cardiomyopathy.** Happens when the heart muscle becomes enlarged, thick, or rigid.

- **Congenital heart defects.** Problems with the heart's structure are present at birth.

- **Heart valve disease.** Occurs if one or more of your heart valves doesn't work properly, which can be present at birth or caused by infection, other heart conditions, and age.

Other Factors

Other factors also can injure the heart muscle and lead to heart failure. Examples include:

- Alcohol abuse or cocaine and other illegal drug use

- HIV/AIDS

- Thyroid disorders (having either too much or too little thyroid hormone in the body)

- Too much vitamin E

- Treatments for cancer, such as radiation and chemotherapy

Who Is at Risk for Heart Failure?

About 5.7 million people in the United States have heart failure. The number of people who have this condition is growing.

Heart failure is more common in:

- People who are age 65 or older. Aging can weaken the heart muscle. Older people also may have had diseases for many years that led to heart failure. Heart failure is a leading cause of hospital stays among people on Medicare.

- Blacks are more likely to have heart failure than people of other races. They're also more likely to have symptoms at a younger age, have more hospital visits due to heart failure, and die from heart failure.

- People who are overweight. Excess weight puts strain on the heart. Being overweight also increases your risk of heart disease and type 2 diabetes. These diseases can lead to heart failure.

- People who have had a heart attack. Damage to the heart muscle from a heart attack and can weaken the heart muscle.

Children who have congenital heart defects also can develop heart failure. These defects occur if the heart, heart valves, or blood vessels near the heart don't form correctly while a baby is in the womb. Congenital heart defects can make the heart work harder. This weakens the heart muscle, which can lead to heart failure. Children don't have the same symptoms of heart failure or get the same treatments as adults. This Health Topic focuses on heart failure in adults.

What Are the Signs and Symptoms of Heart Failure?

The most common signs and symptoms of heart failure are:

- Shortness of breath or trouble breathing

- Fatigue (tiredness)

- Swelling in the ankles, feet, legs, abdomen, and veins in the neck

All of these symptoms are the result of fluid buildup in your body. When symptoms start, you may feel tired and short of breath after routine physical effort, like climbing stairs.

As your heart grows weaker, symptoms get worse. You may begin to feel tired and short of breath after getting dressed or walking across the room. Some people have shortness of breath while lying flat.

Fluid buildup from heart failure also causes weight gain, frequent urination, and a cough that's worse at night and when you're lying down. This cough may be a sign of acute pulmonary edema. This is a condition in which too much fluid builds up in your lungs. The condition requires emergency treatment.

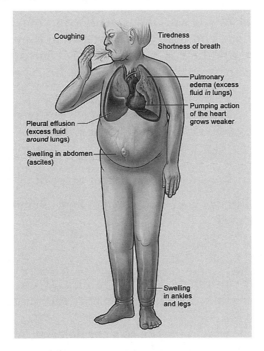

Coughing

Tiredness
Shortness of breath

Pulmonary
edema (excess
fluid *in* lungs)

Pumping action
of the heart
grows weaker

Pleural effusion
(excess fluid
around lungs)

Swelling in abdomen
(ascites)

Swelling
in ankles
and legs

Figure 17.1. *Heart Failure Signs and Symptoms*

How Is Heart Failure Diagnosed?

Your doctor will diagnose heart failure based on your medical and family histories, a physical exam, and test results. The signs and symptoms of heart failure also are common in other conditions. Thus, your doctor will:

- Find out whether you have a disease or condition that can cause heart failure, such as coronary heart disease (CHD), high blood pressure, or diabetes

- Rule out other causes of your symptoms

- Find any damage to your heart and check how well your heart pumps blood

Early diagnosis and treatment can help people who have heart failure live longer, more active lives.

Medical and Family Histories

Your doctor will ask whether you or others in your family have or have had a disease or condition that can cause heart failure.

Your doctor also will ask about your symptoms. He or she will want to know which symptoms you have, when they occur, how long you've had them, and how severe they are. Your answers will help show whether and how much your symptoms limit your daily routine.

Physical Exam

During the physical exam, your doctor will:

- Listen to your heart for sounds that aren't normal

- Listen to your lungs for the sounds of extra fluid buildup

- Look for swelling in your ankles, feet, legs, abdomen, and the veins in your neck

Diagnostic Tests

No single test can diagnose heart failure. If you have signs and symptoms of heart failure, your doctor may recommend one or more tests.

Your doctor also may refer you to a cardiologist. A cardiologist is a doctor who specializes in diagnosing and treating heart diseases and conditions.

- EKG (Electrocardiogram)
- Chest X-Ray
- BNP Blood Test
- Echocardiography
- Doppler Ultrasound
- Holter Monitor
- Nuclear Heart Scan
- Cardiac Catheterization
- Coronary Angiography
- Stress Test
- Cardiac MRI
- Thyroid Function Tests

How Is Heart Failure Treated?

Early diagnosis and treatment can help people who have heart failure live longer, more active lives. Treatment for heart failure depends on the type and severity of the heart failure.

The goals of treatment for all stages of heart failure include:

- Treating the condition's underlying cause, such as coronary heart disease, high blood pressure, or diabetes

- Reducing symptoms

- Stopping the heart failure from getting worse
- Increasing your lifespan and improving your quality of life

Treatments usually include lifestyle changes, medicines, and ongoing care. If you have severe heart failure, you also may need medical procedures or surgery.

Heart-Healthy Lifestyle Changes

Your doctor may recommend heart-healthy lifestyle changes if you have heart failure. Heart-healthy lifestyle changes include:

- Heart-healthy eating
- Maintaining a healthy weight
- Physical activity
- Quitting smoking

Medicines

Your doctor will prescribe medicines based on the type of heart failure you have, how severe it is, and your response to certain medicines. The following medicines are commonly used to treat heart failure:

- **ACE inhibitors** lower blood pressure and reduce strain on your heart. They also may reduce the risk of a future heart attack.
- **Aldosterone antagonists** trigger the body to remove excess sodium through urine. This lowers the volume of blood that the heart must pump.
- **Angiotensin receptor blockers** relax your blood vessels and lower blood pressure to decrease your heart's workload.
- **Beta blockers** slow your heart rate and lower your blood pressure to decrease your heart's workload.
- **Digoxin** makes the heart beat stronger and pump more blood.
- **Diuretics** (fluid pills) help reduce fluid buildup in your lungs and swelling in your feet and ankles.
- **Isosorbide dinitrate/hydralazine hydrochloride** helps relax your blood vessels so your heart doesn't work as hard to pump blood. Studies have shown that this medicine can reduce the risk

of death in blacks. More studies are needed to find out whether this medicine will benefit other racial groups.

Take all medicines regularly, as your doctor prescribes. Don't change the amount of your medicine or skip a dose unless your doctor tells you to. You should still follow a heart healthy lifestyle, even if you take medicines to treat your heart failure.

Medical Procedures and Surgery

As heart failure worsens, lifestyle changes and medicines may no longer control your symptoms. You may need a medical procedure or surgery.

In heart failure, the right and left sides of the heart may no longer contract at the same time. This disrupts the heart's pumping. To correct this problem, your doctor might implant a cardiac resynchronization therapy device (a type of pacemaker) near your heart. This device helps both sides of your heart contract at the same time, which can decrease heart failure symptoms.

Some people who have heart failure have very rapid, irregular heartbeats. Without treatment, these heartbeats can cause sudden cardiac arrest. Your doctor might implant an implantable cardioverter defibrillator (ICD) near your heart to solve this problem. An ICD checks your heart rate and uses electrical pulses to correct irregular heart rhythms.

People who have severe heart failure symptoms at rest, despite other treatments, may need:

- A mechanical heart pump, such as a left ventricular assist device. This device helps pump blood from the heart to the rest of the body. You may use a heart pump until you have surgery or as a long-term treatment.

- Heart transplant. A heart transplant is an operation in which a person's diseased heart is replaced with a healthy heart from a deceased donor. Heart transplants are done as a life-saving measure for end-stage heart failure when medical treatment and less drastic surgery have failed.

How Can Heart Failure Be Prevented?

You can take steps to prevent heart failure. The sooner you start, the better your chances of preventing or delaying the condition.

For People Who Have Healthy Hearts

If you have a healthy heart, you can take action to prevent heart disease and heart failure. To reduce your risk of heart disease:

- Avoid using illegal drugs.

- Be physically active. The more active you are, the more you will benefit.

- Follow a heart-healthy eating plan.

- If you smoke, make an effort to quit. Talk with your doctor about programs and products that can help you quit smoking. Also, try to avoid secondhand smoke.

- Maintain a healthy weight. Work with your healthcare team to create a reasonable weight-loss plan.

For People Who Are at High Risk for Heart Failure

Even if you're at high risk for heart failure, you can take steps to reduce your risk. People at high risk include those who have coronary heart disease, high blood pressure, or diabetes.

- Follow all of the steps listed above. Talk with your doctor about what types and amounts of physical activity are safe for you.

- Treat and control any conditions that can cause heart failure. Take medicines as your doctor prescribes.

- Avoid drinking alcohol.

- See your doctor for ongoing care.

For People Who Have Heart Damage but No Signs of Heart Failure

If you have heart damage but no signs of heart failure, you can still reduce your risk of developing the condition. In addition to the steps above, take your medicines as prescribed to reduce your heart's workload.

Chapter 18

Arrhythmias

Chapter Contents

Section 18.1

What Is an Arrhythmia?

Text in this section is excerpted from "Arrhythmias," ©1995–2016.
The Nemours Foundation/KidsHealth®. Reprinted with permission.

An arrhythmia is an abnormal heart rhythm usually caused by an electrical "short circuit" in the heart.

The heart normally beats in a consistent pattern, but an arrhythmia can make it beat too slowly, too quickly, or irregularly. This can cause the heart muscle's pumping function to work erratically, which can lead to a variety of symptoms, including fatigue, dizziness, and chest pain.

What Causes Arrhythmias?

The heart has its own conduction system, or electrical system, that sends electrical signals around the heart, telling it when to contract and pump blood throughout the body. The electrical signals originate from a group of cells in the **right atrium**, called the **sinus node**. The sinus node functions as the heart's **pacemaker** and makes sure the heart is beating at a normal and consistent rate. The sinus node normally increases the heart rate in response to factors like exercise, emotions, and stress, and slows the heart rate during sleep.

However, sometimes the electrical signals flowing through the heart don't "communicate" properly with the heart muscle, and the heart can start beating in an abnormal pattern—an arrhythmia (also called dysrhythmia).

Arrhythmias can be temporary or permanent. They can be caused by several things, but also can occur for no apparent reason. Arrhythmias can be congenital (meaning kids are born with it), sometimes due to a birth defect of the heart but sometimes even when the heart has formed normally.

Other causes of arrhythmias in kids include chemical imbalances in the blood, infections, or other diseases that cause irritation or inflammation of the heart, medications (prescription or over-the-counter), and injuries to the heart from chest trauma or heart surgery. Other factors (such as illegal drugs, alcohol, tobacco, caffeine, stress, and some herbal remedies) also can cause arrhythmias.

Signs and Symptoms

Because arrhythmias can cause the heart to beat less effectively, blood flow to the brain and to the rest of the body can be interrupted. If the heart is beating too fast, its chambers can't fill with the proper amount of blood. If it's beating too slowly or irregularly, the proper amount of blood can't be pumped out to the body.

If the body doesn't get the supply of blood it needs to run smoothly, these symptoms can occur:

- dizziness

- fatigue

- lightheadedness

- weakness

- palpitations (a feeling of fluttering or pounding in the chest)

- shortness of breath

- chest pain

- fainting

Arrhythmias can be constant, but usually come and go at random. Sometimes arrhythmias can cause no detectable symptoms at all. In these cases, the arrhythmia can only be discovered during a physical examination or a heart function test.

What's a Normal Heart Rate?

Heart rate is measured by counting the number of beats per minute. Normal heart rate varies depending on factors like age and whether the person leads an active lifestyle or not. (For example, athletes often have a lower resting heart rate).

The resting heart rate decreases as kids get older. Typical normal resting heart rate ranges are:

- babies (birth to 3 months of age): 100–150 beats per minute

- kids 1–3 years old: 70–110 beats per minute

- kids by age 12: 55–85 beats per minute

Your doctor should help you determine whether or not your child's heart rate is abnormally fast or slow, since the significance of an abnormal heart rate depends on the situation. For example, an older child or adult with a slow heart rate might begin to show symptoms when his or her heart rate drops below 50 beats per minute. However, trained athletes have a lower resting heart rate—so a slow heart rate in them isn't considered abnormal if no symptoms are associated with it.

Types of Arrhythmias

There are several types of arrhythmias, including:

Premature Atrial Contraction (PAC) and Premature Ventricular Contraction (PVC)

Premature contractions are usually considered minor arrhythmias, in which the person may feel a fluttering or pounding in the chest caused by an early or extra beat. PACs and PVCs are very common, and are what happens when it feels like your heart "skips" a beat. It doesn't skip a beat—an extra beat actually comes sooner than normal. Occasional premature beats are common and considered normal, but in some cases they can indicate an underlying medical problem or heart condition.

Tachycardias

Tachycardias are arrhythmias that involve an abnormally rapid heartbeat. They fall into two major categories—**supraventricular** and **ventricular:**

1. **Supraventricular tachycardia (SVT):** is the most common significant arrhythmia, it's characterized by bursts of fast heartbeats that originate in the upper chambers of the heart. The bursts can happen suddenly, and episodes can last anywhere from a few seconds to several days. Specific treatment is usually recommended if incidents of SVT are long-lasting or happen often.

2. **Ventricular tachycardia:** is a serious but relatively uncommon condition that originates in the lower chambers of the heart and can be dangerous.

Bradycardias

Bradycardias—arrhythmias characterized by an abnormally slow heartbeat—include:

- **Sinus node dysfunction:** is when the heart's sinus node isn't working correctly, most commonly following surgery to correct a congenital heart defect. An abnormally slow heartbeat is typically seen in this condition; however, episodes of rapid heartbeat due to SVT also can occur.

- **Heart block:** is often caused by a congenital heart defect, but also can be the result of disease or injury. Heart block happens when electrical impulses can't make their way from the upper to lower chambers of the heart. When this happens, another node in the lower chambers takes over and acts as the heart's pacemaker. Although it sends out electrical impulses to keep the heart beating, the transmission of the signals is much slower, leading to a slower heart rate.

Diagnosing Arrhythmias

Doctors use several tools to diagnose arrhythmias. It's very important to know your child's medical history and give this information to your doctor, who will use it, along with a physical examination, to begin the evaluation.

If an arrhythmia is suspected, the doctor will probably recommend an electrocardiogram (EKG) to measures the heart's electrical activity. There is nothing painful about an EKG—a series of electrodes (small metal tabs) are fixed to the skin with sticky papers, then information about the electrical activity of the heart is transferred to a computer, where it's interpreted and drawn as a graph.

The doctor might recommend the following types of EKG tests:

- **Resting EKG.** This measures resting heart rate and rhythm, and lasts about a minute.

- **Exercise EKG** (also called a **stress test**). This measures heart rate and rhythm while exercising, like riding a stationary bicycle or walking on a treadmill.

- **Signal-average EKG.** This measures heart rate much like a resting EKG. The only difference is the signal-average EKG monitors the heartbeat over a longer time period (around 15–20 minutes).

- **Holter monitor.** This is an EKG done over a long period of time, usually 24 hours or more. The electrodes are connected to the chest, and the wires are attached to a portable EKG recorder. The child is encouraged to continue normal daily activities, but must be careful to not get the electrodes wet (for example, no swimming, showering, or activities that cause a lot of sweating). The two kinds of Holter monitoring are: **continuous recording**, which means the EKG is on throughout the entire monitoring period; and **event monitoring**, which means data is recorded only when the child feels symptoms and then turns the Holter monitor on.

Treating Arrhythmias

Many arrhythmias don't require treatment; however, some can pose a health problem and need to be evaluated and treated by a doctor.

Depending on the type and severity of the arrhythmia, one of these options might be recommended:

- **Medications.** Many types of prescription anti-arrhythmic medications are available to treat arrhythmias. The doctor will determine which is best by considering the type of arrhythmia, possible underlying medical causes, and any medications a child is taking. Sometimes, anti-arrhythmic medications can increase symptoms and cause unwanted side effects, so their use and effectiveness should be closely monitored by the doctor, you, and your child.

- **Pacemakers.** A pacemaker is a small, battery-operated device implanted into the body (near the collarbone) through a surgical procedure. Connected to the heart by a wire, pacemakers can help treat bradycardia. Through a sensing device, a pacemaker can detect if the heart rate is too slow and sends electrical signals to the heart to speed up the heartbeat.

- **Defibrillators.** Like a pacemaker, a defibrillator can deliver electrical impulses to the heart. A small battery-operated implantable cardioverter defibrillator (ICD) can be implanted near the left collarbone through a surgical procedure. Wires run from the defibrillator to the heart. It senses if the heart has developed a dangerously fast or irregular rhythm and delivers an electrical shock to restore a normal heartbeat.

- **Catheter ablation.** "Ablation" literally means removal or elimination. In the case of catheter ablation, a catheter (a long, thin wire) is guided through a vein in the leg to the heart. Arrhythmias are often caused by microscopic defects in the heart muscle. Once the problem area of the heart is pinpointed, the catheter heats or freezes the muscle cells and destroys them.

- **Surgery.** Surgery is usually recommended only if all other options have failed. In this case, the child is put under anesthesia, the chest is opened, and the heart is exposed. Then, the tissue causing the arrhythmia is removed.

Section 18.2

Atrial Fibrillation

This section includes text excerpted from "Atrial Fibrillation," National Heart, Lung, and Blood Institute (NHLBI), September 18, 2014.

What Is Atrial Fibrillation?

Atrial fibrillation, or AF, is the most common type of arrhythmia. An arrhythmia is a problem with the rate or rhythm of the heartbeat. During an arrhythmia, the heart can beat too fast, too slow, or with an irregular rhythm.

AF occurs if rapid, disorganized electrical signals cause the heart's two upper chambers—called the atri—to fibrillate. The term "fibrillate" means to contract very fast and irregularly.

In AF, blood pools in the atria. It isn't pumped completely into the heart's two lower chambers, called the ventricles. As a result, the heart's upper and lower chambers don't work together as they should.

People who have AF may not feel symptoms. However, even when AF isn't noticed, it can increase the risk of stroke. In some people, AF can cause chest pain or heart failure, especially if the heart rhythm is very rapid.

AF may happen rarely or every now and then, or it may become an ongoing or long-term heart problem that lasts for years.

Understanding the Heart's Electrical System

To understand AF, it helps to understand the heart's internal electrical system. The heart's electrical system controls the rate and rhythm of the heartbeat.

With each heartbeat, an electrical signal spreads from the top of the heart to the bottom. As the signal travels, it causes the heart to contract and pump blood.

Each electrical signal begins in a group of cells called the sinus node or sinoatrial (SA) node. The SA node is located in the right atrium. In a healthy adult heart at rest, the SA node sends an electrical signal to begin a new heartbeat 60 to 100 times a minute. (This rate may be slower in very fit athletes.)

From the SA node, the electrical signal travels through the right and left atria. It causes the atria to contract and pump blood into the ventricles.

The electrical signal then moves down to a group of cells called the atrioventricular (AV) node, located between the atria and the ventricles. Here, the signal slows down slightly, allowing the ventricles time to finish filling with blood.

The electrical signal then leaves the AV node and travels to the ventricles. It causes the ventricles to contract and pump blood to the lungs and the rest of the body. The ventricles then relax, and the heartbeat process starts all over again in the SA node.

Understanding the Electrical Problem in Atrial Fibrillation

In AF, the heart's electrical signals don't begin in the SA node. Instead, they begin in another part of the atria or in the nearby pulmonary veins. The signals don't travel normally. They may spread throughout the atria in a rapid, disorganized way. This can cause the atria to fibrillate.

The faulty signals flood the AV node with electrical impulses. As a result, the ventricles also begin to beat very fast. However, the AV node can't send the signals to the ventricles as fast as they arrive. So, even though the ventricles are beating faster than normal, they aren't beating as fast as the atria.

Thus, the atria and ventricles no longer beat in a coordinated way. This creates a fast and irregular heart rhythm. In AF, the ventricles may beat 100 to 175 times a minute, in contrast to the normal rate of 60 to 100 beats a minute.

If this happens, blood isn't pumped into the ventricles as well as it should be. Also, the amount of blood pumped out of the ventricles to the body is based on the random atrial beats.

The body may get rapid, small amounts of blood and occasional larger amounts of blood. The amount will depend on how much blood has flowed from the atria to the ventricles with each beat.

Most of the symptoms of AF are related to how fast the heart is beating. If medicines or age slow the heart rate, the symptoms are minimized.

AF may be brief, with symptoms that come and go and end on their own. Or, the condition may be ongoing and require treatment. Sometimes AF is permanent, and medicines or other treatments can't restore a normal heart rhythm.

Types of Atrial Fibrillation

Paroxysmal Atrial Fibrillation

In paroxysmal atrial fibrillation (AF), the faulty electrical signals and rapid heart rate begin suddenly and then stop on their own. Symptoms can be mild or severe. They stop within about a week, but usually in less than 24 hours.

Persistent Atrial Fibrillation

Persistent AF is a condition in which the abnormal heart rhythm continues for more than a week. It may stop on its own, or it can be stopped with treatment.

Permanent Atrial Fibrillation

Permanent AF is a condition in which a normal heart rhythm can't be restored with treatment. Both paroxysmal and persistent AF may become more frequent and, over time, result in permanent AF.

Other Names for Atrial Fibrillation

- A fib
- Auricular fibrillation

What Causes Atrial Fibrillation?

Atrial fibrillation (AF) occurs if the heart's electrical signals don't travel through the heart in a normal way. Instead, they become very rapid and disorganized.

Damage to the heart's electrical system causes AF. The damage most often is the result of other conditions that affect the health of the heart, such as high blood pressure and coronary heart disease.

The risk of AF increases as you age. Inflammation also is thought to play a role in causing AF.

Sometimes, the cause of AF is unknown.

Who Is at Risk for Atrial Fibrillation?

Atrial fibrillation (AF) affects millions of people, and the number is rising. Men are more likely than women to have the condition. In the United States, AF is more common among Whites than African Americans or Hispanic Americans.

The risk of AF increases as you age. This is mostly because your risk for heart disease and other conditions that can cause AF also increases as you age. However, about half of the people who have AF are younger than 75.

AF is uncommon in children.

Major Risk Factors

AF is more common in people who have:

- High blood pressure

- Coronary heart disease (CHD)

- Heart failure

- Rheumatic heart disease

- Structural heart defects, such as mitral valve prolapse

- Pericarditis; a condition in which the membrane, or sac, around your heart is inflamed)

- Congenital heart defects

- Sick sinus syndrome (a condition in which the heart's electrical signals don't fire properly and the heart rate slows down; sometimes the heart will switch back and forth between a slow rate and a fast rate)

AF also is more common in people who are having heart attacks or who have just had surgery.

Other Risk Factors

Other conditions that raise your risk for AF include hyperthyroidism (too much thyroid hormone), obesity, diabetes, and lung disease.

Certain factors also can raise your risk for AF. For example, drinking large amounts of alcohol, especially binge drinking, raises your risk. Even modest amounts of alcohol can trigger AF in some people. Caffeine or psychological stress also may trigger AF in some people.

Some data suggest that people who have sleep apnea are at greater risk for AF. Sleep apnea is a common disorder that causes one or more pauses in breathing or shallow breaths while you sleep.

Metabolic syndrome also raises your risk for AF. Metabolic syndrome is the name for a group of risk factors that raises your risk for CHD and other health problems, such as diabetes and stroke.

Research suggests that people who receive high-dose steroid therapy are at increased risk for AF. This therapy is used for asthma and some inflammatory conditions. It may act as a trigger in people who have other AF risk factors.

Genetic factors also may play a role in causing AF. However, their role isn't fully known.

What Are the Signs and Symptoms of Atrial Fibrillation?

Atrial fibrillation (AF) usually causes the heart's lower chambers, the ventricles, to contract faster than normal.

When this happens, the ventricles can't completely fill with blood. Thus, they may not be able to pump enough blood to the lungs and body. This can lead to signs and symptoms, such as:

- Palpitations (feelings that your heart is skipping a beat, fluttering, or beating too hard or fast)
- Shortness of breath
- Weakness or problems exercising
- Chest pain
- Dizziness or fainting
- Fatigue (tiredness)
- Confusion

Atrial Fibrillation Complications

AF has two major complications—stroke and heart failure.

Stroke

During AF, the heart's upper chambers, the atria, don't pump all of their blood to the ventricles. Some blood pools in the atria. When this happens, a blood clot (also called a thrombus) can form.

If the clot breaks off and travels to the brain, it can cause a stroke. (A clot that forms in one part of the body and travels in the bloodstream to another part of the body is called an embolus.)

Blood-thinning medicines that reduce the risk of stroke are an important part of treatment for people who have AF.

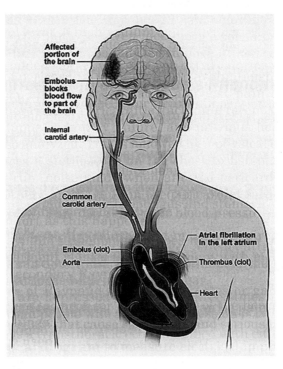

Figure 18.1 Atrial Fibrillation and Stroke

The illustration shows how a stroke can occur during atrial fibrillation. A blood clot (thrombus) can form in the left atrium of the heart. If a piece of the clot breaks off and travels to an artery in the brain, it can block blood flow through the artery. The lack of blood flow to the portion of the brain fed by the artery causes a stroke.

Heart Failure

Heart failure occurs if the heart can't pump enough blood to meet the body's needs. AF can lead to heart failure because the ventricles are beating very fast and can't completely fill with blood. Thus, they may not be able to pump enough blood to the lungs and body.

Fatigue and shortness of breath are common symptoms of heart failure. A buildup of fluid in the lungs causes these symptoms. Fluid also can build up in the feet, ankles, and legs, causing weight gain.

Lifestyle changes, medicines, and procedures or surgery (rarely, a mechanical heart pump or heart transplant) are the main treatments for heart failure.

How Is Atrial Fibrillation Diagnosed?

Atrial fibrillation (AF) is diagnosed based on your medical and family histories, a physical exam, and the results from tests and procedures.

Sometimes AF doesn't cause signs or symptoms. Thus, it may be found during a physical exam or EKG (electrocardiogram) test done for another purpose.

If you have AF, your doctor will want to find out what is causing it. This will help him or her plan the best way to treat the condition.

Medical and Family Histories

Your doctor will likely ask questions about your:

- Signs and symptoms. What symptoms are you having? Have you had palpitations? Are you dizzy or short of breath? Are your feet or ankles swollen (a possible sign of heart failure)? Do you have any chest pain?

- Medical history. Do you have other health problems, such as a history of heart disease, high blood pressure, lung disease, diabetes, or thyroid problems?

- Family's medical history. Does anyone in your family have a history of AF? Has anyone in your family ever had heart disease or high blood pressure? Has anyone had thyroid problems? Does your family have a history of other illnesses or health problems?

- Health habits. Do you smoke or use alcohol or caffeine?

Physical Exam

Your doctor will do a complete cardiac exam. He or she will listen to the rate and rhythm of your heartbeat and take your pulse and blood pressure reading. Your doctor will likely check for any signs of heart muscle or heart valve problems. He or she will listen to your lungs to check for signs of heart failure.

Your doctor also will check for swelling in your legs or feet and look for an enlarged thyroid gland or other signs of hyperthyroidism (too much thyroid hormone).

Diagnostic Tests and Procedures

- EKG

- Holter and Event Monitors

- Stress Test

- Echocardiography

- Transesophageal Echocardiography

- Chest X-Ray

- Blood Tests

How Is Atrial Fibrillation Treated?

Treatment for atrial fibrillation (AF) depends on how often you have symptoms, how severe they are, and whether you already have heart disease. General treatment options include medicines, medical procedures, and lifestyle changes.

Goals of Treatment

The goals of treating AF include:

- Preventing blood clots from forming, thus lowering the risk of stroke.

- Controlling how many times a minute the ventricles contract. This is called rate control. Rate control is important because it allows the ventricles enough time to completely fill with blood. With this approach, the abnormal heart rhythm continues, but you feel better and have fewer symptoms.

- Restoring a normal heart rhythm. This is called rhythm control. Rhythm control allows the atria and ventricles to work together to efficiently pump blood to the body.

- Treating any underlying disorder that's causing or raising the risk of AF—for example, hyperthyroidism (too much thyroid hormone).

Who Needs Treatment for Atrial Fibrillation?

People who have AF but don't have symptoms or related heart problems may not need treatment. AF may even go back to a normal heart rhythm on its own. (This also can occur in people who have AF with symptoms.)

In some people who have AF for the first time, doctors may choose to use an electrical procedure or medicine to restore a normal heart rhythm.

Repeat episodes of AF tend to cause changes to the heart's electrical system, leading to persistent or permanent AF. Most people who have persistent or permanent AF need treatment to control their heart rate and prevent complications.

Specific Types of Treatment

Blood Clot Prevention

People who have AF are at increased risk for stroke. This is because blood can pool in the heart's upper chambers (the atria), causing a blood clot to form. If the clot breaks off and travels to the brain, it can cause a stroke.

Preventing blood clots from forming is probably the most important part of treating AF. The benefits of this type of treatment have been proven in multiple studies.

Doctors prescribe blood-thinning medicines to prevent blood clots. These medicines include warfarin (Coumadin®), dabigatran, heparin, and aspirin.

People taking blood-thinning medicines need regular blood tests to check how well the medicines are working.

Rate Control

Doctors can prescribe medicines to slow down the rate at which the ventricles are beating. These medicines help bring the heart rate to a normal level.

Rate control is the recommended treatment for most patients who have AF, even though an abnormal heart rhythm continues and the heart doesn't work as well as it should. Most people feel better and can function well if their heart rates are well-controlled.

Medicines used to control the heart rate include beta blockers (for example, metoprolol and atenolol), calcium channel blockers (diltiazem and verapamil), and digitalis (digoxin). Several other medicines also are available.

Rhythm Control

Restoring and maintaining a normal heart rhythm is a treatment approach recommended for people who aren't doing well with rate control treatment. This treatment also may be used for people who have only recently started having AF. The long-term benefits of rhythm control have not been proven conclusively yet.

Doctors use medicines or procedures to control the heart's rhythm. Patients often begin rhythm control treatment in a hospital so that their hearts can be closely watched.

The longer you have AF, the less likely it is that doctors can restore a normal heart rhythm. This is especially true for people who have had AF for 6 months or more.

Restoring a normal rhythm also becomes less likely if the atria are enlarged or if any underlying heart disease worsens. In these cases, the chance that AF will recur is high, even if you're taking medicine to help convert AF to a normal rhythm.

Medicines used to control the heart rhythm include amiodarone, sotalol, flecainide, propafenone, dofetilide, and ibutilide. Sometimes older medicines—such as quinidine, procainamide, and disopyramide—are used.

Approaches to Treating Underlying Causes and Reducing Risk Factors

Your doctor may recommend treatments for an underlying cause of AF or to reduce AF risk factors. For example, he or she may prescribe medicines to treat an overactive thyroid, lower high blood pressure, or manage high blood cholesterol.

Your doctor also may recommend lifestyle changes, such as following a healthy diet, cutting back on salt intake (to help lower blood pressure), quitting smoking, and reducing stress.

Limiting or avoiding alcohol, caffeine, or other stimulants that may increase your heart rate also can help reduce your risk for AF.

How Can Atrial Fibrillation Be Prevented?

Following a healthy lifestyle and taking steps to lower your risk for heart disease may help you prevent atrial fibrillation (AF). These steps include:

- Following a heart healthy diet that's low in saturated fat, trans fat, and cholesterol. A healthy diet includes a variety of whole grains, fruits, and vegetables daily.
- Not smoking.

- Being physically active.

- Maintaining a healthy weight.

If you already have heart disease or other AF risk factors, work with your doctor to manage your condition. In addition to adopting the healthy habits above, which can help control heart disease, your doctor may advise you to:

- Follow the DASH eating plan to help lower your blood pressure.

- Keep your cholesterol and triglycerides at healthy levels with dietary changes and medicines (if prescribed).

- Limit or avoid alcohol.

- Control your blood sugar level if you have diabetes.

- Get ongoing medical care and take your medicines as prescribed.

Section 18.3

Brugada Syndrome

This section includes text excerpted from "Brugada Syndrome," Genetics Home Reference (GHR), April 20, 2016.

What Is Brugada Syndrome?

Brugada syndrome is a condition that causes a disruption of the heart's normal rhythm. Specifically, this disorder can lead to irregular heartbeats in the heart's lower chambers (ventricles), which is an abnormality called ventricular arrhythmia. If untreated, the irregular heartbeats can cause fainting (syncope), seizures, difficulty breathing, or sudden death. These complications typically occur when an affected person is resting or asleep.

Brugada syndrome usually becomes apparent in adulthood, although it can develop any time throughout life. Signs and symptoms related to arrhythmias, including sudden death, can occur from early infancy to late adulthood. Sudden death typically occurs around age 40. This condition may explain some cases of sudden infant death syndrome (SIDS), which is a major cause of death in babies younger than 1 year. SIDS is characterized by sudden and unexplained death, usually during sleep.

Sudden unexplained nocturnal death syndrome (SUNDS) is a condition characterized by unexpected cardiac arrest in young adults, usually at night during sleep. This condition was originally described in Southeast Asian populations, where it is a major cause of death. Researchers have determined that SUNDS and Brugada syndrome are the same disorder.

Frequency

The exact prevalence of Brugada syndrome is unknown, although it is estimated to affect 5 in 10,000 people worldwide. This condition occurs much more frequently in people of Asian ancestry, particularly in Japanese and Southeast Asian populations.

Although Brugada syndrome affects both men and women, the condition appears to be 8 to 10 times more common in men. Researchers suspect that testosterone, a sex hormone present at much higher levels in men, may account for this difference.

Genetic Changes

Brugada syndrome can be caused by mutations in one of several genes. The most commonly mutated gene in this condition is *SCN5A*, which is altered in approximately 30 percent of affected individuals. This gene provides instructions for making a sodium channel, which normally transports positively charged sodium atoms (ions) into heart muscle cells. This type of ion channel plays a critical role in maintaining the heart's normal rhythm. Mutations in the *SCN5A* gene alter the structure or function of the channel, which reduces the flow of sodium ions into cells. A disruption in ion transport alters the way the heart beats, leading to the abnormal heart rhythm characteristic of Brugada syndrome.

Mutations in other genes can also cause Brugada syndrome. Together, these other genetic changes account for less than two percent of cases of the condition. Some of the additional genes involved in Brugada syndrome provide instructions for making proteins that ensure the correct location or function of sodium channels in heart muscle cells. Proteins produced by other genes involved in the condition form or help regulate ion channels that transport calcium or potassium into or out of heart muscle cells. As with sodium channels, proper flow of ions through calcium and potassium channels in the heart muscle helps maintain a regular heartbeat. Mutations in these genes disrupt the flow of ions, impairing the heart's normal rhythm.

In affected people without an identified gene mutation, the cause of Brugada syndrome is often unknown. In some cases, certain drugs may cause a nongenetic (acquired) form of the disorder. Drugs that can induce an altered heart rhythm include medications used to treat some forms of arrhythmia, a condition called angina (which causes chest pain), high blood pressure, depression, and other mental illnesses. Abnormally high blood levels of calcium (hypercalcemia) or potassium (hyperkalemia), as well as unusually low potassium levels (hypokalemia), also have been associated with acquired Brugada syndrome. In addition to causing a nongenetic form of this disorder, these factors may trigger symptoms in people with an underlying mutation in *SCN5A* or another gene.

Inheritance Pattern

This condition is inherited in an autosomal dominant pattern, which means one copy of the altered gene in each cell is sufficient to cause the disorder. In most cases, an affected person has one parent with the condition. Other cases may result from new mutations in the gene. These cases occur in people with no history of the disorder in their family.

Section 18.4

Heart Block

Heart block—also known as atrioventricular (AV) block—is a condition where the electrical signals that normally cause the heart muscle to contract are prevented from performing this function, resulting in an abnormally slow heartbeat. Ordinarily, a heartbeat begins with an electrical signal generated by the sinus node, a group of specialized cells located in the upper right atrium chamber of the heart. This signal travels downward to the atrioventricular node, an electrical relay station located between the heart's upper and lower chambers. Finally, the current passes through special fibers into the lower chambers or ventricles, causing the heart muscle to contract and pump blood through the body. When the conduction of electrical signals through the heart is delayed or interrupted, partial or total heart block occurs.

Causes and Symptoms

Although some people are born with congenital heart block, most cases are acquired later in life. In fact, the risk of acquired heart block increases as people get older and become more susceptible to heart disease. Heart block can be caused by many different types of heart disease as well as by certain other types of medical conditions. Some of the most common causes of acquired heart block include the following:

- heart attack
- coronary artery disease
- heart failure
- cardiomyopathy (enlarged heart)
- rheumatic heart disease
- heart valve abnormalities or structural heart disorders
- injury during open heart surgery
- side effects of some medications
- exposure to toxic substances
- Lyme disease

Although people with some types of heart block do not experience any symptoms, others may experience fainting, dizziness, fatigue, shortness of breath, or chest pain. These symptoms sometimes indicate other heart problems, so emergency medical attention may be warranted if they appear suddenly.

Diagnosis and Treatment

Heart block is often diagnosed as part of a regular medical examination, when a doctor detects an arrhythmia while listening to the patient's heartbeat or an abnormally slow heart rhythm while taking their pulse. If heart block is suspected, the patient will likely be referred to a cardiologist for further evaluation. The specialist will typically inquire about the patient's symptoms, family history of heart disease, and any medications they may be taking. The doctor may then order an electrocardiogram (EKG) to monitor electrical activity in the patient's heart, as well as perform tests to rule out other types of arrhythmias.

There are several different types of heart block that differ in terms of severity, symptoms, and treatment.

- **First-degree heart block:** This condition is fairly common and rarely causes symptoms or requires treatment. It often occurs in well-trained athletes and healthy teenagers, as well as people who take certain medications. In first-degree heart block, all of the electrical signals reach the ventricles, although their progress is slowed as they pass through the conduction system.

- **Type I second-degree heart block:** This condition sometimes causes dizziness or other symptoms and may require monitoring or treatment. It can occur in people with normal conduction systems during sleep. In this type of heart block, the delay before electrical impulses reach the ventricles grows longer and longer until conduction failure occurs, resulting in a brief pause in the heartbeat.

- **Type II second-degree heart block:** In this condition, some electrical signals fail to reach the ventricles. Although it is less common than Type I, it typically causes more severe symptoms and is considered a more serious condition. A pacemaker is often recommended to regulate the heartbeat in people with Type II heart block.

- **Third-degree or complete heart block:** This condition occurs when no electrical signals successfully reach the ventricles. In the absence of impulses from the right atrium, the lower chambers typically generate ventricular escape beats, which serve as a sort of backup system. Since these beats occur very slowly, people with third-degree heart block usually experience severe symptoms of fatigue, lightheadedness, and fainting.

Most cases of first-degree heart block do not require treatment. In addition, some cases of acquired heart block may improve with treatment of the underlying medical condition. For instance, heart block that occurs following a heart attack may resolve itself during recovery, or heart block that is caused by medication may go away if the dosage is lowered or the prescription is changed.

The main form of treatment for third-degree heart block—and some cases of second-degree heart block—is a pacemaker. A pacemaker is a small device that is inserted beneath the skin of the chest or abdomen. It generates electrical impulses to help regulate the heartbeat. Although people with pacemakers can usually pursue normal activities, it is important to avoid things that may prevent the pacemaker from working properly. Examples include devices that produce strong electrical currents or magnetic fields, such as airport screening devices and magnetic resonance imaging (MRI) scanners. Most people with pacemakers wear a medical ID bracelet or carry a card that describes their pacemaker and lists things that may interfere with its operation.

References

1.   "Heart Block," Cleveland Clinic, 2016.

2.   "Heart Block," Heart Rhythm Society, 2016.

Section 18.5

Long QT Syndrome

This section includes text excerpted from "Long QT Syndrome,"
National Heart, Lung, and Blood Institute (NHLBI),
September 21, 2011. Reviewed June 2016.

What Is Long QT Syndrome?

Long QT syndrome (LQTS) is a disorder of the heart's electrical activity. It can cause sudden, uncontrollable, dangerous arrhythmias in response to exercise or stress. Arrhythmias are problems with the rate or rhythm of the heartbeat.

People who have LQTS also can have arrhythmias for no known reason. However, not everyone who has LQTS has dangerous heart rhythms. When they do occur, though, they can be fatal.

What Does "Long QT" Mean?

The term "long QT" refers to an abnormal pattern seen on an EKG (electrocardiogram). An EKG is a test that detects and records the heart's electrical activity.

With each heartbeat, an electrical signal spreads from the top of your heart to the bottom. As it travels, the signal causes the heart to contract and pump blood. An EKG records electrical signals as they move through your heart.

Data from the EKG are mapped on a graph so your doctor can study your heart's electrical activity. Each heartbeat is mapped as five distinct electrical waves: P, Q, R, S, and T.

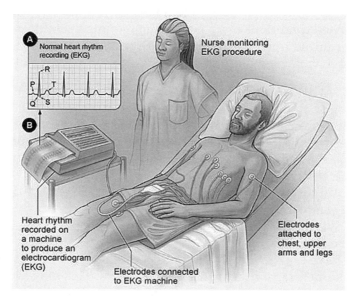

Figure 18.2. *EKG*

The image shows the standard setup for an EKG. In (A), a normal heart rhythm recording shows the electrical pattern of a regular heartbeat. In (B), a patient lies in a bed with EKG electrodes attached to his chest, upper arms, and legs. A nurse monitors the painless procedure.

The electrical activity that occurs between the Q and T waves is called the QT interval. This interval shows electrical activity in the heart's lower chambers, the ventricles.

The timing of the heart's electrical activity is complex, and the body carefully controls it. Normally the QT interval is about a third of each heartbeat cycle. However, in people who have LQTS, the QT interval lasts longer than normal.

A long QT interval can upset the careful timing of the heartbeat and trigger dangerous heart rhythms.

Other Names for Long QT Syndrome

- Jervell and Lange-Nielsen syndrome
- Romano-Ward syndrome

What Causes Long QT Syndrome?

Long QT syndrome (LQTS) can be inherited or acquired. "Inherited" means you're born with the condition and have it your whole life. Inherited conditions are passed from parents to children through genes. "Acquired" means you aren't born with the condition, but you develop it during your lifetime.

Inherited Long QT Syndrome

Faulty genes cause inherited LQTS. These genes control the production of certain types of ion channels in your heart. Faulty genes may cause the body to make too few ion channels, ion channels that don't work well, or both.

There are seven known types of inherited LQTS (types 1 though 7). The most common types are LQTS 1, 2, and 3.

Some types of LQTS involve faulty or lacking potassium ion or sodium ion channels.

If you have LQTS 1 or LQTS 2, the flow of potassium ions through the ion channels in your heart cells isn't normal. This may cause problems when you exercise or when you have strong emotions.

You may develop a rapid, uncontrollable heart rhythm that prevents your heart from pumping blood. This type of heart rhythm can be fatal if it's not quickly brought under control.

If you have LQTS 3, the flow of sodium ions through ion channels in your heart cells isn't normal. This can trigger a rapid, uncontrollable heart rhythm that can be fatal. In LQTS 3, problems usually occur when your heart beats slower than normal, such as during sleep.

Acquired Long QT Syndrome

Some medicines and conditions can cause acquired LQTS.

Medication-Induced Long QT Syndrome

More than 50 medicines have been found to cause LQTS. Some common medicines that may cause the disorder include:

- Antihistamines and decongestants

- Diuretics (pills that remove excess water from your body)

- Antibiotics

- Antiarrhythmic medicines

- Antidepressant and antipsychotic medicines

- Cholesterol-lowering medicines and some diabetes medicines

Some people who have medication-induced LQTS also may have an inherited form of the disorder. They may not have symptoms unless they take medicines that lengthen the QT interval or lower potassium levels in the blood. When LQTS doesn't cause symptoms, it's called silent LQTS.

Other Causes of Acquired Long QT Syndrome

Severe diarrhea or vomiting that causes a major loss of potassium or sodium ions from the bloodstream may cause LQTS. The disorder lasts until these ion levels return to normal.

The eating disorders anorexia nervosa and bulimia and some thyroid disorders may cause a drop in potassium ion levels in the blood, causing LQTS.

Who Is at Risk for Long QT Syndrome?

Long QT syndrome (LQTS) is a rare disorder. Experts think that about 1 in 7,000 people has LQTS. But no one knows for sure, because LQTS often goes undiagnosed.

LQTS causes about 3,000 to 4,000 sudden deaths in children and young adults each year in the United States. Unexplained sudden deaths in children are rare. When they do occur, LQTS often is the cause.

Inherited LQTS usually is first detected during childhood or young adulthood. Half of all people who have LQTS have their first abnormal heart rhythm by the time they're 12 years old, and 90 percent by the time they're 40 years old. The condition rarely is diagnosed after age 40.

In boys who have LQTS, the QT interval (which can be seen on an EKG test) often returns toward normal after puberty. If this happens, the risk of LQTS symptoms and complications goes down.

LQTS is more common in women than men. Women who have LQTS are more likely to faint or die suddenly from the disorder during menstruation and shortly after giving birth.

Children who are born deaf also are at increased risk for LQTS. This is because the same genetic problem that affects hearing also affects the function of ion channels in the heart.

Major Risk Factors

You're at risk of having LQTS if anyone in your family has ever had it. Unexplained fainting or seizures, drowning or near drowning, and unexplained sudden death are all possible signs of LQTS.

You're also at risk for LQTS if you take medicines that make the QT interval longer. Your doctor can tell you whether your prescription or over-the-counter medicines might do this.

You also may develop LQTS if you have excessive vomiting or diarrhea or other conditions that cause low blood levels of potassium or sodium. These conditions include the eating disorders anorexia nervosa and bulimia, as well as some thyroid disorders.

What Are the Signs and Symptoms of Long QT Syndrome?

Major Signs and Symptoms

If you have long QT syndrome (LQTS), you can have sudden and dangerous arrhythmias (abnormal heart rhythms). Signs and symptoms of LQTS-related arrhythmias often first occur during childhood and include:

- Unexplained fainting. This happens because the heart isn't pumping enough blood to the brain. Fainting may occur during physical or emotional stress. Fluttering feelings in the chest may occur before fainting.

- Unexplained drowning or near drowning. This may be due to fainting while swimming.

- Unexplained sudden cardiac arrest (SCA) or death. SCA is a condition in which the heart suddenly stops beating for no obvious reason. People who have SCA die within minutes unless they receive treatment. In about 1 out of 10 people who have LQTS, SCA or sudden death is the first sign of the disorder.

Other Signs and Symptoms

Often, people who have LQTS 3 develop an abnormal heart rhythm during sleep. This may cause noisy gasping while sleeping.

Silent Long QT Syndrome

Sometimes long QT syndrome doesn't cause any signs or symptoms. This is called silent LQTS. For this reason, doctors often advise family members of people who have LQTS to be tested for the disorder, even if they have no symptoms.

Medical and genetic tests may reveal whether these family members have LQTS and what type of the condition they have.

How Is Long QT Syndrome Diagnosed?

Cardiologists diagnose and treat long QT syndrome (LQTS). Cardiologists are doctors who specialize in diagnosing and treating heart diseases and conditions. To diagnose LQTS, your cardiologist will consider your:

- EKG (electrocardiogram) results
- Medical history and the results from a physical exam
- Genetic test results

Types of Inherited Long QT Syndrome

If you have inherited LQTS, it may be helpful to know which type you have. This will help you and your doctor plan your treatment and decide which lifestyle changes you should make.

To find out what type of LQTS you have, your doctor will consider:

- Genetic test results
- The types of situations that trigger an abnormal heart rhythm
- How well you respond to medicine

How Is Long QT Syndrome Treated?

The goal of treating long QT syndrome (LQTS) is to prevent life-threatening, abnormal heart rhythms and fainting spells.

Treatment isn't a cure for the disorder and may not restore a normal QT interval on an EKG (electrocardiogram). However, treatment greatly improves the chances of survival.

Specific Types of Treatment

Your doctor will recommend the best treatment for you based on:

- Whether you've had symptoms, such as fainting or sudden cardiac arrest (SCA)

- What type of LQTS you have

- How likely it is that you'll faint or have SCA

- What treatment you feel most comfortable with

People who have LQTS without symptoms may be advised to:

- Make lifestyle changes that reduce the risk of fainting or SCA. Lifestyle changes may include avoiding certain sports and strenuous exercise, such as swimming, which can cause abnormal heart rhythms.

- Avoid medicines that may trigger abnormal heart rhythms. This may include some medicines used to treat allergies, infections, high blood pressure, high blood cholesterol, depression, and arrhythmias.

- Take medicines such as beta-blockers, which reduce the risk of symptoms by slowing the heart rate.

The type of medicine you take will depend on the type of LQTS you have. For example, doctors usually will prescribe sodium channel blocker medicines only for people who have LQTS 3.

If your doctor thinks you're at increased risk for LQTS complications, he or she may suggest more aggressive treatments (in addition to medicines and lifestyle changes). These treatments may include:

- A surgically implanted device, such as a pacemaker or implantable cardioverter defibrillator (ICD). These devices help control abnormal heart rhythms.

- Surgery on the nerves that regulate your heartbeat.

People at increased risk are those who have fainted or who have had dangerous heart rhythms from their LQTS.

Lifestyle Changes

If possible, try to avoid things that can trigger abnormal heart rhythms. For example, people who have LQTS should avoid medicines that lengthen the QT interval or lower potassium blood levels.

Many people who have LQTS also benefit from adding more potassium to their diets. Check with your doctor about eating more potassium-rich foods (such as bananas) or taking potassium supplements daily.

Medicines

Beta blockers are medicines that prevent the heart from beating faster in response to physical or emotional stress. Most people who have LQTS are treated with beta blockers.

Doctors may suggest that people who have LQTS 3 take sodium channel blockers, such as mexiletine. These medicines make sodium ion channels less active.

Medical Devices

Pacemakers and ICDs are small devices that help control abnormal heart rhythms. Both devices use electrical currents to prompt the heart to beat normally. Surgeons implant pacemakers and ICDs in the chest or belly with a minor procedure.

The use of these devices is similar in children and adults. However, because children are still growing, other issues may arise. For example, as children grow, they may need to have their devices replaced.

Surgery

People who are at high risk of death from LQTS sometimes are treated with surgery. During surgery, the nerves that prompt the heart to beat faster in response to physical or emotional stress are cut.

This type of surgery keeps the heart beating at a steady pace and lowers the risk of dangerous heart rhythms in response to stress or exercise.

Living with Long QT Syndrome

Long QT syndrome (LQTS) usually is a lifelong condition. The risk of having an abnormal heart rhythm that leads to fainting or sudden cardiac arrest may lessen as you age. However, the risk never completely goes away.

You'll need to take certain steps for the rest of your life to prevent abnormal heart rhythms. You can:

- Avoid things that trigger abnormal heart rhythms

- Let others know you might faint or your heart might stop beating, and tell them what steps they can take

- Have a plan in place for how to handle abnormal heart rhythms

If an abnormal heart rhythm does occur, you'll need to seek treatment right away.

Avoid Triggers

If exercise triggers an abnormal heart rhythm, your doctor may tell you to avoid any strenuous exercise, especially swimming. Ask your doctor what types and amounts of exercise are safe for you.

If you have a pacemaker or implantable cardioverter defibrillator, avoid contact sports that may dislodge these devices. You may want to exercise in public or with a friend who can help you if you faint.

Avoid medicines that can trigger an abnormal heart rhythm. This includes some medicines used to treat allergies, infections, high blood pressure, high blood cholesterol, depression, and arrhythmias. Talk with your doctor before taking any prescription, over-the-counter, or other medicines or drugs.

Seek medical care right away for conditions that lower the sodium or potassium level in your blood. These conditions include the eating disorders anorexia nervosa and bulimia, excessive vomiting or diarrhea, and certain thyroid disorders.

If you have LQTS 2, try to avoid unexpected noises, such as loud or jarring alarm clock buzzers and telephone ringers.

Inform Others

You may want to wear a medical ID necklace or bracelet that states that you have LQTS. This will help alert medical personnel and others about your condition if you have an emergency.

Let your roommates, coworkers, or other people with whom you have regular contact know that you have a condition that might cause you to faint or go into cardiac arrest. Tell them to call 9–1–1 right away if you faint.

Consider asking a family member and/or coworker to learn cardiopulmonary resuscitation (CPR) in case your heart stops beating.

You also may want to keep an automated external defibrillator (AED) with you at home or at work. This device uses electric shocks to restore a normal heart rhythm.

Someone at your home and/or workplace should be trained on how to use the AED, just in case your heart stops beating. If a trained person isn't available, an untrained person also can use the AED to help save your life.

If you have LQTS 3 and you sleep alone, you may want to have an intercom in your bedroom that's connected to someone else's bedroom. This will let others detect the noisy gasping that often occurs if you have an abnormal heart rhythm while lying down.

Section 18.6

Sick Sinus Syndrome

This section includes text excerpted from "Sick Sinus Syndrome," Genetics Home Reference (GHR), August 2013.

What Is Sick Sinus Syndrome?

Sick sinus syndrome (also known as sinus node dysfunction) is a group of related heart conditions that can affect how the heart beats. "Sick sinus" refers to the sino-atrial (SA) node, which is an area of specialized cells in the heart that functions as a natural pacemaker. The SA node generates electrical impulses that start each heartbeat. These signals travel from the SA node to the rest of the heart, signaling the heart (cardiac) muscle to contract and pump blood. In people with sick sinus syndrome, the SA node does not function normally. In some cases, it does not produce the right signals to trigger a regular heartbeat. In others, abnormalities disrupt the electrical impulses and prevent them from reaching the rest of the heart.

Sick sinus syndrome tends to cause the heartbeat to be too slow (bradycardia), although occasionally the heartbeat is too fast (tachycardia). In some cases, the heartbeat rapidly switches from being too fast to being too slow, a condition known as tachycardia-bradycardia syndrome. Symptoms related to abnormal heartbeats can include dizziness, light-headedness, fainting (syncope), a sensation of fluttering or pounding in the chest (palpitations), and confusion or memory problems. During exercise, many affected individuals experience chest pain, difficulty breathing, or excessive tiredness (fatigue). Once symptoms of sick sinus syndrome appear, they usually worsen with time. However, some people with the condition never experience any related health problems.

Sick sinus syndrome occurs most commonly in older adults, although it can be diagnosed in people of any age. The condition increases the risk of several life-threatening problems involving the heart and blood vessels. These include a heart rhythm abnormality called atrial fibrillation, heart failure, cardiac arrest, and stroke.

Frequency

Sick sinus syndrome accounts for 1 in 600 patients with heart disease who are over age 65. The incidence of this condition increases with age.

Genetic Changes

Sick sinus syndrome can result from genetic or environmental factors. In many cases, the cause of the condition is unknown.

Genetic changes are an uncommon cause of sick sinus syndrome. Mutations in two genes, *SCN5A* and HCN4, have been found to cause the condition in a small number of families. These genes provide instructions for making proteins called ion channels that transport positively charged atoms (ions) into cardiac cells, including cells that make up the SA node. The flow of these ions is essential for creating the electrical impulses that start each heartbeat and coordinate contraction of the cardiac muscle. Mutations in these genes reduce the flow of ions, which alters the SA node's ability to create and spread electrical signals. These changes lead to abnormal heartbeats and the other symptoms of sick sinus syndrome.

A particular variation in another gene, MYH6, appears to increase the risk of developing sick sinus syndrome. The protein produced from the MYH6 gene forms part of a larger protein called myosin, which generates the mechanical force needed for cardiac muscle to contract. Researchers believe that the MYH6 gene variation changes the structure of myosin, which can affect cardiac muscle contraction and increase the likelihood of developing an abnormal heartbeat.

More commonly, sick sinus syndrome is caused by other factors that alter the structure or function of the SA node. These include a variety of heart conditions, other disorders such as muscular dystrophy, abnormal inflammation, or a shortage of oxygen (hypoxia). Certain medications, such as drugs given to treat abnormal heart rhythms or high blood pressure, can also disrupt SA node function. One of the most common causes of sick sinus syndrome in children is trauma to the SA node, such as damage that occurs during heart surgery.

In older adults, sick sinus syndrome is often associated with age-related changes in the heart. Over time, the SA node may harden and develop scar-like damage (fibrosis) that prevents it from working properly.

Inheritance Pattern

Most cases of sick sinus syndrome are not inherited. They are described as sporadic, which means they occur in people with no history of the disorder in their family.

When sick sinus syndrome results from mutations in the HCN4 gene, it has an autosomal dominant pattern of inheritance. Autosomal dominant inheritance means that one copy of the altered gene in each cell is sufficient to cause the disorder. In most cases, an affected person has one parent with the condition.

When sick sinus syndrome is caused by mutations in the *SCN5A* gene, it is inherited in an autosomal recessive pattern. Autosomal recessive inheritance means both copies of the gene in each cell have mutations. The parents of an individual with an autosomal recessive condition each carry one copy of the mutated gene, but they typically do not show signs and symptoms of the condition.

Chapter 19

Heart Valve Disease

Chapter Contents

Section 19.1

Heart Valve Disease: Overview

This section includes text excerpted from "Heart Valve Disease," National Heart, Lung, and Blood Institute (NHLBI), October 30, 2015.

What Is Heart Valve Disease?

Heart valve disease occurs if one or more of your heart valves don't work well. The heart has four valves: the tricuspid, pulmonary, mitral, and aortic valves.

These valves have tissue flaps that open and close with each heartbeat. The flaps make sure blood flows in the right direction through your heart's four chambers and to the rest of your body.

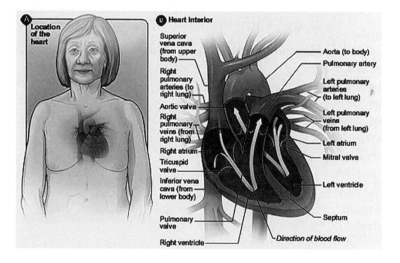

Figure 19.1. *Healthy Heart Cross-Section*

(A) shows the location of the heart in the body. (B) shows a cross-section of a healthy heart and its inside structures. The blue arrow shows the direction in which oxygen-poor blood flows through the heart to the lungs. The red arrow shows the direction in which oxygen-rich blood flows from the lungs into the heart and then out to the body.

Birth defects, age-related changes, infections, or other conditions can cause one or more of your heart valves to not open fully or to let blood leak back into the heart chambers. This can make your heart work harder and affect its ability to pump blood.

Other Names for Heart Valve Disease

- Aortic regurgitation
- Aortic stenosis
- Aortic sclerosis
- Aortic valve disease
- Bicuspid aortic valve
- Congenital heart defect
- Congenital valve disease
- Mitral regurgitation
- Mitral stenosis
- Mitral valve disease
- Mitral valve prolapse
- Pulmonic regurgitation
- Pulmonic stenosis
- Pulmonic valve disease
- Tricuspid regurgitation
- Tricuspid stenosis
- Tricuspid valve disease

What Causes Heart Valve Disease?

Heart conditions and other disorders, age-related changes, rheumatic fever, or infections can cause acquired heart valve disease. These factors change the shape or flexibility of once-normal heart valves.

The cause of congenital heart valve disease isn't known. It occurs before birth as the heart is forming. Congenital heart valve disease can occur alone or with other types of congenital heart defects.

Heart Conditions and Other Disorders

Certain conditions can stretch and distort the heart valves. These conditions include:

- Advanced high blood pressure and heart failure, this can enlarge the heart or the main arteries.

- Atherosclerosis in the aorta. Atherosclerosis is a condition in which a waxy substance called plaque builds up inside the arteries. The aorta is the main artery that carries oxygen-rich blood to the body.

- Damage and scar tissue due to a heart attack or injury to the heart.

Rheumatic Fever

Untreated strep throat or other infections with strep bacteria that progress to rheumatic fever can cause heart valve disease.

When the body tries to fight the strep infection, one or more heart valves may be damaged or scarred in the process. The aortic and mitral valves most often are affected. Symptoms of heart valve damage often don't appear until many years after recovery from rheumatic fever.

Currently, most people who have strep infections are treated with antibiotics before rheumatic fever occurs. If you have strep throat, take all of the antibiotics your doctor prescribes, even if you feel better before the medicine is gone.

Heart valve disease caused by rheumatic fever mainly affects older adults who had strep infections before antibiotics were available. It also affects people from developing countries, where rheumatic fever is more common.

Infections

Common germs that enter the bloodstream and get carried to the heart can sometimes infect the inner surface of the heart, including the heart valves. This rare but serious infection is called infective endocarditis.

The germs can enter the bloodstream through needles, syringes, or other medical devices and through breaks in the skin or gums. Often, the body's defenses fight off the germs and no infection occurs. Sometimes these defenses fail, which leads to infective endocarditis.

Infective endocarditis can develop in people who already have abnormal blood flow through a heart valve as the result of congenital or acquired heart valve disease. The abnormal blood flow causes blood clots to form on the surface of the valve. The blood clots make it easier for germs to attach to and infect the valve.

Infective endocarditis can worsen existing heart valve disease.

Other Conditions and Factors Linked to Heart Valve Disease

Many other conditions and factors are linked to heart valve disease. However, the role they play in causing heart valve disease often isn't clear.

- **Autoimmune disorders.** Autoimmune disorders, such as lupus, can affect the aortic and mitral valves.

- **Carcinoid syndrome.** Tumors in the digestive tract that spread to the liver or lymph nodes can affect the tricuspid and pulmonary valves.

- **Diet medicines.** The use of fenfluramine and phentermine sometimes has been linked to heart valve problems. These problems typically stabilize or improve after the medicine is stopped.

- **Marfan syndrome.** Congenital disorders, such as Marfan syndrome and other connective tissue disorders, can affect the heart valves.

- **Metabolic disorders.** Relatively uncommon diseases (such as Fabry disease) and other metabolic disorders (such as high blood cholesterol) can affect the heart valves.

- **Radiation therapy.** Radiation therapy to the chest area can cause heart valve disease. This therapy is used to treat cancer. Heart valve disease due to radiation therapy may not cause symptoms until years after the therapy.

Who Is at Risk for Heart Valve Disease?

Older age is a risk factor for heart valve disease. As you age, your heart valves thicken and become stiffer. Also, people are living longer now than in the past. As a result, heart valve disease has become an increasing problem.

People who have a history of infective endocarditis (IE), rheumatic fever, heart attack, or heart failure—or previous heart valve disease—also are at higher risk for heart valve disease. In addition, having risk factors for IE, such as intravenous drug use, increases the risk of heart valve disease.

You're also at higher risk for heart valve disease if you have risk factors for coronary heart disease. These risk factors include high blood cholesterol, high blood pressure, smoking, insulin resistance, diabetes, overweight or obesity, lack of physical activity, and a family history of early heart disease.

Some people are born with an aortic valve that has two flaps instead of three. Sometimes an aortic valve may have three flaps, but two flaps are fused together and act as one flap. This is called a bicuspid or bicommissural aortic valve. People who have this congenital condition are more likely to develop aortic heart valve disease.

What Are the Signs and Symptoms of Heart Valve Disease?

Major Signs and Symptoms

The main sign of heart valve disease is an unusual heartbeat sound called a heart murmur. Your doctor can hear a heart murmur with a stethoscope.

However, many people have heart murmurs without having heart valve disease or any other heart problems. Others may have heart murmurs due to heart valve disease, but have no other signs or symptoms.

Heart valve disease often worsens over time, so signs and symptoms may occur years after a heart murmur is first heard. Many people who have heart valve disease don't have any symptoms until they're middle-aged or older.

Other common signs and symptoms of heart valve disease relate to heart failure, which heart valve disease can cause. These signs and symptoms include:

- Unusual fatigue (tiredness)

- Shortness of breath, especially when you exert yourself or when you're lying down

- Swelling in your ankles, feet, legs, abdomen, and veins in the neck

Other Signs and Symptoms

Heart valve disease can cause chest pain that may happen only when you exert yourself. You also may notice a fluttering, racing, or irregular heartbeat. Some types of heart valve disease, such as aortic or mitral valve stenosis, can cause dizziness or fainting.

How Is Heart Valve Disease Diagnosed?

Your primary care doctor may detect a heart murmur or other signs of heart valve disease. However, a cardiologist usually will diagnose the condition. A cardiologist is a doctor who specializes in diagnosing and treating heart problems.

To diagnose heart valve disease, your doctor will ask about your signs and symptoms. He or she also will do a physical exam and look at the results from tests and procedures.

Physical Exam

Your doctor will listen to your heart with a stethoscope. He or she will want to find out whether you have a heart murmur that's likely caused by a heart valve problem.

Your doctor also will listen to your lungs as you breathe to check for fluid buildup. He or she will check for swollen ankles and other signs that your body is retaining water.

Tests and Procedures

Echocardiography (echo) is the main test for diagnosing heart valve disease. But an EKG (electrocardiogram) or chest X-ray commonly is used to reveal certain signs of the condition. If these signs are present, echo usually is done to confirm the diagnosis.

Your doctor also may recommend other tests and procedures if you're diagnosed with heart valve disease. For example, you may have cardiac catheterization, stress testing, or cardiac MRI (magnetic resonance imaging). These tests and procedures help your doctor assess how severe your condition is so he or she can plan your treatment.

- EKG
- Chest X-ray
- Echocardiography
- Cardiac Catheterization
- Stress Test
- Cardiac MRI

How Is Heart Valve Disease Treated?

Currently, no medicines can cure heart valve disease. However, lifestyle changes and medicines often can treat symptoms successfully and delay problems for many years. Eventually, though, you may need surgery to repair or replace a faulty heart valve.

The goals of treating heart valve disease might include:

- Medicines
- Repairing or replacing faulty valves
- Lifestyle changes to treat other related heart conditions

Medicines

In addition to heart-healthy lifestyle changes, your doctor may prescribe medicines to:

- Lower high blood pressure or high blood cholesterol.

- Prevent arrhythmias (irregular heartbeats).

- Thin the blood and prevent clots (if you have a man-made replacement valve). Doctors also prescribe these medicines for mitral stenosis or other valve defects that raise the risk of blood clots.

- Treat coronary heart disease. Medicines for coronary heart disease can reduce your heart's workload and relieve symptoms.

- Treat heart failure. Heart failure medicines widen blood vessels and rid the body of excess fluid.

Repairing or Replacing Heart Valves

Your doctor may recommend repairing or replacing your heart valve(s), even if your heart valve disease isn't causing symptoms. Repairing or replacing a valve can prevent lasting damage to your heart and sudden death.

The decision to repair or replace heart valves depends on many factors, including:

- The severity of your valve disease

- Whether you need heart surgery for other conditions, such as bypass surgery to treat coronary heart disease. Bypass surgery and valve surgery can be performed at the same time.

- Your age and general health

When possible, heart valve repair is preferred over heart valve replacement. Valve repair preserves the strength and function of the heart muscle. People who have valve repair also have a lower risk of infective endocarditis after the surgery, and they don't need to take blood-thinning medicines for the rest of their lives.

However, heart valve repair surgery is harder to do than valve replacement. Also, not all valves can be repaired. Mitral valves often can be repaired. Aortic and pulmonary valves often have to be replaced.

Repairing Heart Valves

Heart surgeons can repair heart valves by:

- Adding tissue to patch holes or tears or to increase the support at the base of the valve

- Removing or reshaping tissue so the valve can close tighter

- Separating fused valve flaps

Sometimes cardiologists repair heart valves using cardiac catheterization. Although catheter procedures are less invasive than surgery, they may not work as well for some patients. Work with your doctor to decide whether repair is appropriate. If so, your doctor can advise you on the best procedure.

Heart valves that cannot open fully (stenosis) can be repaired with surgery or with a less invasive catheter procedure called balloon valvuloplasty. This procedure also is called balloon valvotomy.

During the procedure, a catheter (thin tube) with a balloon at its tip is threaded through a blood vessel to the faulty valve in your heart. The balloon is inflated to help widen the opening of the valve. Your doctor then deflates the balloon and removes both it and the tube. You're awake during the procedure, which usually requires an overnight stay in a hospital.

Balloon valvuloplasty relieves many symptoms of heart valve disease, but may not cure it. The condition can worsen over time. You still may need medicines to treat symptoms or surgery to repair or replace the faulty valve. Balloon valvuloplasty has a shorter recovery time than surgery. The procedure may work as well as surgery for some patients who have mitral valve stenosis. For these people, balloon valvuloplasty often is preferred over surgical repair or replacement.

Balloon valvuloplasty doesn't work as well as surgery for adults who have aortic valve stenosis. Doctors often use balloon valvuloplasty to repair valve stenosis in infants and children.

Replacing Heart Valves

Sometimes heart valves can't be repaired and must be replaced. This surgery involves removing the faulty valve and replacing it with a man-made or biological valve.

Biological valves are made from pig, cow, or human heart tissue and may have man-made parts as well. These valves are specially treated, so you won't need medicines to stop your body from rejecting the valve.

Man-made valves last longer than biological valves and usually don't have to be replaced. Biological valves usually have to be replaced after about 10 years, although newer ones may last 15 years or longer. Unlike biological valves, however, man-made valves require you to take blood-thinning medicines for the rest of your life. These medicines prevent blood clots from forming on the valve. Blood clots can cause a heart attack or stroke. Man-made valves also raise your risk of infective endocarditis.

You and your doctor will decide together whether you should have a man-made or biological replacement valve.

If you're a woman of childbearing age or if you're athletic, you may prefer a biological valve so you don't have to take blood-thinning medicines. If you're elderly, you also may prefer a biological valve, as it will likely last for the rest of your life.

Ross Procedure

Doctors also can treat faulty aortic valves with the Ross procedure. During this surgery, your doctor removes your faulty aortic valve and replaces it with your pulmonary valve. Your pulmonary valve is then replaced with a pulmonary valve from a deceased human donor.

This is more involved surgery than typical valve replacement, and it has a greater risk of complications. The Ross procedure may be especially useful for children because the surgically replaced valves continue to grow with the child. Also, lifelong treatment with blood-thinning medicines isn't required. But in some patients, one or both valves fail to work well within a few years of the surgery. Researchers continue to study the use of this procedure.

Other Approaches for Repairing and Replacing Heart Valves

Some forms of heart valve repair and replacement surgery are less invasive than traditional surgery. These procedures use smaller incisions (cuts) to reach the heart valves. Hospital stays for these newer types of surgery usually are 3 to 5 days, compared with a 5-day stay for traditional heart valve surgery.

New surgeries tend to cause less pain and have a lower risk of infection. Recovery time also tends to be shorter—2 to 4 weeks versus 6 to 8 weeks for traditional surgery.

Transcatheter Valve Therapy

Interventional cardiologists perform procedures that involve threading clips or other devices to repair faulty heart valves using a catheter (tube) inserted through a large blood vessel. The clips or devices are used to reshape the valves and stop the backflow of blood. People who receive these clips recover more easily than people who have surgery. However, the clips may not treat backflow as well as surgery.

Doctors also may use a catheter to replace faulty aortic valves. This procedure is called transcatheter aortic valve replacement (TAVR). For this procedure, the catheter usually is inserted into an artery in the groin (upper thigh) and threaded to the heart. A deflated balloon with a folded replacement valve around it is at the end of the catheter.

Once the replacement valve is placed properly, the balloon is used to expand the new valve so it fits securely within the old valve. The balloon is then deflated, and the balloon and catheter are removed.

A replacement valve also can be inserted in an existing replacement valve that is failing. This is called a valve-in-valve procedure.

Lifestyle Changes to Treat Other Related Heart Valve Diseases

To help treat heart conditions related to heart valve disease, your doctor may advise you to make heart-healthy lifestyle changes, such as:

* Heart-healthy eating
* Maintaining a healthy weight
* Managing stress
* Physical activity
* Quitting smoking

How Can Heart Valve Disease Be Prevented?

To prevent heart valve disease caused by rheumatic fever, see your doctor if you have signs of a strep infection. These signs include a painful sore throat, fever, and white spots on your tonsils. If you do have a strep infection, be sure to take all medicines prescribed to treat it. Prompt treatment of strep infections can prevent rheumatic fever, which damages the heart valves.

It's possible that exercise, a heart-healthy diet, and medicines that lower cholesterol might prevent aortic stenosis (thickening and stiffening of the aortic valve). Researchers continue to study this possibility.

Heart-healthy eating, physical activity, other heart-healthy lifestyle changes, and medicines aimed at preventing a heart attack, high blood pressure, or heart failure also may help prevent heart valve disease.

Section 19.2

Aortic Stenosis

Aortic Stenosis

May also be called: Aortic Valve Stenosis

The aortic valve is one of two valves that control the flow of blood as it leaves the heart. (The other is the pulmonary valve.) These valves work to keep the blood flowing forward. They open up to let the blood move ahead, then close quickly to keep the blood from flowing backward.

In aortic stenosis, the aortic valve is too narrow and can't open all the way.

More to Know

The aorta, the body's largest blood vessel, starts from the left ventricle of the heart and carries oxygen-rich blood to the body. Blood flows from the left ventricle into the aorta through the aortic valve, one of the four valves in the heart.

In aortic stenosis, the aortic valve is narrow. This decreases the amount of blood flowing into the aorta and out to the rest of the body. Aortic stenosis is most common in adults over 50, but can be present at birth (congenital).

Aortic stenosis makes the heart work harder to pump blood to the body. Over time, this added stress can weaken the heart and lead to life-threatening heart problems.

Aortic stenosis can be identified before birth, allowing babies born with severe cases to be treated right away. Babies with aortic stenosis can have trouble gaining weight, problems with feeding, and serious breathing problems that develop soon after birth. Older children also may have a heart murmur. These children may be sent for an echocardiogram, a type of heart ultrasound that will show how the valves are working.

People with severe aortic stenosis may have chest pain and shortness of breath, feel tired or dizzy, and have abnormal heartbeats. Mild cases of aortic stenosis may not need treatment. Medicines sometimes can treat the symptoms of aortic stenosis, but it can only be corrected through surgery.

Keep in Mind

Many people with aortic stenosis have no symptoms. Others have mild symptoms that never become a problem. In severe cases, however, the valve needs to be surgically repaired or replaced. Aortic stenosis often can be treated without open-heart surgery through a less invasive procedure called a cardiac catheterization. In young children with a severe problem, this usually involves a procedure called balloon valvuloplasty, in which an unopened balloon is threaded through the aortic valve and inflated to open the valve.

Kids and teens with moderate or severe aortic stenosis should avoid sports. Physical activity can increase blood flow, which can put added stress on the heart and lead to a medical emergency.

Section 19.3

Mitral Valve Prolapse

This section includes text excerpted from "Mitral Valve Prolapse," National Heart, Lung, and Blood Institute (NHLBI), October 29, 2015.

What Is Mitral Valve Prolapse?

Mitral valve prolapse (MVP) is a condition in which the heart's mitral valve doesn't work well. The flaps of the valve are "floppy" and may not close tightly. These flaps normally help seal or open the valve.

Much of the time, MVP doesn't cause any problems. Rarely, blood can leak the wrong way through the floppy valve. This can lead to palpitations, shortness of breath, chest pain, and other symptoms. (Palpitations are feelings that your heart is skipping a beat, fluttering, or beating too hard or too fast.)

Normal Mitral Valve

The mitral valve controls blood flow between the upper and lower chambers of the left side of the heart. The upper chamber is called the left atrium. The lower chamber is called the left ventricle.

The mitral valve allows blood to flow from the left atrium into the left ventricle, but not back the other way. The heart also has a right atrium and ventricle, separated by the tricuspid valve.

With each heartbeat, the atria contract and push blood into the ventricles. The flaps of the mitral and tricuspid valves open to let blood through. Then, the ventricles contract to pump the blood out of the heart.

When the ventricles contract, the flaps of the mitral and tricuspid valves close. They form a tight seal that prevents blood from flowing back into the atria.

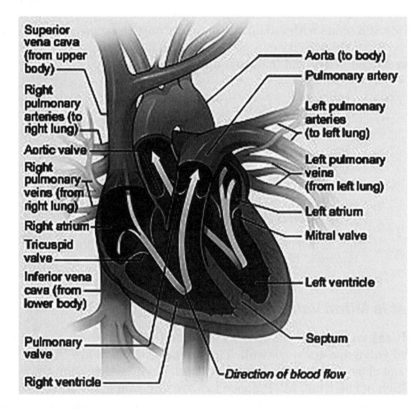

Figure 19.2. *Heart Interior*

Source: "Heart Valve Disease", National Heart, Lung, and Blood Institute (NHLBI), June 22, 2015.

Mitral Valve Prolapse

In MVP, when the left ventricle contracts, one or both flaps of the mitral valve flop or bulge back (prolapse) into the left atrium. This can prevent the valve from forming a tight seal. As a result, blood may leak from the ventricle back into the atrium. The backflow of blood is called regurgitation.

MVP doesn't always cause backflow. In fact, most people who have MVP don't have backflow and never have any related symptoms or problems. When backflow occurs, it can get worse over time and it can change the heart's size and raise pressure in the left atrium and lungs. Backflow also raises the risk of heart valve infections.

Medicines can treat troublesome MVP symptoms and help prevent complications. Some people will need surgery to repair or replace their mitral valves.

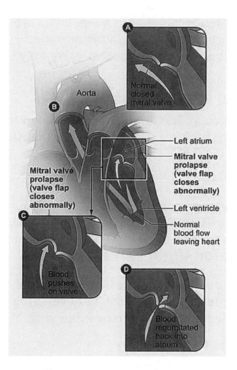

Figure 19.3. *Mitral Valve Prolapse*

(A) shows a normal mitral valve. The valve separates the left atrium from the left ventricle. (B) shows a heart with mitral valve prolapse. (C) shows a closeup view of mitral valve prolapse. (D) shows a mitral valve that allows blood to flow back into the left atrium.

Other Names for Mitral Valve Prolapse

- Balloon mitral valve
- Barlow syndrome
- Billowing mitral valve
- Click-murmur syndrome
- Floppy valve syndrome
- Myxomatous mitral valve
- Prolapsing mitral valve syndrome

What Causes Mitral Valve Prolapse?

The exact cause of mitral valve prolapse (MVP) isn't known. Most people who have the condition are born with it. MVP tends to run in families. Also, it's more common in people who are born with connective tissue disorders, such as Marfan syndrome.

In people who have MVP, the mitral valve may be abnormal in the following ways:

- The valve flaps may be too large and thick.
- The valve flaps may be "floppy." The tissue of the flaps and their supporting "strings" are too stretchy, and parts of the valve flop or bulge back into the atrium.
- The opening of the valve may stretch.

These problems can keep the valve from making a tight seal. Some people's valves are abnormal in more than one way.

Who Is at Risk for Mitral Valve Prolapse?

Mitral valve prolapse (MVP) affects people of all ages and both sexes; however, aging raises the risk of developing the disease.

Certain conditions have been associated with MVP, including:

- A history of rheumatic fever
- Connective tissue disorders, such as Marfan syndrome or Ehlers-Danlos syndrome
- Graves' disease
- Scoliosis and other skeletal problems
- Some types of muscular dystrophy

What Are the Signs and Symptoms of Mitral Valve Prolapse?

Most people who have mitral valve prolapse (MVP) aren't affected by the condition. They don't have any symptoms or major mitral valve backflow.

When MVP does cause signs and symptoms, they may include:

- Palpitations (feelings that your heart is skipping a beat, fluttering, or beating too hard or too fast)
- Shortness of breath
- Cough
- Fatigue (tiredness), dizziness, or anxiety
- Migraine headaches
- Chest discomfort

MVP symptoms can vary from one person to another. They tend to be mild but can worsen over time, mainly when complications occur.

Mitral Valve Prolapse Complications

MVP complications are rare. When present, they're most often caused by the backflow of blood through the mitral valve.

Mitral valve backflow is most common among men and people who have high blood pressure. People who have severe backflow may need valve surgery to prevent complications.

Mitral valve backflow causes blood to flow from the left ventricle back into the left atrium. Blood can even back up from the atrium into the lungs, causing shortness of breath.

The backflow of blood strains the muscles of both the atrium and the ventricle. Over time, the strain can lead to arrhythmias. Backflow also increases the risk of infective endocarditis (IE). IE is an infection of the inner lining of your heart chambers and valves.

Arrhythmias

Arrhythmias are problems with the rate or rhythm of the heartbeat. The most common types of arrhythmias are harmless. Other arrhythmias can be serious or even life threatening, such as ventricular arrhythmias.

If the heart rate is too slow, too fast, or irregular, the heart may not be able to pump enough blood to the body. Lack of blood flow can damage the brain, heart, and other organs.

One troublesome arrhythmia that MVP can cause is atrial fibrillation (AF). In AF, the walls of the atria quiver instead of beating normally. As a result, the atria aren't able to pump blood into the ventricles the way they should.

AF is bothersome but rarely life threatening, unless the atria contract very fast or blood clots form in the atria. Blood clots can occur because some blood "pools" in the atria instead of flowing into the ventricles. If a blood clot breaks off and travels through the bloodstream, it can reach the brain and cause a stroke.

Infection of the Mitral Valve

A deformed mitral valve flap can attract bacteria in the bloodstream. The bacteria attach to the valve and can cause a serious infection called infective endocarditis (IE). Signs and symptoms of a bacterial infection include fever, chills, body aches, and headaches.

IE doesn't happen often, but when it does, it's serious. MVP is the most common heart condition that puts people at risk for this infection.

If you have MVP, you can take steps to prevent IE. Floss and brush your teeth regularly. Gum infections and tooth decay can cause IE.

How Is Mitral Valve Prolapse Diagnosed?

Mitral valve prolapse (MVP) most often is detected during a routine physical exam. During the exam, your doctor will listen to your heart with a stethoscope.

Stretched valve flaps can make a clicking sound as they shut. If the mitral valve is leaking blood back into the left atrium, your doctor may heart a heart murmur or whooshing sound.

However, these abnormal heart sounds may come and go. Your doctor may not hear them at the time of an exam, even if you have MVP. Thus, you also may have tests and procedures to diagnose MVP.

Diagnostic Tests and Procedures

- Echocardiography

- Doppler Ultrasound

- Chest X-ray

- EKG

How Is Mitral Valve Prolapse Treated?

Most people who have mitral valve prolapse (MVP) don't need treatment because they don't have symptoms and complications.

Even people who do have symptoms may not need treatment. The presence of symptoms doesn't always mean that the backflow of blood through the valve is significant.

People who have MVP and troublesome mitral valve backflow may be treated with medicines, surgery, or both.

The goals of treating MVP include:

- Correcting the underlying mitral valve problem, if necessary
- Preventing infective endocarditis, arrhythmias, and other complications
- Relieving symptoms

Medicines

Medicines called beta blockers may be used to treat palpitations and chest discomfort in people who have little or no mitral valve backflow.

If you have significant backflow and symptoms, your doctor may prescribe:

- Blood-thinning medicines to reduce the risk of blood clots forming if you have atrial fibrillation.
- Digoxin to strengthen your heartbeat.
- Diuretics (fluid pills) to remove excess sodium and fluid in your body and lungs.
- Medicines such as flecainide and procainamide to regulate your heart rhythms.
- Vasodilators to widen your blood vessels and reduce your heart's workload. Examples of vasodilators are isosorbide dinitrate and hydralazine.

Take all medicines regularly, as your doctor prescribes. Don't change the amount of your medicine or skip a dose unless your doctor tells you to.

Surgery

Surgery is done only if the mitral valve is very abnormal and blood is flowing back into the atrium. The main goal of surgery is to improve symptoms and reduce the risk of heart failure.

The timing of the surgery is important. If it's done too early and your leaking valve is working fairly well, you may be put at needless risk from surgery. If it's done too late, you may have heart damage that can't be fixed.

Surgical Approaches

Traditionally, heart surgeons repair or replace a mitral valve by making an incision (cut) in the breastbone and exposing the heart.

A small but growing number of surgeons are using another approach that involves one or more small cuts through the side of the chest wall. This results in less cutting, reduced blood loss, and a shorter hospital stay. However, not all hospitals offer this method.

• Valve Repair and Valve Replacement

In mitral valve surgery, the valve is repaired or replaced. Valve repair is preferred when possible. Repair is less likely than replacement to weaken the heart. Repair also lowers the risk of infection and decreases the need for lifelong use of blood-thinning medicines.

If repair isn't an option, the valve can be replaced. Mechanical and biological valves are used as replacement valves.

Mechanical valves are man-made and can last a lifetime. People who have mechanical valves must take blood-thinning medicines for the rest of their lives.

Biological valves are taken from cows or pigs or made from human tissue. Many people who have biological valves don't need to take blood-thinning medicines for the rest of their lives. The major drawback of biological valves is that they weaken over time and often last only about 10 years.

After surgery, you'll likely stay in the hospital's intensive care unit for 2 to 3 days. Overall, most people who have mitral valve surgery spend about 1 to 2 weeks in the hospital. Complete recovery takes a few weeks to several months, depending on your health before surgery.

If you've had valve repair or replacement, you may need antibiotics before dental work and surgery. These procedures can allow bacteria to enter your bloodstream. Antibiotics can help prevent infective endocarditis, a serious heart valve infection. Discuss with your doctor whether you need to take antibiotics before such procedures.

• Transcatheter Valve Therapy

Interventional cardiologists may be able to repair leaky mitral valves by implanting a device using a catheter (tube) inserted through a large blood vessel. This approach is less invasive and can prevent a person from having open-heart surgery. At present, the device is only approved for people with severe mitral regurgitation who cannot undergo surgery.

How Can Mitral Valve Prolapse Be Prevented?

You can't prevent mitral valve prolapse (MVP). Most people who have the condition are born with it.

Complications from MVP, such as arrhythmias (irregular heartbeats) and infective endocarditis (IE), are rare. IE is an infection of the inner lining of your heart chambers and valves.

People at high risk for IE may be given antibiotics before some types of surgery and dental work. Antibiotics can help prevent IE. Your doctor will tell you whether you need this type of treatment.

People at high risk for IE may include those who've had valve repair or replacement or who have some types of underlying heart disease.

Section 19.4

Pulmonic Valvular Stenosis

Text in this section is excerpted from "A to Z: Pulmonic Valvular Stenosis," ©1995–2016. The Nemours Foundation/ KidsHealth®. Reprinted with permission.

May also be called: Pulmonary Stenosis; PS; Pulmonary Valve Stenosis; PVS; Valvular Pulmonary Stenosis; Heart Valve Pulmonary Stenosis

Pulmonic Valvular Stenosis

Pulmonic valvular stenosis is a condition in which a deformity of the pulmonic valve causes less blood than normal to flow from the heart to the lungs.

More to Know

The heart has four chambers; the right ventricle and left ventricle are on the bottom, and the right atrium and left atrium are on the top:

- Oxygen-poor blood returning from the body enters the heart in the right atrium and then flows into the right ventricle.

- When the heart beats, the ventricle pushes blood through the pulmonic valve into the pulmonary artery, which carries blood to the lungs so it can pick up oxygen.

When someone has pulmonic valvular stenosis (also called pulmonary stenosis), it means that a deformity on or near the pulmonic valve is narrowing the passage for blood. This slows down the flow of blood to the lungs.

Deformities that affect the pulmonic valve are usually caused by congenital heart defects (heart problems that kids are born with). Sometimes tumors or other heart disorders cause problems with the pulmonic valve. Pulmonic valvular stenosis is most common in newborns, but can affect people of any age.

Some people with pulmonic valvular stenosis have no problems, while others might have a range of problems, such as heart murmurs or rapid heartbeat (palpitations), shortness of breath, chest pain, fatigue, and in some cases, a bluish color to the skin. In severe cases, children may have growth problems and enlarged abdomens from the backup of blood.

Not all cases of pulmonic valvular stenosis need treatment, but doctors may use medicines depending on how the heart is working.

More serious cases usually are treated with a surgical procedure called a **balloon valvuloplasty.** In this treatment, an uninflated balloon is placed in the pulmonic valve and then inflated to open the valve wider. Then the balloon is removed. In rare cases, doctors may use open-heart surgery to repair the pulmonic valve and pulmonary artery.

Keep in Mind

Mild cases of pulmonic valvular stenosis may never require any treatment. If needed, treatments like balloon valvuloplasty or open-heart surgery have great results and in most cases the stenosis does not return.

Chapter 20

Heart Murmurs

What Is a Heart Murmur?

A heart murmur is an extra or unusual sound heard during a heartbeat. Murmurs range from very faint to very loud. Sometimes they sound like a whooshing or swishing noise.

Normal heartbeats make a "lub-DUPP" or "lub-DUB" sound. This is the sound of the heart valves closing as blood moves through the heart. Doctors can hear these sounds and heart murmurs using a stethoscope.

Overview

The two types of heart murmurs are innocent (harmless) and abnormal.

Innocent heart murmurs aren't caused by heart problems. These murmurs are common in healthy children. Many children will have heart murmurs heard by their doctors at some point in their lives.

People who have abnormal heart murmurs may have signs or symptoms of heart problems. Most abnormal murmurs in children are caused by congenital heart defects. These defects are problems with the heart's structure that are present at birth.

In adults, abnormal heart murmurs most often are caused by acquired heart valve disease. This is heart valve disease that develops as the result of another condition. Infections, diseases, and aging can cause heart valve disease.

This chapter includes text excerpted from "Heart Murmurs," National Heart, Lung, and Blood Institute (NHLBI), September 20, 2012. Reviewed June 2016.

Outlook

A heart murmur isn't a disease, and most murmurs are harmless. Innocent murmurs don't cause symptoms. Having one doesn't require you to limit your physical activity or do anything else special. Although you may have an innocent murmur throughout your life, you won't need treatment for it.

The outlook and treatment for abnormal heart murmurs depend on the type and severity of the heart problem causing them.

What Causes Heart Murmurs?

Innocent Heart Murmurs

Why some people have innocent heart murmurs and others do not isn't known. Innocent murmurs are simply sounds made by blood flowing through the heart's chambers and valves, or through blood vessels near the heart.

Extra blood flow through the heart also may cause innocent heart murmurs. After childhood, the most common cause of extra blood flow through the heart is pregnancy. This is because during pregnancy, women's bodies make extra blood. Most heart murmurs that occur in pregnant women are innocent.

Abnormal Heart Murmurs

Congenital heart defects or acquired heart valve disease often are the cause of abnormal heart murmurs.

Congenital Heart Defects

Congenital heart defects are the most common cause of abnormal heart murmurs in children. These defects are problems with the heart's structure that are present at birth. They change the normal flow of blood through the heart.

Congenital heart defects can involve the interior walls of the heart, the valves inside the heart, or the arteries and veins that carry blood to and from the heart. Some babies are born with more than one heart defect.

Heart valve problems, septal defects (also called holes in the heart), and diseases of the heart muscle such as hypertrophic cardiomyopathy are common heart defects that cause abnormal heart murmurs.

Examples of valve problems are narrow valves that limit blood flow or leaky valves that don't close properly. Septal defects are holes in the wall that separates the right and left sides of the heart. This wall is called the septum.

A hole in the septum between the heart's two upper chambers is called an atrial septal defect. A hole in the septum between the heart's two lower chambers is called a ventricular septal defect.

Hypertrophic cardiomyopathy (HCM) occurs if heart muscle cells enlarge and cause the walls of the ventricles (usually the left ventricle) to thicken. The thickening may block blood flow out of the ventricle. If a blockage occurs, the ventricle must work hard to pump blood to the body. HCM also can affect the heart's mitral valve, causing blood to leak backward through the valve.

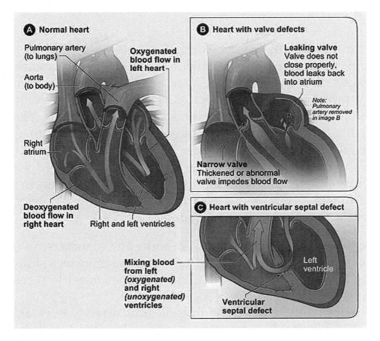

Figure 20.1. *Heart Defects That Can Cause Abnormal Heart Murmurs*

(A) shows the structure and blood flow insidhttps://wcms.nhlbi.nih.gov/node/4390/edite a normal heart. (B) shows a heart with leaking and narrowed valves. (C) shows a heart with a ventricular septal defect.

Acquired Heart Valve Disease

Acquired heart valve disease often is the cause of abnormal heart murmurs in adults. This is heart valve disease that develops as the result of another condition.

Many conditions can cause heart valve disease. Examples include heart conditions and other disorders, age-related changes, rheumatic fever, and infections.

Heart conditions and other disorders. Certain conditions can stretch and distort the heart valves, such as:

Damage and scar tissue from a heart attack or injury to the heart.

Advanced high blood pressure and heart failure. These conditions can enlarge the heart or its main arteries.

Age-related changes. As you get older, calcium deposits or other deposits may form on your heart valves. These deposits stiffen and thicken the valve flaps and limit blood flow. This stiffening and thickening of the valve is called sclerosis.

Rheumatic fever. The bacteria that cause strep throat, scarlet fever, and, in some cases, impetigo also can cause rheumatic fever. This serious illness can develop if you have an untreated or not fully treated streptococcal (strep) infection.

Rheumatic fever can damage and scar the heart valves. The symptoms of this heart valve damage often don't occur until many years after recovery from rheumatic fever.

Today, most people who have strep infections are treated with antibiotics before rheumatic fever develops. It's very important to take all of the antibiotics your doctor prescribes for strep throat, even if you feel better before the medicine is gone.

Infections. Common germs that enter the bloodstream and get carried to the heart can sometimes infect the inner surface of the heart, including the heart valves. This rare but sometimes life-threatening infection is called infective endocarditis, or IE.

IE is more likely to develop in people who already have abnormal blood flow through a heart valve because of heart valve disease. The abnormal blood flow causes blood clots to form on the surface of the valve. The blood clots make it easier for germs to attach to and infect the valve.

IE can worsen existing heart valve disease.

Other Causes

Some heart murmurs occur because of an illness outside of the heart. The heart is normal, but an illness or condition can cause blood flow that's faster than normal. Examples of this type of illness include fever, anemia, and hyperthyroidism.

Anemia is a condition in which the body has a lower than normal number of red blood cells. Hyperthyroidism is a condition in which the body has too much thyroid hormone.

What Are the Signs and Symptoms of a Heart Murmur?

People who have innocent (harmless) heart murmurs don't have any signs or symptoms other than the murmur itself. This is because innocent heart murmurs aren't caused by heart problems.

People who have abnormal heart murmurs may have signs or symptoms of the heart problems causing the murmurs. These signs and symptoms may include:

- Poor eating and failure to grow normally (in infants)
- Shortness of breath, which may occur only with physical exertion
- Excessive sweating with minimal or no exertion
- Chest pain
- Dizziness or fainting
- A bluish color on the skin, especially on the fingertips and lips
- Chronic cough
- Swelling or sudden weight gain
- Enlarged liver
- Enlarged neck veins

Signs and symptoms depend on the problem causing the heart murmur and its severity.

How Is a Heart Murmur Diagnosed?

Doctors use a stethoscope to listen to heart sounds and hear heart murmurs. They may detect heart murmurs during routine checkups or while checking for another condition.

If a congenital heart defect causes a murmur, it's often heard at birth or during infancy. Abnormal heart murmurs caused by other heart problems can be heard in patients of any age.

Specialists Involved

Primary care doctors usually refer people who have abnormal heart murmurs to cardiologists or pediatric cardiologists for further care and testing.

Cardiologists are doctors who specialize in diagnosing and treating heart problems in adults. Pediatric cardiologists specialize in diagnosing and treating heart problems in children.

Physical Exam

Your doctor will carefully listen to your heart or your child's heart with a stethoscope to find out whether a murmur is innocent or abnormal. He or she will listen to the loudness, location, and timing of the murmur. This will help your doctor diagnose the cause of the murmur.

Your doctor also may:

- Ask about your medical and family histories.

- Do a complete physical exam. He or she will look for signs of illness or physical problems. For example, your doctor may look for a bluish color on your skin. In infants, doctors may look for delayed growth and feeding problems.

- Ask about your symptoms, such as chest pain, shortness of breath (especially with physical exertion), dizziness, or fainting.

Evaluating Heart Murmurs

When evaluating a heart murmur, your doctor will pay attention to many things, such as:

- How faint or loud the sound is. Your doctor will grade the murmur on a scale of 1 to 6 (1 is very faint and 6 is very loud).

- When the sound occurs in the cycle of the heartbeat.

- Where the sound is heard in the chest and whether it also can be heard in the neck or back.

- Whether the sound has a high, medium, or low pitch.

- How long the sound lasts.

- How breathing, physical activity, or a change in body position affects the sound.

Diagnostic Tests and Procedures

If your doctor thinks you or your child has an abnormal heart murmur, he or she may recommend one or more of the following tests.

Chest X-Ray

A chest X-ray is a painless test that creates pictures of the structures inside your chest, such as your heart, lungs, and blood vessels. This test is done to find the cause of symptoms, such as shortness of breath and chest pain.

EKG

An EKG (electrocardiogram) is a simple test that detects and records the heart's electrical activity. An EKG shows how fast the heart is beating and its rhythm (steady or irregular). An EKG also records the strength and timing of electrical signals as they pass through each part of the heart.

This test is used to detect and locate the source of heart problems. The results from an EKG also may be used to rule out certain heart problems.

Echocardiography

Echocardiography, or echo, is a painless test that uses sound waves to create pictures of your heart. The test shows the size and shape of your heart and how well your heart's chambers and valves are working.

Echo also can show areas of poor blood flow to the heart, areas of heart muscle that aren't contracting normally, and previous injury to the heart muscle caused by poor blood flow.

There are several types of echo, including a stress echo. This test is done both before and after a stress test. During this test, you exercise to make your heart work hard and beat fast. If you can't exercise, you may be given medicine to make your heart work hard and beat fast. Echo is used to take pictures of your heart before you exercise and as soon as you finish.

Stress echo shows whether you have decreased blood flow to your heart (a sign of coronary heart disease).

How Is a Heart Murmur Treated?

A heart murmur isn't a disease. It's an extra or unusual sound heard during the heartbeat. Thus, murmurs themselves don't require treatment. However, if an underlying condition is causing a heart murmur, your doctor may recommend treatment for that condition.

Innocent (Harmless) Heart Murmurs

Healthy children who have innocent (harmless) heart murmurs don't need treatment. Their heart murmurs aren't caused by heart problems or other conditions.

Pregnant women who have innocent heart murmurs due to extra blood volume also don't need treatment. Their heart murmurs should go away after pregnancy.

Abnormal Heart Murmurs

If you or your child has an abnormal heart murmur, your doctor will recommend treatment for the disease or condition causing the murmur.

Some medical conditions, such as anemia or hyperthyroidism, can cause heart murmurs that aren't related to heart disease. Treating these conditions should make the heart murmur go away.

If a congenital heart defect is causing a heart murmur, treatment will depend on the type and severity of the defect. Treatment may include medicines or surgery.

If acquired heart valve disease is causing a heart murmur, treatment usually will depend on the type, amount, and severity of the disease.

Currently, no medicines can cure heart valve disease. However, lifestyle changes and medicines can treat symptoms and help delay complications. Eventually, though, you may need surgery to repair or replace a faulty heart valve.

Chapter 21

Infectious Diseases
of the Heart

Chapter Contents

Section 21.1

Endocarditis

"Endocarditis," © 2016 Omnigraphics. Reviewed June 2016.

Endocarditis is an inflammation of the endocardium, the membrane that lines the inner chambers of the heart. It generally occurs when bacteria or, less commonly, fungi travel through the bloodstream and cause an infection in this lining or in a heart valve. If left untreated, endocarditis can be deadly.

What Are the Causes?

Endocarditis is not common in healthy hearts. It occurs most often in a diseased heart or one with damaged valves, in which the roughened tissue can provide an ideal spot for bacteria or other microorganisms to settle, multiply, and cause an infection. Endocarditis can, on occasion, also be caused by fungi, such as Candida.

Microorganisms can enter bloodstream through:

- regular activities, such as eating or drinking

- poor oral hygiene or gum disease

- certain dental procedures

- using infected needles for body piercings, tattoos, or to inject drugs

- the use of a catheter

- cuts on skin or infections, such as a skin sore

- other medical conditions, including sexually transmitted diseases and intestinal disorders

What Are the Signs and Symptoms?

Symptoms of endocarditis differ from person to person and usually develop slowly over a period of time. In the initial stages, they can be similar to the symptoms of many other illnesses, such as pneumonia or flu. Some more severe symptoms can occur suddenly and may result from damage or inflammation in the heart.

Some of the symptoms of endocarditis include:

- pale skin
- night sweats
- fever and chills
- joint and muscle pain
- decreased appetite
- a full feeling in the upper left part of the stomach
- nausea
- weight loss
- swollen feet, legs, or stomach
- shortness of breath
- cough
- new or changed heart murmur
- enlarged spleen, which may be tender to touch
- blood in urine

   Endocarditis may also cause changes to the skin, such as:

- red or purple spots under or on fingers or toes
- broken blood vessels that appear as red spots, called petechiae, usually found on the whites of the eyes, inside the mouth, or on the chest

These symptoms depend on what causes the infection and whether there are any other underlying heart problems. A person with previous heart surgery, or a history of endocarditis or other heart issues should contact a doctor immediately if any of these symptoms occur, especially if they last for more than three days or if the person feels unusually tired.

What Are the Risk Factors?

   The following are some of the risk factors for developing endocarditis:

- Past history of endocarditis

- Certain types of heart defects, such as congenital defects

- Scarring of a heart valve caused by certain medical conditions, such as rheumatic fever

- Artificial heart valve or pacemaker

- HIV

- Use of needles to inject drugs, or for tattoos or body piercings

What Are the Complications?

Endocarditis can lead to numerous complications, including:

- Scarred or otherwise damaged heart valves

- Abnormal heart rhythm, such as atrial fibrillation

- Blood clots that may travel to the lungs or other parts of the body

- Jaundice, a yellowing of the skin and whites of the eyes

- Stroke or organ damage, often caused by clumps of bacteria and cell fragments that travel to the brain and other organs

- Abscesses (collection of pus) in other parts of body, including the brain, liver, spleen or kidneys

- Heart failure, especially when endocarditis is left untreated causing the heart to work harder to pump blood

How Is It Diagnosed?

A review of medical history and physical signs and symptoms, such as fever, will help the doctor diagnose endocarditis. A change in heart murmur, identified using a stethoscope, is another possible sign of the condition.

Some of the following tests may also be requested to make the diagnosis:

- A **blood test** will confirm the presence of bacteria, fungi, or other organisms that could cause endocarditis. It can also reveal if other conditions, such as anemia, are causing the infection.

- An **echocardiogram**, which creates an image of the heart using ultrasound waves, can be used by the doctor to spot signs of damage or abnormal movements in the heart.

- A **transesophageal echocardiogram** provides another image of the heart by means of an ultrasound device passed through the throat into the esophagus.

- If the doctor thinks that an irregular heartbeat is caused by endocarditis, an **electrocardiogram** may be ordered to analyze electrical activity of the heart.

- A **chest X-ray** will help reveal the condition of the heart and lungs, allowing the doctor to determine whether the infection has caused enlargement of the heart or if it has spread to the lungs. X-ray images also help differentiate between endocarditis and a collapsed lung.

- The doctor may order a **Magnetic Resonance Imaging (MRI)** or **Computerized Tomography (CT)** scan of other parts of the body, such as the brain or chest, to see if infection has spread to those areas.

How Is It Treated?

Endocarditis is usually treated with antibiotics, and in some cases, in which infection has damaged the heart valves or caused complications, surgery may be required.

Antibiotics

Antibiotics are prescribed if endocarditis is caused by a bacterial infection. This treatment would continue until the infection subsides, which may take up to six weeks. In some cases, hospitalization may be required so that high doses of intravenous (IV) antibiotics can be administered until the worst of the symptoms have passed.

Surgery

Surgery to treat endocarditis may be required if the heart valves are damaged because of the infection or if infection persists. The valve may either be repaired or replaced with an artificial valve that is made of animal tissue or synthetic materials. Surgery is sometimes also required if a fungal infection caused the endocarditis, since this is more difficult to treat than a bacterial infection.

How Can It Be Prevented?

- It is important to practice good oral hygiene to eliminate some of the germs in the mouth. Brush and floss teeth and gums often and have regular dental check-ups.

- Watch out for symptoms of endocarditis, such as unexplained fatigue and fever, especially if there is a history of endocarditis, heart disease, or heart surgery.

- Avoid procedures that may allow transfer of germs to the bloodstream, such as tattooing, body piercing, or IV drug use.

- Seek immediate medical attention if any skin infection develops or if open sores or cuts don't heal properly.

- If antibiotics have been prescribed by a doctor after certain dental or medical procedures, the medication should be taken exactly as directed. Preventive antibiotics may be required for:
  - previous endocarditis infection
  - certain heart surgery procedures
  - artificial heart valve surgery
  - certain types of congenital heart defects
  - procedures that involve the respiratory tract, infected skin, or tissue connecting muscle to bone

References

1. Sullivan, Debra Henline. "Endocarditis," Healthline, January 28, 2016.

2. "Endocarditis," Mayo Clinic, June 14, 2014.

Section 21.2

Myocarditis

Myocarditis is a disease characterized by inflammation of the heart muscle, called the myocardium. It is estimated to affect thousands of Americans each year and is caused by a wide variety of factors, including viral and bacterial infections, environmental toxins, autoimmune diseases, and allergic reactions to certain toxins and medications. Myocarditis often produces no symptoms, and because it is relatively uncommon, the best ways to diagnose and treat the condition are still being studied. It usually affects people who are otherwise healthy, including a significant number of young adults. The best way to prevent myocarditis is by seeking immediate medical attention for infections.

What Are the Causes?

Myocarditis is primarily caused by viral infections, the most common among them being those that affect the upper respiratory tract. Other less common causes include contagious infections, such as Lyme disease.

Some of the viral infections that can cause myocarditis include hepatitis C, herpes, HIV, and parvovirus. Bacterial infections that can lead to myocarditis include chlamydia (a common sexually transmitted disease), streptococcus (strep), staphylococcus (staph), mycoplasma (bacteria that cause a lung infection), and treponema (the cause of syphilis). The condition can also be brought on by such factors as allergic reactions to certain medicines and toxins like drugs, alcohol, spider or snake bites, wasp stings, lead, radiation, and chemotherapy.

Myocarditis can also be caused by autoimmune diseases (in which the immune system attacks the body), such as lupus or rheumatoid arthritis.

What Are the Signs and Symptoms?

Some of the symptoms of myocarditis include:

- Shortness of breath during exercise, which may lead to breathing troubles at night, as well

- Irregular heartbeat and, in some cases, fainting

- Heart palpitations

- Light-headedness

- Sharp or stabbing chest pain or pressure

- Fatigue

- Swelling in joints, legs, or neck veins

- Indications of infection, such as fever, sore throat, muscle aches, headache, or diarrhea

These symptoms often follow a respiratory infection, and if they occur it is important to seek medical attention promptly.

What Are the Complications?

Not treating myocarditis can cause the heart to work harder to pump blood. This can lead to symptoms of heart failure and in serious cases may be fatal. Cardiomyopathy and pericarditis are other possible complications of this infection, both of which are leading causes of heart transplants in the United States. Cardiomyopathy is an increase in size, thickness, or rigidity of the heart muscle. Pericarditis is the inflammation of pericardium, or the sac covering the heart.

How Is It Diagnosed?

In many cases, myocarditis has no symptoms and is not diagnosed. However, when there are symptoms, the doctor will conduct a physical exam to check for abnormal heartbeat, fluid in lungs, or swelling in legs. Some of the following tests may also be conducted:

- **Blood test** to analyze blood cell count and check for infection or antibodies

- An **electrocardiogram** to evaluate the electrical activity of the heart

- A **chest X-ray** to study the shape and size of the heart

- An **echocardiogram** to inspect the structure of the heart and measure blood flow

- Occasionally, a **cardiac magnetic resonance imaging (MRI)** scan or a **heart biopsy** may be performed to confirm the diagnosis

How Is It Treated?

When a person has myocarditis, treatment will be provided for its underlying cause. This will typically include medication to take the load off the heart, improve heart function, and prevent or control further complications.

In the presence of an abnormal heart rhythm, additional treatment such as a pacemaker or defibrillator could be required. Hospitalization may be necessary in case of serious complications, such as a blood clots or a weakened heart. ACE (Angiotensin Converting Enzyme) inhibitors, calcium channel blockers, and diuretics are some medicines that may be prescribed to help the heart function better. Steroids and other medications may also be used to treat heart inflammation. Often, reduced physical activity for at least six months, rest, and a low-salt diet are recommended.

The cause of myocarditis, overall health of the person, and complications, if any, determine the outlook. The infected person could either recover completely or develop a chronic condition. There is a small possibility that myocarditis may recur and could, in rare cases, lead to dilated cardiomyopathy, an enlargement and weakening of the ventricles, the heart's pumping chambers.

References

1. "Discover Myocarditis Causes, Symptoms, Diagnosis and Treatment," Myocarditis Foundation, n.d.

2. Beckerman, James, "Myocarditis," WebMD, July 14, 2014.

Section 21.3

Pericarditis

Pericarditis is the swelling and irritation that occurs on the thin sac-like membrane called the pericardium, that surrounds the heart. It is characterized by symptoms such as sharp chest pains that occur when inflamed layers of the pericardium brush against each other.

When pericarditis is acute, it usually develops suddenly and may last for a few months. It is considered chronic when the symptoms appear more gradually or persist for a longer period of time. In some cases, excess fluid builds up in the space between the pericardial layers, resulting in pericardial effusion, which can affect heart function.

Most cases of pericarditis are mild, and improvement occurs gradually. For more severe cases, medication and, rarely, surgery will be needed. Risks of long-term complications can be reduced by diagnosing and treating the condition in its early stages.

What Are the Causes?

It is often difficult to determine what causes pericarditis. When the cause is unknown, it is called idiopathic pericarditis. In most cases, it occurs due to one of the following causes:

- infections that are viral, bacterial, fungal, or parasitic in nature

- traumatic events causing injury to the chest

- health complications, such as kidney failure, tumors, AIDS, tuberculosis, or genetic diseases like Familial Mediterranean Fever (FMF)

- autoimmune diseases, such as lupus, rheumatoid arthritis, and scleroderma

- Dressler syndrome, in which pericarditis can occur a few weeks after a major heart attack or heart surgery

- procedures like radiation therapy or those performed through the skin, such as radiofrequency ablation (RFA) or cardiac catheterization

- in rare cases, certain medications that suppress the immune system

What Are the Signs and Symptoms?

Symptoms of acute pericarditis include:

- a sharp, stabbing chest pain that increases when coughing, swallowing or breathing deeply

- pain in the shoulder and neck that spreads from the chest

- trouble breathing when lying down

- dry cough

- fatigue

- heart palpitations

- swelling in the feet, legs, ankles, or abdomen (a symptom of constrictive pericarditis)

Chronic pericarditis is characterized by continued inflammation that sometimes results in fluid buildup around the heart (pericardial effusion), and chest pain is the most common symptom.

Also called recurring pericarditis, the chronic form often results from autoimmune disorders. The attacks can extend over a long period of time and are of two types. The incessant type occurs within six weeks of discontinuing treatment for acute infection, while the intermittent type occurs after six weeks.

Since most symptoms mimic those of other lung and heart conditions, it is important to consult a doctor as soon as symptoms of pericarditis develop. This enables proper diagnosis and treatment and could possibly help identify other health problems, as well. If not treated, pericarditis can lead to fatal conditions, such as cardiac tamponade, which compresses the heart so much that it affects its functioning.

What Are the Complications?

Constrictive Pericarditis is a severe condition in people with long-term inflammation and chronic recurrent episodes. It is characterized by stiff, thickened pericardial layers, which make the pericardium less elastic and restrict the heart from expanding as it normally would when filling up with blood. Eventually the condition results in symptoms of heart failure, such as swelling of the heart, feet, or legs, labored breathing, water retention, and abnormal heartbeat. These symptoms should improve when constrictive pericarditis is treated.

Pericardial Effusion is a condition that occurs when excess fluid builds up in the space between the two pericardial layers. When fluid accumulates rapidly, it leads to *cardiac tamponade*—a severe compression of heart that affects its normal functioning and causes a sudden drop in blood pressure. This is a life-threatening condition that requires immediate removal of the fluid using a catheter.

How Is It Diagnosed?

Diagnosis of pericarditis begins with an evaluation of the patient's medical history and symptoms, such as chest pain and difficulty breathing. Other risks of pericarditis, including recent viral illnesses, diseases like lupus or kidney failure, and previous heart disease or surgery are also analyzed. This is followed by a physical exam in which the doctor places a stethoscope on the chest to listen for such signs as pericardial rub (noise made when affected pericardial layers rub against each other), excess fluid in the pericardial sac, or indications of fluid in the space around lungs.

Some of the diagnostic procedures that may be required are:

- **Blood tests** to determine whether viral, bacterial, or other types of infections are present.

- **Chest X-rays** to check for enlargement of the heart or congestion in the lungs.

- An **electrocardiogram** to measure electrical impulses and identify changes in the normal rhythm of the heart.

- An **echocardiogram** to analyze signs of constrictive pericarditis or pericardial effusion.

- **Cardiac Magnetic Resonance Imaging (MRI)** and **Computerized Tomography (CT)** scans to reveal abnormal changes in the pericardium and to exclude other causes of acute chest pain.

- **Cardiac catheterization** to study the pressure and flow of blood and confirm diagnosis of constrictive pericarditis.

- **Other laboratory tests** to assess heart function, which may include testing for autoimmune diseases and examining the fluid in the pericardium to evaluate sedimentation rate (ESR) and C-reactive protein levels.

How Is It Treated?

Treatment for pericarditis depends on what causes it and its severity. Mild cases of pericarditis may not require any treatment.

Medication for acute pericarditis typically includes over-the-counter pain relievers and nonsteroidal anti-inflammatory drugs to reduce pain and inflammation and to prevent the infection from recurring weeks or months later. The small number of patients who develop chronic pericarditis may need to take these medications for a number of years.

Frequent follow-up care to assess changes in liver and kidney function may be required for people taking high doses of nonsteroidal anti-inflammatory drugs. Antibiotics or antifungal medication may be prescribed depending on what causes the infection. Previously, steroids were prescribed to prevent infection from recurring, but in some cases these caused dependency on the medication to prevent recurrence.

For most people, pericarditis does not usually require surgery. In the case of cardiac tamponade, a procedure called pericardiocentesis will be required to drain excess fluid by means of a needle and catheter. A surgical procedure called pericardial window is performed if the fluid cannot be drained using the needle. In severe cases, such as constrictive pericarditis, the doctor might suggest a surgical procedure called pericardiectomy to surgically remove a portion of the pericardium that has thickened and affects the normal functioning of the heart.

References

1.   "Pericarditis," Cleveland Clinic, n.d.

2.   "Pericarditis," Mayo Clinic, April 6, 2014.

Chapter 22

Cardiac Tumors

What Are Cardiac Tumors?

Cardiac tumors are abnormal growths that occur within the heart, heart valves, or lining of the heart. Primary heart tumors originate in the heart, while secondary or metastatic heart tumors develop elsewhere in the body and spread to the heart. Primary tumors are usually noncancerous (benign), while metastatic tumors are always cancerous (malignant). Although cardiac tumors are rare, the condition can be serious or even fatal.

Types of Cardiac Tumors

Primary cardiac tumors are quite rare, occurring an estimated once in every 2,000 people. Yet there are many different types—including some that are noncancerous and some that are cancerous—that grow in different parts of the heart. Some of the recognized types of primary cardiac tumors include the following:

- **Myxoma** is the most common type, accounting for about half of all noncancerous primary heart tumors in adults, although it can affect people of any age. It occurs most frequently at the atrial septum, which divides the two upper chambers of the heart. Inherited genetic conditions such as Carney complex cause around 10 percent of myxomas.

- **Rhabdomyoma** is the most common type of noncancerous primary cardiac tumor in infants and children. These tumors usually develop within the heart wall from the heart's muscle cells, and they most often occur in groups.

- **Fibromas** also primarily appear in infants and children. These noncancerous primary tumors typically affect the heart valves and develop from the heart's fibrous tissue cells.

- **Lipomas** are noncancerous tumors that can grow in the lining of the heart chambers, on the heart wall, or on the outer surface of the heart.

- **Papillary fibroelastoma** is a benign primary tumor that grows on the heart valves.

- **Paraganglionoma** and teratoma are benign tumors that occur where the major blood vessels attach at the base of the heart.

- Pericardial cysts are noncancerous primary growths that affect the pericardium membrane that covers the heart.

- **Sarcomas** are the most common type of cancerous primary heart tumor, ranking second only to myxoma in overall prevalence. They tend to develop in the right or left atrium, where they can block blood flow through the heart or spread to the lungs.

- **Mesothelioma** is a type of cancerous primary heart tumor that can develop in the pericardium and spread to the spine or brain.

- **Lymphoma**, or cancer of the white blood cells, occasionally develops in the hearts of people who have acquired immune deficiency syndrome (AIDS).

Secondary cardiac tumors are cancerous growths that develop in the lungs, breasts, kidneys, liver, blood, or skin and then spread to the heart. Although they are rare, they are between 30 and 40 times more common than primary heart tumors.

Symptoms of Cardiac Tumors

The symptoms of cardiac tumors vary widely depending on the tumor's location, size, and the extent to which it impedes blood flow through the heart. Some people experience no symptoms at all, and their tumors are only discovered when they undergo an echocardiogram or chest X-ray for another reason. Some patients have minor symptoms such as:

- lightheadedness

- shortness of breath

- fatigue

- joint pain or inflammation

- unexplained fever

- small red spots on the skin

Some people with cardiac tumors may experience these symptoms only when they are in a certain physical position—such as standing up or lying down—that causes the tumor to block blood flow.

Around half of people with tumors on a heart valve will develop a heart murmur due to restricted blood flow through the valve. Finally, some patients with cardiac tumors present with symptoms of severe heart malfunction, such as abnormal heart rhythms, extremely low blood pressure (hypotension), or heart failure.

Diagnosis of Cardiac Tumors

Diagnosing primary heart tumors can be difficult because they are relatively rare. In addition, the symptoms vary widely and often resemble those of other health conditions. Doctors are more likely to suspect secondary heart tumors in cancer patients who begin experiencing heart problems.

The diagnosis of a cardiac tumor is typically confirmed through an echocardiogram, which involves using ultrasound to produce an image of the heart. Doctors may seek additional information about the tumor by using a computed tomography (CT) scan, magnetic resonance imaging (MRI), or radionuclide imaging. Since imaging results usually enable doctors to determine whether cardiac tumors are benign or malignant, heart biopsies are seldom performed.

Risks of Cardiac Tumors

Depending on their size and location, cardiac tumors can interfere with the function of the heart and cause serious health risks. Both noncancerous and cancerous tumors can block blood flow and create life-threatening heart problems such as heart failure or atrial fibrillation. Another risk related to cardiac tumors is embolism. Small pieces of tumor can break loose, be carried through the bloodstream to distant parts of the body, and block arteries that supply blood to vital organs.

Similarly, blood clots that form on the surface of cardiac tumors may break off to form emboli and lodge in arteries.

Treatment of Cardiac Tumors

Treatment of primary cardiac tumors depends on their size and type, as well as the patient's symptoms and overall health. Small, noncancerous tumors that do not impede blood flow may not require treatment. Infants born with rhabdomyomas, for instance, usually do not need treatment. About half of these tumors regress on their own, while those that remain in place seldom grow any larger.

The preferred treatment for noncancerous primary heart tumors is surgical removal. Although removal often requires complicated open-heart surgery, it can sometimes be performed robotically or through minimally invasive techniques. The patient typically must spend several days in the hospital followed by several weeks in recovery. Follow-up treatment includes an annual echocardiogram to ensure that the tumor does not return and that no new growths appear.

In cases where a noncancerous primary heart tumor is large, blocks blood flow, or grows into the surrounding tissue, heart transplantation may be the only surgical option available. However, this procedure is performed only in rare circumstances.

Surgery is not an option for primary cancerous heart tumors because they have usually already spread to other parts of the body. Such tumors are usually fatal, although chemotherapy or radiation therapy may help slow the progression of disease. These treatment options may also be used for metastatic cardiac tumors, depending on the type of cancer and the other organs affected.

References

1. "Cardiac Tumors," Cleveland Clinic, 2016.

2. Howlett, Jonathan G. "Overview of Heart Tumors," Merck and Co., Inc., n.d.

Part Three

Blood Vessel Disorders

Chapter 23

Atherosclerosis

What Is Atherosclerosis?

Atherosclerosis is a disease in which plaque builds up inside your arteries. Arteries are blood vessels that carry oxygen-rich blood to your heart and other parts of your body.

Plaque is made up of fat, cholesterol, calcium, and other substances found in the blood. Over time, plaque hardens and narrows your arteries. This limits the flow of oxygen-rich blood to your organs and other parts of your body.

Atherosclerosis can lead to serious problems, including heart attack, stroke, or even death.

Atherosclerosis-Related Diseases

Atherosclerosis can affect any artery in the body, including arteries in the heart, brain, arms, legs, pelvis, and kidneys. As a result, different diseases may develop based on which arteries are affected.

Coronary Heart Disease

Coronary heart disease (CHD), also called coronary artery disease, occurs when plaque builds up in the coronary arteries. These arteries supply oxygen-rich blood to your heart.

Plaque narrows the coronary arteries and reduces blood flow to your heart muscle. Plaque buildup also makes it more likely that blood

---

This chapter includes text excerpted from "Atherosclerosis," National Heart, Lung, and Blood Institute (NHLBI), September 22, 2015.

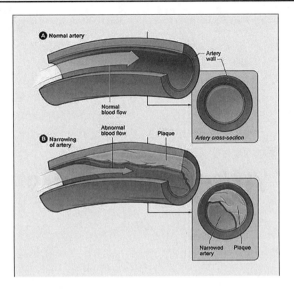

Figure 23.1. *Atherosclerosis*

(A) shows a normal artery with normal blood flow. The inset image shows a cross-section of a normal artery. (B) shows an artery with plaque buildup. The inset image shows a cross-section of an artery with plaque buildup.

clots will form in your arteries. Blood clots can partially or completely block blood flow.

If blood flow to your heart muscle is reduced or blocked, you may have angina (chest pain or discomfort) or a heart attack.

Plaque also can form in the heart's smallest arteries. This disease is called coronary microvascular disease (MVD). In coronary MVD, plaque doesn't cause blockages in the arteries as it does in CHD.

Carotid Artery Disease

Carotid artery disease occurs if plaque builds up in the arteries on each side of your neck (the carotid arteries). These arteries supply oxygen-rich blood to your brain. If blood flow to your brain is reduced or blocked, you may have a stroke.

Peripheral Artery Disease

Peripheral artery disease (P.A.D.) occurs if plaque builds up in the major arteries that supply oxygen-rich blood to your legs, arms, and pelvis.

If blood flow to these parts of your body is reduced or blocked, you may have numbness, pain, and, sometimes, dangerous infections.

Chronic Kidney Disease

Chronic kidney disease can occur if plaque builds up in the renal arteries. These arteries supply oxygen-rich blood to your kidneys.

Over time, chronic kidney disease causes a slow loss of kidney function. The main function of the kidneys is to remove waste and extra water from the body.

Other Names for Atherosclerosis

- Arteriosclerosis

- Hardening of the arteries

What Causes Atherosclerosis?

The exact cause of atherosclerosis isn't known. However, studies show that atherosclerosis is a slow, complex disease that may start in childhood. It develops faster as you age.

Atherosclerosis may start when certain factors damage the inner layers of the arteries. These factors include:

- Smoking

- High amounts of certain fats and cholesterol in the blood

- High blood pressure

- High amounts of sugar in the blood due to insulin resistance or diabetes

Plaque may begin to build up where the arteries are damaged. Over time, plaque hardens and narrows the arteries. Eventually, an area of plaque can rupture (break open).

When this happens, blood cell fragments called platelets stick to the site of the injury. They may clump together to form blood clots. Clots narrow the arteries even more, limiting the flow of oxygen-rich blood to your body.

Depending on which arteries are affected, blood clots can worsen angina (chest pain) or cause a heart attack or stroke.

Researchers continue to look for the causes of atherosclerosis. They hope to find answers to questions such as:

- Why and how do the arteries become damaged?

- How does plaque develop and change over time?
- Why does plaque rupture and lead to blood clots?

Who Is at Risk for Atherosclerosis?

The exact cause of atherosclerosis isn't known. However, certain traits, conditions, or habits may raise your risk for the disease. These conditions are known as risk factors. The more risk factors you have, the more likely it is that you'll develop atherosclerosis.

You can control most risk factors and help prevent or delay atherosclerosis. Other risk factors can't be controlled.

Major Risk Factors

- **Unhealthy blood cholesterol levels.** This includes high LDL cholesterol (sometimes called "bad" cholesterol) and low HDL cholesterol (sometimes called "good" cholesterol).

- **High blood pressure.** Blood pressure is considered high if it stays at or above 140/90 mmHg over time. If you have diabetes or chronic kidney disease, high blood pressure is defined as 130/80 mmHg or higher. (The mmHg is millimeters of mercury— the units used to measure blood pressure.)

- **Smoking.** Smoking can damage and tighten blood vessels, raise cholesterol levels, and raise blood pressure. Smoking also doesn't allow enough oxygen to reach the body's tissues.

- **Insulin resistance.** This condition occurs if the body can't use its insulin properly. Insulin is a hormone that helps move blood sugar into cells where it's used as an energy source. Insulin resistance may lead to diabetes.

- **Diabetes.** With this disease, the body's blood sugar level is too high because the body doesn't make enough insulin or doesn't use its insulin properly.

- **Overweight or obesity.** The terms "overweight" and "obesity" refer to body weight that's greater than what is considered healthy for a certain height.

- **Lack of physical activity.** A lack of physical activity can worsen other risk factors for atherosclerosis, such as unhealthy blood cholesterol levels, high blood pressure, diabetes, and overweight and obesity.

- **Unhealthy diet.** An unhealthy diet can raise your risk for atherosclerosis. Foods that are high in saturated and *trans* fats, cholesterol, sodium (salt), and sugar can worsen other atherosclerosis risk factors.

- **Older age.** As you get older, your risk for atherosclerosis increases. Genetic or lifestyle factors cause plaque to build up in your arteries as you age. By the time you're middle-aged or older, enough plaque has built up to cause signs or symptoms. In men, the risk increases after age 45. In women, the risk increases after age 55.

- **Family history of early heart disease.** Your risk for atherosclerosis increases if your father or a brother was diagnosed with heart disease before 55 years of age, or if your mother or a sister was diagnosed with heart disease before 65 years of age.

Although age and a family history of early heart disease are risk factors, it doesn't mean that you'll develop atherosclerosis if you have one or both. Controlling other risk factors often can lessen genetic influences and prevent atherosclerosis, even in older adults.

Studies show that an increasing number of children and youth are at risk for atherosclerosis. This is due to a number of causes, including rising childhood obesity rates.

Emerging Risk Factors

Scientists continue to study other possible risk factors for atherosclerosis.

High levels of a protein called C-reactive protein (CRP) in the blood may raise the risk for atherosclerosis and heart attack. High levels of CRP are a sign of inflammation in the body.

Inflammation is the body's response to injury or infection. Damage to the arteries' inner walls seems to trigger inflammation and help plaque grow.

People who have low CRP levels may develop atherosclerosis at a slower rate than people who have high CRP levels. Research is under way to find out whether reducing inflammation and lowering CRP levels also can reduce the risk for atherosclerosis.

High levels of triglycerides in the blood also may raise the risk for atherosclerosis, especially in women. Triglycerides are a type of fat.

Studies are under way to find out whether genetics may play a role in atherosclerosis risk.

Other Factors That Affect Atherosclerosis

Other factors also may raise your risk for atherosclerosis, such as:

- **Sleep apnea.** Sleep apnea is a disorder that causes one or more pauses in breathing or shallow breaths while you sleep. Untreated sleep apnea can raise your risk for high blood pressure, diabetes, and even a heart attack or stroke.

- **Stress.** Research shows that the most commonly reported "trigger" for a heart attack is an emotionally upsetting event, especially one involving anger.

- **Alcohol.** Heavy drinking can damage the heart muscle and worsen other risk factors for atherosclerosis. Men should have no more than two drinks containing alcohol a day. Women should have no more than one drink containing alcohol a day.

What Are the Signs and Symptoms of Atherosclerosis?

Atherosclerosis usually doesn't cause signs and symptoms until it severely narrows or totally blocks an artery. Many people don't know they have the disease until they have a medical emergency, such as a heart attack or stroke.

Some people may have signs and symptoms of the disease. Signs and symptoms will depend on which arteries are affected.

Coronary Arteries

The coronary arteries supply oxygen-rich blood to your heart. If plaque narrows or blocks these arteries (a disease called coronary heart disease, or CHD), a common symptom is angina. Angina is chest pain or discomfort that occurs when your heart muscle doesn't get enough oxygen-rich blood.

Angina may feel like pressure or squeezing in your chest. You also may feel it in your shoulders, arms, neck, jaw, or back. Angina pain may even feel like indigestion. The pain tends to get worse with activity and go away with rest. Emotional stress also can trigger the pain.

Other symptoms of CHD are shortness of breath and arrhythmias. Arrhythmias are problems with the rate or rhythm of the heartbeat.

Plaque also can form in the heart's smallest arteries. This disease is called coronary microvascular disease (MVD). Symptoms of coronary MVD include angina, shortness of breath, sleep problems, fatigue (tiredness), and lack of energy.

Carotid Arteries

The carotid arteries supply oxygen-rich blood to your brain. If plaque narrows or blocks these arteries (a disease called carotid artery disease), you may have symptoms of a stroke. These symptoms may include:

- Sudden weakness

- Paralysis (an inability to move) or numbness of the face, arms, or legs, especially on one side of the body

- Confusion

- Trouble speaking or understanding speech

- Trouble seeing in one or both eyes

- Problems breathing

- Dizziness, trouble walking, loss of balance or coordination, and unexplained falls

- Loss of consciousness

- Sudden and severe headache

Peripheral Arteries

Plaque also can build up in the major arteries that supply oxygen-rich blood to the legs, arms, and pelvis (a disease called peripheral artery disease).

If these major arteries are narrowed or blocked, you may have numbness, pain, and, sometimes, dangerous infections.

Renal Arteries

The renal arteries supply oxygen-rich blood to your kidneys. If plaque builds up in these arteries, you may develop chronic kidney disease. Over time, chronic kidney disease causes a slow loss of kidney function.

Early kidney disease often has no signs or symptoms. As the disease gets worse it can cause tiredness, changes in how you urinate (more often or less often), loss of appetite, nausea (feeling sick to the stomach), swelling in the hands or feet, itchiness or numbness, and trouble concentrating.

How Is Atherosclerosis Diagnosed?

Your doctor will diagnose atherosclerosis based on your medical and family histories, a physical exam, and test results.

Physical Exam

During the physical exam, your doctor may listen to your arteries for an abnormal whooshing sound called a bruit. Your doctor can hear a bruit when placing a stethoscope over an affected artery. A bruit may indicate poor blood flow due to plaque buildup.

Your doctor also may check to see whether any of your pulses (for example, in the leg or foot) are weak or absent. A weak or absent pulse can be a sign of a blocked artery.

Diagnostic Tests

Your doctor may recommend one or more tests to diagnose atherosclerosis. These tests also can help your doctor learn the extent of your disease and plan the best treatment.

Blood Tests

Blood tests check the levels of certain fats, cholesterol, sugar, and proteins in your blood. Abnormal levels may be a sign that you're at risk for atherosclerosis.

EKG (Electrocardiogram)

An EKG is a simple, painless test that detects and records the heart's electrical activity. The test shows how fast the heart is beating and its rhythm (steady or irregular). An EKG also records the strength and timing of electrical signals as they pass through the heart.

An EKG can show signs of heart damage caused by CHD. The test also can show signs of a previous or current heart attack.

Chest X-ray

A chest X-ray takes pictures of the organs and structures inside your chest, such as your heart, lungs, and blood vessels. A chest x ray can reveal signs of heart failure.

Ankle/Brachial Index

This test compares the blood pressure in your ankle with the blood pressure in your arm to see how well your blood is flowing. This test can help diagnose P.A.D.

Echocardiography

Echocardiography (echo) uses sound waves to create a moving picture of your heart. The test provides information about the size and shape of your heart and how well your heart chambers and valves are working.

Echo also can identify areas of poor blood flow to the heart, areas of heart muscle that aren't contracting normally, and previous injury to the heart muscle caused by poor blood flow.

Computed Tomography Scan

A computed tomography (CT) scan creates computer-generated pictures of the heart, brain, or other areas of the body. The test can show hardening and narrowing of large arteries.

A cardiac CT scan also can show whether calcium has built up in the walls of the coronary (heart) arteries. This may be an early sign of CHD.

Stress Testing

During stress testing, you exercise to make your heart work hard and beat fast while heart tests are done. If you can't exercise, you may be given medicine to make your heart work hard and beat fast.

When your heart is working hard, it needs more blood and oxygen. Plaque-narrowed arteries can't supply enough oxygen-rich blood to meet your heart's needs.

A stress test can show possible signs and symptoms of CHD, such as:

• Abnormal changes in your heart rate or blood pressure

• Shortness of breath or chest pain

• Abnormal changes in your heart rhythm or your heart's electrical activity

As part of some stress tests, pictures are taken of your heart while you exercise and while you rest. These imaging stress tests can show

how well blood is flowing in various parts of your heart. They also can show how well your heart pumps blood when it beats.

Angiography

Angiography is a test that uses dye and special X-rays to show the inside of your arteries. This test can show whether plaque is blocking your arteries and how severe the blockage is.

A thin, flexible tube called a catheter is put into a blood vessel in your arm, groin (upper thigh), or neck. Dye that can be seen on an X-ray picture is injected through the catheter into the arteries. By looking at the X-ray picture, your doctor can see the flow of blood through your arteries.

Other Tests

Other tests are being studied to see whether they can give a better view of plaque buildup in the arteries. Examples of these tests include magnetic resonance imaging (MRI) and positron emission tomography (PET).

How Is Atherosclerosis Treated?

Treatments for atherosclerosis may include heart-healthy lifestyle changes, medicines, and medical procedures or surgery. The goals of treatment include:

- Lowering the risk of blood clots forming
- Preventing atherosclerosis-related diseases
- Reducing risk factors in an effort to slow or stop the buildup of plaque
- Relieving symptoms
- Widening or bypassing plaque-clogged arteries

Chapter 24

Carotid Artery Disease

What Is Carotid Artery Disease?

Carotid artery disease is a disease in which a waxy substance called plaque builds up inside the carotid arteries. You have two common carotid arteries, one on each side of your neck. They each divide into internal and external carotid arteries.

The internal carotid arteries supply oxygen-rich blood to your brain. The external carotid arteries supply oxygen-rich blood to your face, scalp, and neck.

Carotid artery disease is serious because it can cause a stroke, also called a "brain attack." A stroke occurs if blood flow to your brain is cut off.

If blood flow is cut off for more than a few minutes, the cells in your brain start to die. This impairs the parts of the body that the brain cells control. A stroke can cause lasting brain damage; long-term disability, such as vision or speech problems or paralysis (an inability to move); or death.

What Causes Carotid Artery Disease?

Carotid artery disease seems to start when damage occurs to the inner layers of the carotid arteries. Major factors that contribute to damage include:

- Smoking

This chapter includes text excerpted from "Carotid Artery Disease," National Heart, Lung, and Blood Institute (NHLBI), October 29, 2015.

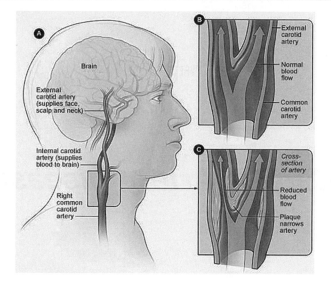

Figure 24.1. *Carotid Arteries*

(A) shows the location of the right carotid artery in the head and neck. (B) shows the inside of a normal carotid artery that has normal blood flow. (C) shows the inside of a carotid artery that has plaque buildup and reduced blood flow.

- High levels of certain fats and cholesterol in the blood
- High blood pressure
- High levels of sugar in the blood due to insulin resistance or diabetes

When damage occurs, your body starts a healing process. The healing may cause plaque to build up where the arteries are damaged.

The plaque in an artery can crack or rupture. If this happens, blood cell fragments called platelets will stick to the site of the injury and may clump together to form blood clots.

The buildup of plaque or blood clots can severely narrow or block the carotid arteries. This limits the flow of oxygen-rich blood to your brain, which can cause a stroke.

Who Is at Risk for Carotid Artery Disease?

The major risk factors for carotid artery disease, listed below, also are the major risk factors for coronary heart disease (also called coronary artery disease) and peripheral artery disease.

- **Diabetes.** With this disease, the body's blood sugar level is too high because the body doesn't make enough insulin or doesn't use its insulin properly. People who have diabetes are four times more likely to have carotid artery disease than are people who don't have diabetes.

- **Family history of atherosclerosis.** People who have a family history of atherosclerosis are more likely to develop carotid artery disease.

- **High blood pressure (Hypertension).** Blood pressure is considered high if it stays at or above 140/90 mmHg over time. If you have diabetes or chronic kidney disease, high blood pressure is defined as 130/80 mmHg or higher. (The mmHg is millimeters of mercury—the units used to measure blood pressure.)

- **Lack of physical activity.** Too much sitting (sedentary lifestyle) and a lack of aerobic activity can worsen other risk factors for carotid artery disease, such as unhealthy blood cholesterol levels, high blood pressure, diabetes, and overweight or obesity.

- **Metabolic syndrome.** Metabolic syndrome is the name for a group of risk factors that raise your risk for stroke and other health problems, such as diabetes and heart disease. The five metabolic risk factors are a large waistline (abdominal obesity), a high triglyceride level (a type of fat found in the blood), a low HDL cholesterol level, high blood pressure, and high blood sugar. Metabolic syndrome is diagnosed if you have at least three of these metabolic risk factors.

- **Older age.** As you age, your risk for atherosclerosis increases. The process of atherosclerosis begins in youth and typically progresses over many decades before diseases develop.

- **Overweight or obesity.** The terms "overweight" and "obesity" refer to body weight that's greater than what is considered healthy for a certain height.

- **Smoking.** Smoking can damage and tighten blood vessels, lead to unhealthy cholesterol levels, and raise blood pressure. Smoking also can limit how much oxygen reaches the body's tissues.

- **Unhealthy blood cholesterol levels.** This includes high LDL ("bad") cholesterol) and low HDL ("good") cholesterol.

- **Unhealthy diet.** An unhealthy diet can raise your risk for carotid artery disease. Foods that are high in saturated and trans fats, cholesterol, sodium, and sugar can worsen other risk factors for carotid artery disease.

Having any of these risk factors does not guarantee that you'll develop carotid artery disease. However, if you know that you have one or more risk factors, you can take steps to help prevent or delay the disease.

If you have plaque buildup in your carotid arteries, you also may have plaque buildup in other arteries. People who have carotid artery disease also are at increased risk for coronary heart disease.

What Are the Signs and Symptoms of Carotid Artery Disease?

Carotid artery disease may not cause signs or symptoms until it severely narrows or blocks a carotid artery. Signs and symptoms may include a bruit, a transient ischemic attack (TIA), or a stroke.

Bruit

During a physical exam, your doctor may listen to your carotid arteries with a stethoscope. He or she may hear a whooshing sound called a bruit. This sound may suggest changed or reduced blood flow due to plaque buildup. To find out more, your doctor may recommend tests.

Not all people who have carotid artery disease have bruits.

Stroke

The symptoms of a stroke are the same as those of a mini-stroke, but the results are not. A stroke can cause lasting brain damage; long-term disability, such as vision or speech problems or paralysis (an inability to move); or death. Most people who have strokes have not previously had warning mini-strokes.

Getting treatment for a stroke right away is very important. You have the best chance for full recovery if treatment to open a blocked artery is given within 4 hours of symptom onset. The sooner treatment occurs, the better your chances of recovery.

Call 9–1–1 for emergency help as soon as symptoms occur. Do not drive yourself to the hospital. It's very important to get checked and to get treatment started as soon as possible.

Make those close to you aware of stroke symptoms and the need for urgent action. Learning the signs and symptoms of a stroke will allow you to help yourself or someone close to you lower the risk of brain damage or death due to a stroke.

Medical History

Your doctor will find out whether you have any of the major risk factors for carotid artery disease. He or she also will ask whether you've had any signs or symptoms of a mini-stroke or stroke.

Transient Ischemic Attack (Mini-Stroke)

For some people, having a transient ischemic attack (TIA), or "mini-stroke," is the first sign of carotid artery disease. During a mini-stroke, you may have some or all of the symptoms of a stroke. However, the symptoms usually go away on their own within 24 hours.

Stroke and mini-stroke symptoms may include:

- A sudden, severe headache with no known cause
- Dizziness or loss of balance
- Inability to move one or more of your limbs
- Sudden trouble seeing in one or both eyes
- Sudden weakness or numbness in the face or limbs, often on just one side of the body
- Trouble speaking or understanding speech

Even if the symptoms stop quickly, **call 9–1–1 for emergency help**. Do not drive yourself to the hospital. It's important to get checked and to get treatment started as soon as possible.

A mini-stroke is a warning sign that you're at high risk of having a stroke. You shouldn't ignore these symptoms. Getting medical care can help find possible causes of a mini-stroke and help you manage risk factors. These actions might prevent a future stroke.

Although a mini-stroke may warn of a stroke, it doesn't predict when a stroke will happen. A stroke may occur days, weeks, or even months after a mini-stroke.

How Is Carotid Artery Disease Diagnosed?

Your doctor will diagnose carotid artery disease based on your medical history, a physical exam, and test results.

Physical Exam

To check your carotid arteries, your doctor will listen to them with a stethoscope. He or she will listen for a whooshing sound called a bruit. This sound may indicate changed or reduced blood flow due to plaque buildup. To find out more, your doctor may recommend tests.

Diagnostic Tests

The following tests are common for diagnosing carotid artery disease. If you have symptoms of a mini-stroke or stroke, your doctor may use other tests as well.

Carotid Ultrasound

Carotid ultrasound (also called sonography) is the most common test for diagnosing carotid artery disease. It's a painless, harmless test that uses sound waves to create pictures of the insides of your carotid arteries. This test can show whether plaque has narrowed your carotid arteries and how narrow they are.

A standard carotid ultrasound shows the structure of your carotid arteries. A Doppler carotid ultrasound shows how blood moves through your carotid arteries.

Carotid Angiography

Carotid angiography is a special type of X-ray. This test may be used if the ultrasound results are unclear or don't give your doctor enough information.

For this test, your doctor will inject a substance (called contrast dye) into a vein, most often in your leg. The dye travels to your carotid arteries and highlights them on X-ray pictures.

Magnetic Resonance Angiography

Magnetic resonance angiography (MRA) uses a large magnet and radio waves to take pictures of your carotid arteries. Your doctor can see these pictures on a computer screen.

For this test, your doctor may give you contrast dye to highlight your carotid arteries on the pictures.

Computed Tomography Angiography

Computed tomography angiography, or CT angiography, takes X-ray pictures of the body from many angles. A computer combines the pictures into two- and three-dimensional images.

For this test, your doctor may give you contrast dye to highlight your carotid arteries on the pictures.

How Is Carotid Artery Disease Treated?

Treatments for carotid artery disease may include healthy lifestyle changes, medicines, and medical procedures. The goals of treatment are to stop the disease from getting worse and to prevent a stroke. Your treatment will depend on your symptoms, how severe the disease is, and your age and overall health.

How Can Carotid Artery Disease Be Prevented?

Taking action to control your risk factors can help prevent or delay carotid artery disease and stroke. Your risk for carotid artery disease increases with the number of risk factors you have.

One step you can take is to adopt a heart-healthy lifestyle, which can include:

- Heart-healthy eating
- Maintaining a healthy weight
- Physical activity
- Quit smoking

Chapter 25

Stroke

What Is a Stroke?

A stroke occurs if the flow of oxygen-rich blood to a portion of the brain is blocked. Without oxygen, brain cells start to die after a few minutes. Sudden bleeding in the brain also can cause a stroke if it damages brain cells.

If brain cells die or are damaged because of a stroke, symptoms occur in the parts of the body that these brain cells control. Examples of stroke symptoms include sudden weakness; paralysis or numbness of the face, arms, or legs (paralysis is an inability to move); trouble speaking or understanding speech; and trouble seeing.

A stroke is a serious medical condition that requires emergency care. A stroke can cause lasting brain damage, long-term disability, or even death.

If you think you or someone else is having a stroke, call 9–1–1 right away. Do not drive to the hospital or let someone else drive you. Call an ambulance so that medical personnel can begin life-saving treatment on the way to the emergency room. During a stroke, every minute counts.

This chapter includes text excerpted from "Stroke," National Heart, Lung, and Blood Institute (NHLBI), October 28, 2015.

Types of Stroke

Ischemic Stroke

An ischemic stroke occurs if an artery that supplies oxygen-rich blood to the brain becomes blocked. Blood clots often cause the blockages that lead to ischemic strokes.

The two types of ischemic stroke are thrombotic and embolic. In a thrombotic stroke, a blood clot (thrombus) forms in an artery that supplies blood to the brain.

In an embolic stroke, a blood clot or other substance (such as plaque, a fatty material) travels through the bloodstream to an artery in the brain. (A blood clot or piece of plaque that travels through the bloodstream is called an embolus.)

With both types of ischemic stroke, the blood clot or plaque blocks the flow of oxygen-rich blood to a portion of the brain.

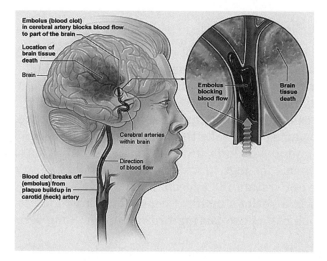

Figure 25.1. *Ischemic Stroke*

The illustration shows how an ischemic stroke can occur in the brain. If a blood clot breaks away from plaque buildup in a carotid (neck) artery, it can travel to and lodge in an artery in the brain. The clot can block blood flow to part of the brain, causing brain tissue death.

Hemorrhagic Stroke

A hemorrhagic stroke occurs if an artery in the brain leaks blood or ruptures (breaks open). The pressure from the leaked blood damages brain cells.

The two types of hemorrhagic stroke are intracerebral and sub-arachnoid. In an intracerebral hemorrhage, a blood vessel inside the brain leaks blood or ruptures.

In a subarachnoid hemorrhage, a blood vessel on the surface of the brain leaks blood or ruptures. When this happens, bleeding occurs between the inner and middle layers of the membranes that cover the brain.

In both types of hemorrhagic stroke, the leaked blood causes swelling of the brain and increased pressure in the skull. The swelling and pressure damage cells and tissues in the brain.

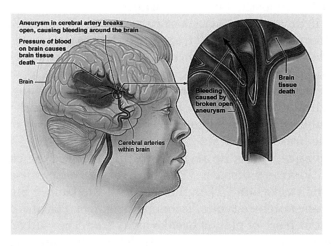

Figure 25.2. *Hemorrhagic Stroke*

The illustration shows how a hemorrhagic stroke can occur in the brain. An aneurysm in a cerebral artery breaks open, which causes bleeding in the brain. The pressure of the blood causes brain tissue death.

Other Names for a Stroke

- Brain attack

- Cerebrovascular accident (CVA)

- Hemorrhagic stroke (includes intracerebral hemorrhage and subarachnoid hemorrhage)

- Ischemic stroke (includes thrombotic stroke and embolic stroke)

A transient ischemic attack sometimes is called a TIA or mini-stroke. A TIA has the same symptoms as a stroke, and it increases your risk of having a stroke.

What Causes a Stroke?

Ischemic Stroke and Transient Ischemic Attack

An ischemic stroke or transient ischemic attack (TIA) occurs if an artery that supplies oxygen-rich blood to the brain becomes blocked. Many medical conditions can increase the risk of ischemic stroke or TIA.

For example, atherosclerosis is a disease in which a fatty substance called plaque builds up on the inner walls of the arteries. Plaque hardens and narrows the arteries, which limits the flow of blood to tissues and organs (such as the heart and brain).

Plaque in an artery can crack or rupture (break open). Blood platelets, which are disc-shaped cell fragments, stick to the site of the plaque injury and clump together to form blood clots. These clots can partly or fully block an artery.

Plaque can build up in any artery in the body, including arteries in the heart, brain, and neck. The two main arteries on each side of the neck are called the carotid arteries. These arteries supply oxygen-rich blood to the brain, face, scalp, and neck.

When plaque builds up in the carotid arteries, the condition is called carotid artery disease. Carotid artery disease causes many of the ischemic strokes and TIAs that occur in the United States.

An embolic stroke (a type of ischemic stroke) or TIA also can occur if a blood clot or piece of plaque breaks away from the wall of an artery. The clot or plaque can travel through the bloodstream and get stuck in one of the brain's arteries. This stops blood flow through the artery and damages brain cells.

Heart conditions and blood disorders also can cause blood clots that can lead to a stroke or TIA. For example, atrial fibrillation, or AF, is a common cause of embolic stroke.

In AF, the upper chambers of the heart contract in a very fast and irregular way. As a result, some blood pools in the heart. The pooling increases the risk of blood clots forming in the heart chambers.

An ischemic stroke or TIA also can occur because of lesions caused by atherosclerosis. These lesions may form in the small arteries of the brain, and they can block blood flow to the brain.

Hemorrhagic Stroke

Sudden bleeding in the brain can cause a hemorrhagic stroke. The bleeding causes swelling of the brain and increased pressure in the skull. The swelling and pressure damage brain cells and tissues.

Examples of conditions that can cause a hemorrhagic stroke include high blood pressure, aneurysms, and arteriovenous malformations (AVMs).

"Blood pressure" is the force of blood pushing against the walls of the arteries as the heart pumps blood. If blood pressure rises and stays high over time, it can damage the body in many ways.

Aneurysms are balloon-like bulges in an artery that can stretch and burst. AVMs are tangles of faulty arteries and veins that can rupture within the brain. High blood pressure can increase the risk of hemorrhagic stroke in people who have aneurysms or AVMs.

Who Is at Risk for a Stroke?

Certain traits, conditions, and habits can raise your risk of having a stroke or transient ischemic attack (TIA). These traits, conditions, and habits are known as risk factors.

The more risk factors you have, the more likely you are to have a stroke. You can treat or control some risk factors, such as high blood pressure and smoking. Other risk factors, such as age and gender, you can't control.

The major risk factors for stroke include:

- **High blood pressure.** High blood pressure is the main risk factor for stroke. Blood pressure is considered high if it stays at or above 140/90 millimeters of mercury (mmHg) over time. If you have diabetes or chronic kidney disease, high blood pressure is defined as 130/80 mmHg or higher.

- **Diabetes.** Diabetes is a disease in which the blood sugar level is high because the body doesn't make enough insulin or doesn't use its insulin properly. Insulin is a hormone that helps move blood sugar into cells where it's used for energy.

- **Heart diseases.** Coronary heart disease, cardiomyopathy, heart failure, and atrial fibrillation can cause blood clots that can lead to a stroke.

- **Smoking.** Smoking can damage blood vessels and raise blood pressure. Smoking also may reduce the amount of oxygen that reaches your body's tissues. Exposure to secondhand smoke also can damage the blood vessels.

- **Age and gender.** Your risk of stroke increases as you get older. At younger ages, men are more likely than women to have strokes. However, women are more likely to die from strokes.

Women who take birth control pills also are at slightly higher risk of stroke.

- **Race and ethnicity.** Strokes occur more often in African American, Alaska Native, and American Indian adults than in white, Hispanic, or Asian American adults.

- **Personal or family history of stroke or TIA.** If you've had a stroke, you're at higher risk for another one. Your risk of having a repeat stroke is the highest right after a stroke. A TIA also increases your risk of having a stroke, as does having a family history of stroke.

- **Brain aneurysms or arteriovenous malformations (AVMs).** Aneurysms are balloon-like bulges in an artery that can stretch and burst. AVMs are tangles of faulty arteries and veins that can rupture (break open) within the brain. AVMs may be present at birth, but often aren't diagnosed until they rupture.

Other risk factors for stroke, many of which of you can control, include:

- Alcohol and illegal drug use, including cocaine, amphetamines, and other drugs

- Certain medical conditions, such as sickle cell disease, vasculitis (inflammation of the blood vessels), and bleeding disorders

- Lack of physical activity

- Overweight and Obesity

- Stress and depression

- Unhealthy cholesterol levels

- Unhealthy diet

- Use of nonsteroidal anti-inflammatory drugs (NSAIDs), but not aspirin, may increase the risk of heart attack or stroke, particularly in patients who have had a heart attack or cardiac bypass surgery. The risk may increase the longer NSAIDs are used. Common NSAIDs include ibuprofen and naproxen.

Following a healthy lifestyle can lower the risk of stroke. Some people also may need to take medicines to lower their risk. Sometimes strokes can occur in people who don't have any known risk factors.

What Are the Signs and Symptoms of a Stroke?

The signs and symptoms of a stroke often develop quickly. However, they can develop over hours or even days.

The type of symptoms depends on the type of stroke and the area of the brain that's affected. How long symptoms last and how severe they are vary among different people.

Signs and symptoms of a stroke may include:

- Sudden weakness

- Paralysis (an inability to move) or numbness of the face, arms, or legs, especially on one side of the body

- Confusion

- Trouble speaking or understanding speech

- Trouble seeing in one or both eyes

- Problems breathing

- Dizziness, trouble walking, loss of balance or coordination, and unexplained falls

- Loss of consciousness

- Sudden and severe headache

A transient ischemic attack (TIA) has the same signs and symptoms as a stroke. However, TIA symptoms usually last less than 1–2 hours (although they may last up to 24 hours). A TIA may occur only once in a person's lifetime or more often.

At first, it may not be possible to tell whether someone is having a TIA or stroke. All stroke-like symptoms require medical care.

If you think you or someone else is having a TIA or stroke, call 9–1–1 right away. Do not drive to the hospital or let someone else drive you. Call an ambulance so that medical personnel can begin life-saving treatment on the way to the emergency room. During a stroke, every minute counts.

Stroke Complications

After you've had a stroke, you may develop other complications, such as:

- Blood clots and muscle weakness. Being immobile (unable to move around) for a long time can raise your risk of developing

291

blood clots in the deep veins of the legs. Being immobile also can lead to muscle weakness and decreased muscle flexibility.

- Problems swallowing and pneumonia. If a stroke affects the muscles used for swallowing, you may have a hard time eating or drinking. You also may be at risk of inhaling food or drink into your lungs. If this happens, you may develop pneumonia.

- Loss of bladder control. Some strokes affect the muscles used to urinate. You may need a urinary catheter (a tube placed into the bladder) until you can urinate on your own. Use of these catheters can lead to urinary tract infections. Loss of bowel control or constipation also may occur after a stroke.

How Is a Stroke Diagnosed?

Your doctor will diagnose a stroke based on your signs and symptoms, your medical history, a physical exam, and test results.

Your doctor will want to find out the type of stroke you've had, its cause, the part of the brain that's affected, and whether you have bleeding in the brain.

If your doctor thinks you've had a transient ischemic attack (TIA), he or she will look for its cause to help prevent a future stroke.

Medical History and Physical Exam

Your doctor will ask you or a family member about your risk factors for stroke. Examples of risk factors include high blood pressure, smoking, heart disease, and a personal or family history of stroke. Your doctor also will ask about your signs and symptoms and when they began.

During the physical exam, your doctor will check your mental alertness and your coordination and balance. He or she will check for numbness or weakness in your face, arms, and legs; confusion; and trouble speaking and seeing clearly.

Your doctor will look for signs of carotid artery disease, a common cause of ischemic stroke. He or she will listen to your carotid arteries with a stethoscope. A whooshing sound called a bruit may suggest changed or reduced blood flow due to plaque buildup in the carotid arteries.

Diagnostic Tests and Procedures

Your doctor may recommend one or more of the following tests to diagnose a stroke or TIA.

Brain Computed Tomography

A brain computed tomography scan, or brain CT scan, is a painless test that uses X-rays to take clear, detailed pictures of your brain. This test often is done right after a stroke is suspected.

A brain CT scan can show bleeding in the brain or damage to the brain cells from a stroke. The test also can show other brain conditions that may be causing your symptoms.

Magnetic Resonance Imaging

Magnetic resonance imaging (MRI) uses magnets and radio waves to create pictures of the organs and structures in your body. This test can detect changes in brain tissue and damage to brain cells from a stroke.

An MRI may be used instead of, or in addition to, a CT scan to diagnose a stroke.

Computed Tomography Arteriogram and Magnetic Resonance Arteriogram

A CT arteriogram (CTA) and magnetic resonance arteriogram (MRA) can show the large blood vessels in the brain. These tests may give your doctor more information about the site of a blood clot and the flow of blood through your brain.

Carotid Ultrasound

Carotid ultrasound is a painless and harmless test that uses sound waves to create pictures of the insides of your carotid arteries. These arteries supply oxygen-rich blood to your brain.

Carotid ultrasound shows whether plaque has narrowed or blocked your carotid arteries.

Your carotid ultrasound test may include a Doppler ultrasound. Doppler ultrasound is a special test that shows the speed and direction of blood moving through your blood vessels.

Carotid Angiography

Carotid angiography is a test that uses dye and special X-rays to show the insides of your carotid arteries.

For this test, a small tube called a catheter is put into an artery, usually in the groin (upper thigh). The tube is then moved up into one of your carotid arteries.

Your doctor will inject a substance (called contrast dye) into the carotid artery. The dye helps make the artery visible on X-ray pictures.

Heart Tests

EKG (Electrocardiogram)

An EKG is a simple, painless test that records the heart's electrical activity. The test shows how fast the heart is beating and its rhythm (steady or irregular). An EKG also records the strength and timing of electrical signals as they pass through each part of the heart.

An EKG can help detect heart problems that may have led to a stroke. For example, the test can help diagnose atrial fibrillation or a previous heart attack.

Echocardiography

Echocardiography, or echo, is a painless test that uses sound waves to create pictures of your heart.

The test gives information about the size and shape of your heart and how well your heart's chambers and valves are working.

Echo can detect possible blood clots inside the heart and problems with the aorta. The aorta is the main artery that carries oxygen-rich blood from your heart to all parts of your body.

Blood Tests

Your doctor also may use blood tests to help diagnose a stroke.

A blood glucose test measures the amount of glucose (sugar) in your blood. Low blood glucose levels may cause symptoms similar to those of a stroke.

A platelet count measures the number of platelets in your blood. Blood platelets are cell fragments that help your blood clot. Abnormal platelet levels may be a sign of a bleeding disorder (not enough clotting) or a thrombotic disorder (too much clotting).

Your doctor also may recommend blood tests to measure how long it takes for your blood to clot. Two tests that may be used are called PT and PTT tests. These tests show whether your blood is clotting normally.

How Is a Stroke Treated?

Treatment for a stroke depends on whether it is ischemic or hemorrhagic. Treatment for a transient ischemic attack (TIA) depends on its cause, how much time has passed since symptoms began, and whether you have other medical conditions.

Strokes and TIAs are medical emergencies. If you have stroke symptoms, call 9–1–1 right away. Do not drive to the hospital or let someone else drive you. Call an ambulance so that medical personnel can begin lifesaving treatment on the way to the emergency room. During a stroke, every minute counts.

Once you receive immediate treatment, your doctor will try to treat your stroke risk factors and prevent complications by recommending heart-healthy lifestyle changes.

Treating an Ischemic Stroke or Transient Ischemic Attack

An ischemic stroke or TIA occurs if an artery that supplies oxygen-rich blood to the brain becomes blocked. Often, blood clots cause the blockages that lead to ischemic strokes and TIAs. Treatment for an ischemic stroke or TIA may include medicines and medical procedures.

Medicines

If you have a stroke caused by a blood clot, you may be given a clot-dissolving, or clot-busting, medication called tissue plasminogen activator (tPA). A doctor will inject tPA into a vein in your arm. This type of medication must be given within 4 hours of symptom onset. Ideally, it should be given as soon as possible. The sooner treatment begins, the better your chances of recovery. Thus, it's important to know the signs and symptoms of a stroke and **to call 9–1–1 right away for emergency care.**

If you can't have tPA for medical reasons, your doctor may give you antiplatelet medicine that helps stop platelets from clumping together to form blood clots or anticoagulant medicine (blood thinner) that keeps existing blood clots from getting larger. Two common medicines are aspirin and clopidogrel.

Medical Procedures

If you have carotid artery disease, your doctor may recommend a carotid endarterectomy or carotid artery angioplasty. Both procedures open blocked carotid arteries.

Researchers are testing other treatments for ischemic stroke, such as intra-arterial thrombolysis and mechanical clot removal in cerebral ischemia (MERCI).

In intra-arterial thrombolysis, a long flexible tube called a catheter is put into your groin (upper thigh) and threaded to the tiny arteries of the brain. Your doctor can deliver medicine through this catheter to break up a blood clot in the brain.

MERCI is a device that can remove blood clots from an artery. During the procedure, a catheter is threaded through a carotid artery to the affected artery in the brain. The device is then used to pull the blood clot out through the catheter.

Treating a Hemorrhagic Stroke

A hemorrhagic stroke occurs if an artery in the brain leaks blood or ruptures. The first steps in treating a hemorrhagic stroke are to find the cause of bleeding in the brain and then control it. Unlike ischemic strokes, hemorrhagic strokes aren't treated with antiplatelet medicines and blood thinners because these medicines can make bleeding worse.

If you're taking antiplatelet medicines or blood thinners and have a hemorrhagic stroke, you'll be taken off the medicine. If high blood pressure is the cause of bleeding in the brain, your doctor may prescribe medicines to lower your blood pressure. This can help prevent further bleeding.

Surgery also may be needed to treat a hemorrhagic stroke. The types of surgery used include aneurysm clipping, coil embolization, and arteriovenous malformation (AVM) repair.

Aneurysm Clipping and Coil Embolization

If an aneurysm (a balloon-like bulge in an artery) is the cause of a stroke, your doctor may recommend aneurysm clipping or coil embolization.

Aneurysm clipping is done to block off the aneurysm from the blood vessels in the brain. This surgery helps prevent further leaking of blood from the aneurysm. It also can help prevent the aneurysm from bursting again. During the procedure, a surgeon will make an incision (cut) in the brain and place a tiny clamp at the base of the aneurysm. You'll be given medicine to make you sleep during the surgery. After the surgery, you'll need to stay in the hospital's intensive care unit for a few days.

Coil embolization is a less complex procedure for treating an aneurysm. The surgeon will insert a tube called a catheter into an artery in the groin. He or she will thread the tube to the site of the aneurysm.

Then, a tiny coil will be pushed through the tube and into the aneurysm. The coil will cause a blood clot to form, which will block blood flow through the aneurysm and prevent it from bursting again. Coil embolization is done in a hospital. You'll be given medicine to make you sleep during the surgery.

Arteriovenous Malformation Repair

If an AVM is the cause of a stroke, your doctor may recommend an AVM repair. (An AVM is a tangle of faulty arteries and veins that can rupture within the brain.) AVM repair helps prevent further bleeding in the brain.

Doctors use several methods to repair AVMs. These methods include:

- Injecting a substance into the blood vessels of the AVM to block blood flow

- Surgery to remove the AVM

- Using radiation to shrink the blood vessels of the AVM

How Can a Stroke Be Prevented?

Taking action to control your risk factors can help prevent or delay a stroke. If you've already had a stroke, these actions can help prevent another one.

- Be physically active. Physical activity can improve your fitness level and health. Talk with your doctor about what types and amounts of activity are safe for you.

- Don't smoke, or if you smoke or use tobacco, quit. Smoking can damage and tighten blood vessels and raise your risk of stroke. Talk with your doctor about programs and products that can help you quit. Also, secondhand smoke can damage the blood vessels.

- Maintain a healthy weight. If you're overweight or obese, work with your doctor to create a reasonable weight loss plan. Controlling your weight helps you control risk factors for stroke.

- Make heart-healthy eating choices. Heart-healthy eating can help lower your risk or prevent a stroke.

- Manage stress. Use techniques to lower your stress levels.

If you or someone in your family has had a stroke, be sure to tell your doctor. By knowing your family history of stroke, you may be able to lower your risk factors and prevent or delay a stroke. If you've had a transient ischemic attack (TIA), don't ignore it. TIAs are warnings, and it's important for your doctor to find the cause of the TIA so you can take steps to prevent a stroke.

Chapter 26

Aortic Disorders

Aortic Aneurysm

An aortic aneurysm is a balloon-like bulge in the aorta, the large artery that carries blood from the heart through the chest and torso. Aortic aneurysms work in two ways:

1. The force of blood pumping can split the layers of the artery wall, allowing blood to leak in between them. This process is called a **dissection**.

2. The aneurysm can burst completely, causing bleeding inside the body. This is called a **rupture**.

Dissections and ruptures are the cause of most deaths from aortic aneurysms.

Aortic Aneurysm in the United States

- Aortic aneurysms were the primary cause of **10,597 deaths** and a contributing cause in more than **17,215 deaths** in the United States in 2009.

This chapter contains text excerpted from the following sources: Text beginning with the heading "Aortic Aneurysm" is excerpted from "Aortic Aneurysm Fact Sheet," Centers for Disease Control and Prevention (CDC), July 22, 2014; Text beginning with the heading "Aortic Dissection" is excerpted from "Dissecting the Presentation," Agency for Healthcare Reasearch and Quality (AHRQ), April 2015.

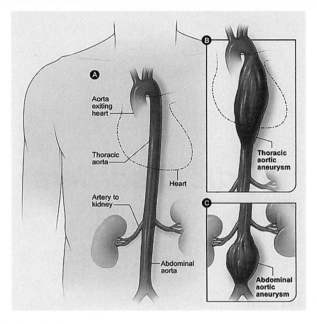

Figure 26.1. *Aortic Aneurysm*

(A) shows a normal aorta. (B) shows a thoracic aortic aneurysm located behind the heart. (C) shows an abdominal aortic aneurysm located below the arteries that supply blood to the kidneys.

- About **two-thirds** of people who have an aortic dissection are male.

- The U.S. Preventive Services Task Force recommends that men aged 65–75 years who have ever smoked should get an ultrasound screening for abdominal aortic aneurysms, even if they have no symptoms.

Types of Aortic Aneurysm

Thoracic Aortic Aneurysms

A thoracic aortic aneurysm occurs in the chest. Men and women are equally likely to get thoracic aortic aneurysms, which become more common with increasing age.

Thoracic aortic aneurysms are usually caused by high blood pressure or sudden injury. Sometimes people with inherited connective tissue disorders, such as Marfan syndrome and Ehlers-Danlos syndrome, get thoracic aortic aneurysms.

Signs and symptoms of thoracic aortic aneurysm can include

- Sharp, sudden pain in the chest or upper back.

- Shortness of breath.

- Trouble breathing or swallowing.

Abdominal Aortic Aneurysms

An abdominal aortic aneurysm occurs below the chest. Abdominal aortic aneurysms happen more often than thoracic aortic aneurysms.

Abdominal aortic aneurysms are more common in men and among people aged 65 years and older. Abdominal aortic aneurysms are less common among blacks compared with whites.

Abdominal aortic aneurysms are usually caused by atherosclerosis (hardened arteries), but infection or injury can also cause them.

Abdominal aortic aneurysms often don't have any symptoms. If an individual does have symptoms, they can include

- Throbbing or deep pain in your back or side.

- Pain in the buttocks, groin, or legs.

Other Types of Aneurysms

Aneurysms can occur in other parts of your body. A ruptured aneurysm in the brain can cause a stroke.

Peripheral aneurysms—those found in arteries other than the aorta—can occur in the neck, in the groin, or behind the knees. These aneurysms are less likely to rupture or dissect than aortic aneurysms, but they can form blood clots. These clots can break away and block blood flow through the artery.

Risk Factors for Aortic Aneurysm

Diseases that damage your heart and blood vessels also increase your risk for aortic aneurysm. These diseases include

- High blood pressure

- High cholesterol

- Atherosclerosis (hardened arteries)

- Smoking

Some inherited connective tissue disorders, such as Marfan syndrome and Ehlers-Danlos syndrome, can also increase your risk for aortic aneurysm. Your family may also have a history of aortic aneurysms that can increase your risk.

Unhealthy behaviors can also increase your risk for aortic aneurysm, especially for people who have one of the diseases listed above. Tobacco use is the most important behavior related to aortic aneurysm. People who have a history of smoking are 3 to 5 times more likely to develop an abdominal aortic aneurysm.

Treating Aortic Aneurysm

The two main treatments for aortic aneurysms are **medicines** and **surgery**. Medicines can lower blood pressure and reduce risk for an aortic aneurysm. Surgery can repair or replace the injured section of the aorta.

Aortic Dissection

What Is an Aortic Dissection?

An aortic dissection is a tear in the wall of the aorta; more specifically, it is a tear of the inner and middle layers of the aortic wall with propagation of a false lumen within the middle layer. Aortic dissection is part of a spectrum often referred to as acute aortic syndrome. This syndrome encompasses not only aortic dissection but also its less common variants, including aortic intramural hematoma and penetrating atherosclerotic ulcer. Aortic dissection is classified using two anatomic systems. The more common (Stanford) classifies dissections that involve the ascending aorta as type A, regardless of the site of intimal tear, and all other dissections as type B.

Epidemiology

Acute aortic dissection (AAD) is rare. The true incidence is difficult to define because dissections can be instantly fatal in the prehospital setting and may be missed on initial presentation. Death is often attributed to other causes, and autopsies may not be performed. We do know that there is a higher incidence of AAD in men (65%) and with increasing age.

Take-Home Points

- Acute aortic dissection is a challenging diagnosis that may not present with the classic sudden onset of tearing or sharp chest pain or pulse deficits but with painless manifestations involving other body systems such as neurological, gastrointestinal, and renal.

- Familiarize yourself with not only the common but the uncommon presentations of acute aortic dissection and keep an open mind when patients present with multiple seemingly unrelated complaints.

- Absence of mediastinal widening on chest radiograph does not rule out aortic dissection.

- Misdiagnosis can occur when patients present with mild illness, when symptoms are suggestive of another disease (e.g., acute coronary syndrome), and when radiographic findings are not typical.

- Providers should be aware of specific pitfalls in the management of acute aortic dissection.

Chapter 27

Disorders of the Peripheral Arteries

Chapter Contents

Section 27.1

Buerger Disease

This section includes text excerpted from "Buerger Disease," Genetic and Rare Diseases Information Center (GARD), June 16, 2015.

Overview

Buerger disease is a disease of the arteries and veins in the arms and legs. The arteries and veins become inflamed which can lead to narrowed and blocked vessels. This reduces blood flow resulting in pain and eventually damage to affected tissues. Buerger disease nearly always occurs in association with cigarette or other tobacco use. Quitting all forms of tobacco is an essential part of treatment.

Signs and Symptoms for Buerger Disease

- Arterial thrombosis
- Gangrene
- Skin ulcer
- Vasculitis
- Acrocyanosis
- Arthralgia

- Paresthesia
- Hyperhidrosis
- Insomnia
- Autosomal recessive inheritance
- Limb pain

What Causes Buerger Disease?

Buerger disease has a strong relationship to cigarette smoking. This association may be due to direct poisioning of cells from some component of tobacco, or by hypersensitivity to the same components. Many people with Buerger disease will show hypersensitivities to injection of tobacco extracts into their skin. There may be a genetic component to susceptibility to Buerger disease as well. It is possible that these genetic influences account for the higher prevalence of Buerger disease in people of Israeli, Indian subcontinent, and Japanese descent.

Certain HLA (human leukocyte antigen) haplotypes have also been found in association with Buerger disease.

How Is Buerger Disease Treated?

Currently there is not a cure for Buerger disease, however there are treatments that can help control it. The most essential part of treatment is to avoid all tobacco and nicotine products. Even one cigarette a day can worsen the disease. A doctor can help a person with Buerger disease learn about safe medications and programs to combat smoking/nicotine addiction. Continued smoking is associated with an overall amputation rate of 40 to 50 percent.

The following treatments may also be helpful, but do not replace smoking/nicotine cessation:

- Medications to dilate blood vessels and improve blood flow (e.g., intravenous Iloprost)

- Medications to dissolve blood clots

- Treatment with calcium channel blockers

- Walking exercises

- Intermittent compression of the arms and legs to increase blood flow to your extremities

- Surgical sympathectomy (a controversial surgery to cut the nerves to the affected area to control pain and increase blood flow)

- Therapeutic angiogenesis (medications to stimulate growth of new blood vessels)

- Spinal cord stimulation

- Amputation, if infection or gangrene occurs.

Section 27.2

Fibromuscular Dysplasia

Fibromuscular dysplasia (FMD) is a rare medical condition in which abnormal cell growth occurs in the walls of medium and large arteries, causing the arteries to become narrowed (stenosis) or enlarged (aneurysm). There are two main types of fibromuscular dysplasia: multifocal and focal. Patients are classified as having one or the other based on the appearance of affected arteries in imaging studies, such as angiography. Multifocal FMD is the most common type, affecting around 90% of patients. The pattern of alternating areas of narrowing and widening in the affected arteries has been described as a "string of beads." Focal FMD is less common, affecting around 10% of patients. The affected arteries have distinct lesions or areas of narrowing.

FMD most commonly affects the renal arteries that supply blood to the kidneys and the carotid arteries in the neck that supply blood to the brain. It occurs more rarely in the mesenteric arteries that supply blood to the intestines, the coronary arteries that supply blood to the heart, and peripheral arteries in the arms and legs. FMD can limit blood flow to vital organs and cause a variety of health complications. Although there is no cure, effective treatments are available.

Causes and Risk Factors

Researchers have not identified a definitive cause of FMD. But they have uncovered several risk factors that appear to increase the likelihood that a person will develop the condition, such as:

- **Hormones**: Since 90% of people who develop FMD are women, many researchers believe that hormones may be a factor.

- **Age**: Most people are diagnosed with FMD between the ages of 40 and 60, although it also affects children and older people.

- **Genetics**: Around 10% of people with FMD have a relative with the condition, leading researchers to believe that there may be a genetic component. In addition, some people who develop FMD have genetic abnormalities in their blood vessels.

- **Abnormal arteries**: Researchers also suspect that FMD may be caused by abnormally formed arteries, which may result from inadequate oxygen supply to the blood vessel walls, pressure due to the position of the arteries, or trauma to the arteries.

- **Smoking**: Smoking affects the arteries and increases the risk of developing FMD.

Symptoms

Many people with fibromuscular dysplasia do not experience symptoms. FMD mainly produces symptoms when stenosis of the arteries restricts blood flow or aneurysms in the arteries tear or rupture. The nature of the symptoms depends on the specific arteries that are affected.

If FMD affects the renal arteries, the symptoms may include high blood pressure or poor kidney function. If FMD affects the carotid arteries, the symptoms are likely to include headaches, dizziness, blurred vision, a swooshing sound in the ears, facial weakness or numbness, or neck pain. FMD in the mesenteric arteries may cause pain in the abdomen, especially after eating, or unexplained weight loss. People with FMD in the peripheral arteries may experience numbness, coldness, weakness, or discomfort in the arms or legs during exercise. When FMD affects the coronary arteries, symptoms may include chest pain, shortness of breath, or occasionally a heart attack.

Diagnosis

Some people are diagnosed with FMD during routine medical exams, when the doctor hears an unusual swooshing noise (bruit) through the stethoscope indicating a problem with blood flow. Other patients are diagnosed with FMD after undergoing an imaging scan for a different medical problem. Several noninvasive tests can help doctors determine whether arteries are affected by FMD, including Doppler ultrasound, magnetic resonance imaging (MRI), and computed tomography angiography (CTA).

Catheter-based angiography is another test that is commonly used to diagnose FMD. In this procedure, a thin tube is inserted into the artery and dye is injected to allow the doctor to examine it. Once a patient is diagnosed with FMD in a particular artery, the doctor will typically scan the rest of the body to see if it is present in other locations. Most patients with FMD also undergo additional tests to check for an aneurysm in the brain or heart that might pose dangerous health complications.

Complications

Fibromuscular dysplasia can cause a variety of health complications, some of which can be life threatening. One of the most common complications is high blood pressure due to the narrowing of the arteries. High blood pressure is a risk factor for heart disease and stroke. FMD can also cause arterial dissection, or tears in the walls of the arteries that allow blood to leak into the artery wall. When this process occurs in the heart it is known as spontaneous coronary artery dissection (SCAD), and it can cause a heart attack. Aneurysms are another complication of FMD that can have serious health consequences. If an aneurysm ruptures in the brain, it can cause a stroke.

Treatment

There are several different options available to treat fibromuscular dysplasia, including medications, procedures like angioplasty, and surgery. The most appropriate treatment depends on the location of the affected artery, the severity of the condition, and the patient's overall health.

People with FMD who do not have symptoms may only need to take medication to prevent blood clots, such as a daily aspirin, or to control high blood pressure. Common blood-pressure medications include angiotensin converting enzyme inhibitors (ACE-inhibitors), angiotensin receptor blockers (ARBs), diuretics, calcium channel blockers, and beta blockers.

The medical procedure most often used to open arteries that become narrowed or blocked due to FMD is percutaneous transluminal angioplasty (PTA). A catheter with a tiny balloon on the end is inserted into the affected artery and inflated to open up the narrowed section. In the angioplasty procedures commonly performed on patients with blocked coronary arteries, a metal mesh tube called a stent is often inserted to keep the artery open. Stents are only used under certain circumstances in patients with FMD, however, such as to prevent an aneurysm from rupturing.

In cases where the artery is blocked or severely damaged, surgery may be required to repair the artery and restore blood flow. Surgical revascularization involves removing the blocked section of the artery or creating a bypass around the blockage. The most commonly performed type of revascularization surgery is an aortorenal bypass, which uses a vein from the leg to replace the renal artery that leads to the kidney.

References

1. "Fibromuscular Dysplasia," Mayo Clinic, 2016.

2. "Fibromuscular Dysplasia (FMD)," Cleveland Clinic, 2016.

Section 27.3

Peripheral Arterial Disease

This section includes text excerpted from "Peripheral Artery Disease," National Heart, Lung, and Blood Institute (NHLBI), November 16, 2015.

What Is Peripheral Artery Disease?

Peripheral artery disease (P.A.D.) is a disease in which plaque builds up in the arteries that carry blood to your head, organs, and limbs. Plaque is made up of fat, cholesterol, calcium, fibrous tissue, and other substances in the blood.

When plaque builds up in the body's arteries, the condition is called atherosclerosis. Over time, plaque can harden and narrow the arteries. This limits the flow of oxygen-rich blood to your organs and other parts of your body.

P.A.D. usually affects the arteries in the legs, but it also can affect the arteries that carry blood from your heart to your head, arms, kidneys, and stomach. This article focuses on P.A.D. that affects blood flow to the legs.

Other Names for Peripheral Artery Disease

- Atherosclerotic peripheral arterial disease

- Claudication

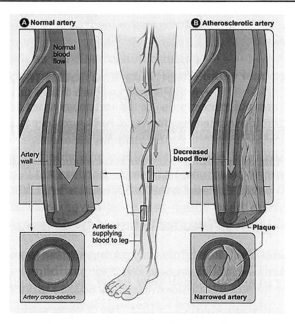

Figure 27.1. *Normal Artery and Artery With Plaque Buildup*

The illustration shows how P.A.D. can affect arteries in the legs. (A) shows a normal artery with normal blood flow. The inset image shows a cross-section of the normal artery. (B) shows an artery with plaque buildup that's partially blocking blood flow. The inset image shows a cross-section of the narrowed artery.

- Hardening of the arteries
- Leg cramps from poor circulation
- Peripheral arterial disease
- Peripheral vascular disease
- Poor circulation
- Vascular disease

What Causes Peripheral Artery Disease?

The most common cause of peripheral artery disease (P.A.D.) is atherosclerosis. Atherosclerosis is a disease in which plaque builds up in your arteries. The exact cause of atherosclerosis isn't known.

The disease may start if certain factors damage the inner layers of the arteries. These factors include:

- Smoking

- High amounts of certain fats and cholesterol in the blood

- High blood pressure

- High amounts of sugar in the blood due to insulin resistance or diabetes

When damage occurs, your body starts a healing process. The healing may cause plaque to build up where the arteries are damaged.

Eventually, a section of plaque can rupture (break open), causing a blood clot to form at the site. The buildup of plaque or blood clots can severely narrow or block the arteries and limit the flow of oxygen-rich blood to your body.

Who Is at Risk for Peripheral Artery Disease?

Peripheral artery disease (P.A.D.) affects millions of people in the United States. The disease is more common in blacks than any other racial or ethnic group. The major risk factors for P.A.D. are smoking, older age, and having certain diseases or conditions.

Smoking

Smoking is the main risk factor for P.A.D. and your risk increases if you smoke or have a history of smoking. Quitting smoking slows the progress of P.A.D. People who smoke and people who have diabetes are at highest risk for P.A.D. complications, such as gangrene (tissue death) in the leg from decreased blood flow.

Older Age

Older age also is a risk factor for P.A.D. Plaque builds up in your arteries as you age. Older age combined with other risk factors, such as smoking or diabetes, also puts you at higher risk for P.A.D.

Diseases and Conditions

Many diseases and conditions can raise your risk of P.A.D., including:

- Diabetes

- High blood pressure

- High blood cholesterol

- Coronary heart disease
- Stroke
- Metabolic syndrome

What Are the Signs and Symptoms of Peripheral Artery Disease?

Many people who have peripheral artery disease (P.A.D.) don't have any signs or symptoms.

Even if you don't have signs or symptoms, ask your doctor whether you should get checked for P.A.D. if you're:

- Aged 70 or older
- Aged 50 or older and have a history of smoking or diabetes
- Younger than 50 and have diabetes and one or more risk factors for atherosclerosis

Other Signs and Symptoms

Other signs and symptoms of P.A.D. include:

- Weak or absent pulses in the legs or feet
- Sores or wounds on the toes, feet, or legs that heal slowly, poorly, or not at all
- A pale or bluish color to the skin
- A lower temperature in one leg compared to the other leg
- Poor nail growth on the toes and decreased hair growth on the legs
- Erectile dysfunction, especially among men who have diabetes

How Is Peripheral Artery Disease Diagnosed?

Peripheral artery disease (P.A.D.) is diagnosed based on your medical and family histories, a physical exam, and test results.

P.A.D. often is diagnosed after symptoms are reported. A correct diagnosis is important because people who have P.A.D. are at higher risk for coronary heart disease (CHD), heart attack, stroke, and transient ischemic attack ("mini-stroke"). If you have P.A.D., your doctor also may want to check for signs of these diseases and conditions.

Specialists Involved

Primary care doctors, such as internists and family doctors, may treat people who have mild P.A.D. For more advanced P.A.D., a vascular specialist may be involved. This is a doctor who specializes in treating blood vessel diseases and conditions.

A cardiologist also may be involved in treating people who have P.A.D. Cardiologists treat heart problems, such as CHD and heart attack, which often affect people who have P.A.D.

Medical and Family Histories

Your doctor may ask:

* Whether you have any risk factors for P.A.D. For example, he or she may ask whether you smoke or have diabetes.
* About your symptoms, including any symptoms that occur when walking, exercising, sitting, standing, or climbing.
* About your diet.
* About any medicines you take, including prescription and over-the-counter medicines.
* Whether anyone in your family has a history of heart or blood vessel diseases.

Physical Exam

During the physical exam, your doctor will look for signs of P.A.D. He or she may check the blood flow in your legs or feet to see whether you have weak or absent pulses.

Your doctor also may check the pulses in your leg arteries for an abnormal whooshing sound called a bruit. He or she can hear this sound with a stethoscope. A bruit may be a warning sign of a narrowed or blocked artery.

Your doctor may compare blood pressure between your limbs to see whether the pressure is lower in the affected limb. He or she also may check for poor wound healing or any changes in your hair, skin, or nails that may be signs of P.A.D.

Diagnostic Tests

Ankle-Brachial Index

A simple test called an ankle-brachial index (ABI) often is used to diagnose P.A.D. The ABI compares blood pressure in your ankle to blood pressure in your arm. This test shows how well blood is flowing in your limbs.

ABI can show whether P.A.D. is affecting your limbs, but it won't show which blood vessels are narrowed or blocked.

A normal ABI result is 1.0 or greater (with a range of 0.90 to 1.30). The test takes about 10 to 15 minutes to measure both arms and both ankles. This test may be done yearly to see whether P.A.D. is getting worse.

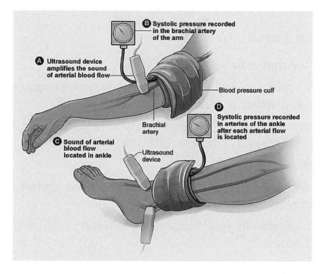

Figure 27.2. *Ankle-Brachial Index*

The illustration shows the ankle-brachial index test. The test compares blood pressure in the ankle to blood pressure in the arm. As the blood pressure cuff deflates, the blood pressure in the arteries is recorded.

Doppler Ultrasound

A Doppler ultrasound looks at blood flow in the major arteries and veins in the limbs. During this test, a handheld device is placed on your body and passed back and forth over the affected area. A computer converts sound waves into a picture of blood flow in the arteries and veins.

The results of this test can show whether a blood vessel is blocked. The results also can help show the severity of P.A.D

Treadmill Test

A treadmill test can show the severity of symptoms and the level of exercise that brings them on. You'll walk on a treadmill for this test. This shows whether you have any problems during normal walking.

You may have an ABI test before and after the treadmill test. This will help compare blood flow in your arms and legs before and after exercise.

Magnetic Resonance Angiogram

A magnetic resonance angiogram (MRA) uses magnetic and radio wave energy to take pictures of your blood vessels. This test is a type of magnetic resonance imaging (MRI).

An MRA can show the location and severity of a blocked blood vessel. If you have a pacemaker, man-made joint, stent, surgical clips, mechanical heart valve, or other metallic devices in your body, you might not be able to have an MRA. Ask your doctor whether an MRA is an option for you.

Arteriogram

An arteriogram provides a "road map" of the arteries. Doctors use this test to find the exact location of a blocked artery.

For this test, dye is injected through a needle or catheter (tube) into one of your arteries. This may make you feel mildly flushed. After the dye is injected, an X-ray is taken. The X-ray can show the location, type, and extent of the blockage in the artery.

Some doctors use a newer method of arteriogram that uses tiny ultrasound cameras. These cameras take pictures of the insides of the blood vessels. This method is called intravascular ultrasound.

Blood Tests

Your doctor may recommend blood tests to check for P.A.D. risk factors. For example, blood tests can help diagnose conditions such as diabetes and high blood cholesterol.

How Is Peripheral Artery Disease Treated?

Treatments for peripheral artery disease (P.A.D.) include lifestyle changes, medicines, and surgery or procedures.

The overall goals of treating P.A.D. include reducing risk of heart attack and stroke; reducing symptoms of claudication; improving mobility and overall quality of life; and preventing complications. Treatment is based on your signs and symptoms, risk factors, and the results of physical exams and tests.

Treatment may slow or stop the progression of the disease and reduce the risk of complications. Without treatment, P.A.D. may progress, resulting in serious tissue damage in the form of sores or gangrene (tissue death) due to inadequate blood flow. In extreme cases of P.A.D., also referred to as critical limb ischemia (CLI), removal (amputation) of part of the leg or foot may be necessary.

Lifestyle Changes

Treatment often includes making long-lasting lifestyle changes, such as:

- Physical activity
- Quitting smoking
- Heart-healthy eating

Medicines

Your doctor may prescribe medicines to:

- Prevent blood clots from forming due to low blood flow with anti-clotting medicines, such as aspirin.
- Treat unhealthy cholesterol levels with statins. Statins control or lower blood cholesterol. By lowering your blood cholesterol level, you can decrease your chance of developing complications from P.A.D.
- Treat high blood pressure with one of many high blood pressure medicines.
- Help ease leg pain that occurs when you walk or climb stairs.
- Reduce the symptoms of intermittent claudication, measured by increased walking distance with certain platelet-aggregation inhibitors.

Surgery or Procedures

Bypass Grafting

Your doctor may recommend bypass grafting surgery if blood flow in your limb is blocked or nearly blocked. For this surgery, your doctor uses a blood vessel from another part of your body or a synthetic tube to make a graft.

This graft bypasses (that is, goes around) the blocked part of the artery. The bypass allows blood to flow around the blockage. This surgery doesn't cure P.A.D., but it may increase blood flow to the affected limb.

Angioplasty and Stent Placement

Your doctor may recommend angioplasty to restore blood flow through a narrowed or blocked artery.

During this procedure, a catheter (thin tube) with a balloon at the tip is inserted into a blocked artery. The balloon is then inflated, which pushes plaque outward against the artery wall. This widens the artery and restores blood flow.

A stent (a small mesh tube) may be placed in the artery during angioplasty. A stent helps keep the artery open after angioplasty is done. Some stents are coated with medicine to help prevent blockages in the artery.

Atherectomy

Atherectomy is a procedure that removes plaque buildup from an artery. During the procedure, a catheter is used to insert a small cutting device into the blocked artery. The device is used to shave or cut off plaque.

The bits of plaque are removed from the body through the catheter or washed away in the bloodstream (if they're small enough).

Doctors also can perform atherectomy using a special laser that dissolves the blockage.

Other Types of Treatment

Researchers are studying cell and gene therapies to treat P.A.D. However, these treatments aren't yet available outside of clinical trials. Read more about clinical trials.

How Can Peripheral Artery Disease Be Prevented?

Taking action to control your risk factors can help prevent or delay peripheral artery disease (P.A.D.) and its complications. Know your family history of health problems related to P.A.D. If you or someone in your family has the disease, be sure to tell your doctor. Controlling risk factors includes the following.

- Be physically active.

- Be screened for P.A.D. A simple office test, called an ankle-brachial index or ABI, can help determine whether you have P.A.D.

- Follow heart-healthy eating.

- If you smoke, quit. Talk with your doctor about programs and products that can help you quit smoking.

If you're overweight or obese, work with your doctor to create a reasonable weight-loss plan.

The lifestyle changes described above can reduce your risk of developing P.A.D. These changes also can help prevent and control conditions that can be associated with P.A.D., such as coronary heart disease, diabetes, high blood pressure, high blood cholesterol, and stroke.

Section 27.4

Raynaud's Phenomenon

This section includes text excerpted from "What Is Raynaud's Phenomenon?" National Institute of Arthritis and Musculoskeletal and Skin Diseases (NIAMS), November 2014.

What Is Raynaud's Phenomenon?

Raynaud's phenomenon is a disorder that affects blood vessels, mostly in the fingers and toes. It causes the blood vessels to narrow when you are:

- Cold

- Feeling stress

Primary Raynaud's phenomenon happens on its own. *Secondary* Raynaud's phenomenon happens along with some other health problem.

Who Gets Raynaud's Phenomenon?

People of all ages can have Raynaud's phenomenon. Raynaud's phenomenon may run in families, but more research is needed.

The primary form is the most common. It most often starts between age 15 and 25. It is most common in:

- Women

- People living in cold places

The secondary form tends to start after age 35 to 40. It is most common in people with connective tissue diseases, such as scleroderma, Sjögren's syndrome, and lupus. Other possible causes include:

- Carpal tunnel syndrome, which affects nerves in the wrists.

- Blood vessel disease.

- Some medicines used to treat high blood pressure, migraines, or cancer.

- Some over-the-counter cold medicines.

- Some narcotics.

People with certain jobs may be more likely to get the secondary form:

- Workers who are around certain chemicals.

- People who use tools that vibrate, such as a jackhammer.

What Are the Symptoms of Raynaud's Phenomenon?

The body saves heat when it is cold by slowing the supply of blood to the skin. It does this by making blood vessels more narrow.

With Raynaud's phenomenon, the body's reaction to cold or stress is stronger than normal. It makes blood vessels narrow faster and tighter than normal. When this happens, it is called an "attack."

During an attack, the fingers and toes can change colors. They may go from white to blue to red. They may also feel cold and numb from lack of blood flow. As the attack ends and blood flow returns, fingers or toes can throb and tingle. After the cold parts of the body warm up, normal blood flow returns in about 15 minutes.

What Is the Difference Between Primary and Secondary Raynaud's Phenomenon?

Primary Raynaud's phenomenon is often so mild a person never seeks treatment. Secondary Raynaud's phenomenon is more serious and complex. It is caused when diseases reduce blood flow to fingers and toes.

How Does a Doctor Diagnose Raynaud's Phenomenon?

It is fairly easy to diagnose Raynaud's phenomenon. But it is harder to find out whether a person has the primary or the secondary form of the disorder.

Doctors will diagnose which form it is using a complete history, an exam, and tests. Tests may include:

- Blood tests

- Looking at fingernail tissue with a microscope

What Is the Treatment for Raynaud's Phenomenon?

Treatment aims to:

- Reduce how many attacks you have

- Make attacks less severe

- Prevent tissue damage

- Prevent loss of finger and toe tissue

Primary Raynaud's phenomenon does not lead to tissue damage, so nondrug treatment is used first. Treatment with medicine is more common with secondary Raynaud's.

Severe cases of Raynaud's can lead to sores or gangrene (tissue death) in the fingers and toes. These cases can be painful and hard to treat. In severe cases that cause skin ulcers and serious tissue damage, surgery may be used.

Nondrug Treatments and Self-Help Measures

To reduce how long and severe attacks are:

- Keep your hands and feet warm and dry

- Warm your hands and feet with warm water

- Avoid air conditioning

- Wear gloves to touch frozen or cold foods

- Wear many layers of loose clothing and a hat when it's cold

- Use chemical warmers, such as small heating pouches that can be placed in pockets, mittens, boots, or shoes

- Talk to your doctor before exercising outside in cold weather

- Don't smoke

- Avoid medicines that make symptoms worse

- Control stress

- Exercise regularly

See a doctor if:

- You worry about attacks

- You have questions about self-care

- Attacks happen on just one side of your body

- You have sores or ulcers on your fingers or toes

Treatment with Medications

People with secondary Raynaud's phenomenon are often treated with:

- Blood pressure medicines

- Medicines that relax blood vessels. One kind can be put on the fingers to heal ulcers.

If blood flow doesn't return and finger loss is a risk, you will need other medicines.

Pregnant woman should not take these medicines. Sometimes Raynaud's phenomenon gets better or goes away when a woman is pregnant.

Chapter 28

Peripheral Venous Disorders

Chapter Contents

325

Section 28.1

Deep Vein Thrombosis

This section includes text excerpted from "Deep Vein
Thrombosis (Blood Clots)," Centers for Disease Control
and Prevention (CDC), March 7, 2016.

Deep vein thrombosis (DVT) and pulmonary embolism (PE) are
serious but preventable medical conditions caused by blood clots that
form in a vein. It is important to know about DVT because it can happen to anyone at any age and can cause serious illness, disability, and
in some cases, death. The good news is that these types of blood clots
are preventable and treatable if discovered early.

Know the Signs and Symptoms

About half of people with DVT have no signs or symptoms at all.
The following are the most common signs and symptoms of DVT that
occur in the affected part of the body:

- Swelling

- Pain

- Tenderness

- Redness of the skin

If you have any of these symptoms, you should see your doctor as
soon as possible.

Tips to Protect Yourself

The following tips can help prevent DVT:

- Move around as soon as possible after having been confined to
  bed, such as after surgery, illness, or injury

- If you're at risk for DVT, talk to your doctor about:

- Compression devices, especially if you are in the hospital

- Medication (anticoagulants) to prevent DVT
- When sitting for long periods of time, such as when traveling for more than four hours:
- Get up and walk around every 2 to 3 hours
- Exercise your legs while you're sitting by
- Raising and lowering your heels while keeping your toes on the floor
- Raising and lowering your toes while keeping your heels on the floor
- Tightening and releasing your leg muscles
- Wearing loose-fitting clothes
- You can reduce your risk by maintaining a healthy weight, being physically active, and following your doctor's recommendations based on your individual risks.

Section 28.2

Varicose Veins

This section includes text excerpted from "Varicose Veins," National Heart, Lung, and Blood Institute (NHLBI), February 13, 2014.

What Are Varicose Veins?

Varicose veins are swollen, twisted veins that you can see just under the surface of the skin. These veins usually occur in the legs, but they also can form in other parts of the body.

Varicose veins are a common condition. They usually cause few signs and symptoms. Sometimes varicose veins cause mild to moderate pain, blood clots, skin ulcers (sores), or other problems.

Overview

Veins are blood vessels that carry blood from your body's tissues to your heart. Your heart pumps the blood to your lungs to pick up oxygen. The oxygen-rich blood then is pumped to your body through blood vessels called arteries.

From your arteries, the blood flows through tiny blood vessels called capillaries, where it gives up its oxygen to the body's tissues. Your blood then returns to your heart through your veins to pick up more oxygen.

Veins have one-way valves that help keep blood flowing toward your heart. If the valves are weak or damaged, blood can back up and pool in your veins. This causes the veins to swell, which can lead to varicose veins.

Many factors can raise your risk for varicose veins. Examples of these factors include family history, older age, gender, pregnancy, overweight or obesity, lack of movement, and leg trauma.

Varicose veins are treated with lifestyle changes and medical procedures. The goals of treatment are to relieve symptoms, prevent complications, and improve appearance.

Outlook

Varicose veins usually don't cause medical problems. If they do, your doctor may simply suggest making lifestyle changes.

Sometimes varicose veins cause pain, blood clots, skin ulcers, or other problems. If this happens, your doctor may recommend one or more medical procedures. Some people choose to have these procedures to improve the way their veins look or to relieve pain.

Many treatments for varicose veins are quick and easy and don't require a long recovery.

Vein Problems Related to Varicose Veins

Many vein problems are related to varicose veins, such as telangiectasias, spider veins, varicoceles, and other vein problems.

Telangiectasias

Telangiectasias are small clusters of blood vessels. They're usually found on the upper body, including the face.

These blood vessels appear red. They may form during pregnancy, and often they develop in people who have certain genetic disorders, viral infections, or other conditions, such as liver disease.

Because telangiectasias can be a sign of a more serious condition, see your doctor if you think you have them.

Spider Veins

Spider veins are a smaller version of varicose veins and a less serious type of telangiectasias. Spider veins involve the capillaries, the smallest blood vessels in the body.

Spider veins often appear on the legs and face. They're red or blue and usually look like a spider web or tree branch. These veins usually aren't a medical concern.

Varicoceles

Varicoceles are varicose veins in the scrotum (the skin over the testicles). Varicoceles may be linked to male infertility. If you think you have varicoceles, see your doctor.

Other Related Vein Problems

Other types of varicose veins include venous lakes, reticular veins, and hemorrhoids. Venous lakes are varicose veins that appear on the face and neck. Reticular veins are flat blue veins often seen behind the knees. Hemorrhoids are varicose veins in and around the anus.

What Causes Varicose Veins?

Weak or damaged valves in the veins can cause varicose veins. After your arteries and capillaries deliver oxygen-rich blood to your body, your veins return the blood to your heart. The veins in your legs must work against gravity to do this.

One-way valves inside the veins open to let blood flow through, and then they shut to keep blood from flowing backward. If the valves are weak or damaged, blood can back up and pool in your veins. This causes the veins to swell.

Weak vein walls may cause weak valves. Normally, the walls of the veins are elastic (stretchy). If these walls become weak, they lose their normal elasticity. They become like an overstretched rubber band. This makes the walls of the veins longer and wider, and it causes the flaps of the valves to separate.

When the valve flaps separate, blood can flow backward through the valves. The backflow of blood fills the veins and stretches the walls even more. As a result, the veins get bigger, swell, and often twist as they try to squeeze into their normal space. These are varicose veins.

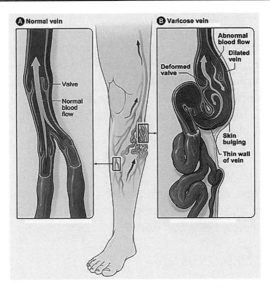

Figure 28.1. *Normal Vein and Varicose Vein*

(A) shows a normal vein with a working valve and normal blood flow. (B) shows a varicose vein with a deformed valve, abnormal blood flow, and thin, stretched walls. The middle image shows where varicose veins might appear in a leg.

Older age or a family history of varicose veins may raise your risk for weak vein walls. You also may be at higher risk if you have increased pressure in your veins due to overweight or obesity or pregnancy.

Who Is at Risk for Varicose Veins?

Many factors may raise your risk for varicose veins, including family history, older age, gender, pregnancy, overweight or obesity, lack of movement, and leg trauma.

Family History

Having family members who have varicose veins may raise your risk for the condition. About half of all people who have varicose veins have a family history of them.

Older Age

Getting older may raise your risk for varicose veins. The normal wear and tear of aging may cause the valves in your veins to weaken and not work well.

Gender

Women tend to get varicose veins more often than men. Hormonal changes that occur during puberty, pregnancy, and menopause (or with the use of birth control pills) may raise a woman's risk for varicose veins.

Pregnancy

During pregnancy, the growing fetus puts pressure on the veins in the mother's legs. Varicose veins that occur during pregnancy usually get better within 3 to 12 months of delivery.

Overweight or Obesity

Being overweight or obese can put extra pressure on your veins. This can lead to varicose veins.

Lack of Movement

Standing or sitting for a long time, especially with your legs bent or crossed, may raise your risk for varicose veins. This is because staying in one position for a long time may force your veins to work harder to pump blood to your heart.

Leg Trauma

Previous blood clots or traumatic damage to the valves in your veins can weaken their ability to move blood back to the heart, increasing the risk for varicose veins.

What Are the Signs and Symptoms of Varicose Veins?

The signs and symptoms of varicose veins include:

- Large veins that you can see just under the surface of your skin.
- Mild swelling of your ankles and feet.
- Painful, achy, or "heavy" legs.
- Throbbing or cramping in your legs.
- Itchy legs, especially on the lower leg and ankle. Sometimes this symptom is incorrectly diagnosed as dry skin.

• Discolored skin in the area around the varicose vein.

Signs of telangiectasias are clusters of red veins that you can see just under the surface of your skin. These clusters usually are found on the upper body, including the face. Signs of spider veins are red or blue veins in a web or tree branch pattern. Often, these veins appear on the legs and face.

See your doctor if you have these signs and symptoms. They also may be signs of other, more serious conditions.

Complications of Varicose Veins

Varicose veins can lead to dermatitis, an itchy rash. If you have varicose veins in your legs, dermatitis may affect your lower leg or ankle. Dermatitis can cause bleeding or skin ulcers (sores) if the skin is scratched or irritated.

Varicose veins also can lead to a condition called superficial thrombophlebitis. Thrombophlebitis is a blood clot in a vein. Superficial thrombophlebitis means that the blood clot occurs in a vein close to the surface of the skin. This type of blood clot may cause pain and other problems in the affected area.

How Are Varicose Veins Diagnosed?

Doctors often diagnose varicose veins based on a physical exam alone. Sometimes tests or procedures are used to find out the extent of the problem or to rule out other conditions.

Specialists Involved

If you have varicose veins, you may see a vascular medicine specialist or vascular surgeon. These doctors specialize in blood vessel conditions. You also may see a dermatologist. This type of doctor specializes in skin conditions.

Physical Exam

To check for varicose veins in your legs, your doctor will look at your legs while you're standing or sitting with your legs dangling. He or she may ask you about your signs and symptoms, including any pain you're having.

Diagnostic Tests and Procedures

Duplex Ultrasound

Your doctor may recommend duplex ultrasound to check blood flow in your veins and to look for blood clots. Duplex ultrasound combines traditional with Doppler ultrasound. Traditional ultrasound uses sound waves to create a picture of the structures in your body, in this case the blood vessels and anything that may be blocking the flow of blood. Doppler ultrasound uses sound waves to create pictures of the flow or movement of the blood through the veins. The two types of ultrasound together paint a picture that helps your doctor diagnose your condition.

During this test, a handheld device will be placed on your body and passed back and forth over the affected area. The device sends and receives sound waves. A computer will convert the sound waves into a picture of the blood flow in your arteries and veins.

Angiogram

Although it is not very common, your doctor may recommend an angiogram to get a more detailed look at the blood flow through your veins.

For this procedure, dye is injected into your veins. The dye outlines your veins on X-ray images.

An angiogram can help your doctor confirm whether you have varicose veins or another condition.

How Are Varicose Veins Treated?

Varicose veins are treated with lifestyle changes and medical procedures. The goals of treatment are to relieve symptoms, prevent complications, and improve appearance.

If varicose veins cause few symptoms, your doctor may simply suggest making lifestyle changes. If your symptoms are more severe, your doctor may recommend one or more medical procedures. For example, you may need a medical procedure if you have a lot of pain, blood clots, or skin disorders caused by your varicose veins.

Some people who have varicose veins choose to have procedures to improve how their veins look.

Although treatment can help existing varicose veins, it can't keep new varicose veins from forming.

Lifestyle Changes

Lifestyle changes often are the first treatment for varicose veins. These changes can prevent varicose veins from getting worse, reduce pain, and delay other varicose veins from forming. Lifestyle changes include the following:

- Avoid standing or sitting for long periods without taking a break. When sitting, avoid crossing your legs. Keep your legs raised when sitting, resting, or sleeping. When you can, raise your legs above the level of your heart.

- Do physical activities to get your legs moving and improve muscle tone. This helps blood move through your veins.

- If you're overweight or obese, try to lose weight. This will improve blood flow and ease the pressure on your veins.

- Avoid wearing tight clothes, especially those that are tight around your waist, groin (upper thighs), and legs. Tight clothes can make varicose veins worse.

- Avoid wearing high heels for long periods. Lower heeled shoes can help tone your calf muscles. Toned muscles help blood move through the veins.

Your doctor may recommend compression stockings. These stockings create gentle pressure up the leg. This pressure keeps blood from pooling and decreases swelling in the legs.

There are three types of compression stockings. One type is support pantyhose. These offer the least amount of pressure. A second type is over-the-counter compression hose. These stockings give a little more pressure than support pantyhose. Over-the-counter compression hose are sold in medical supply stores and pharmacies.

Prescription-strength compression hose are the third type of compression stockings. These stockings offer the greatest amount of pressure. They also are sold in medical supply stores and pharmacies. However, you need to be fitted for them in the store by a specially trained person.

Medical Procedures

Medical procedures are done either to remove varicose veins or to close them. Removing or closing varicose veins usually doesn't cause problems with blood flow because the blood starts moving through other veins.

You may be treated with one or more of the procedures described below. Common side effects right after most of these procedures include bruising, swelling, skin discoloration, and slight pain.

The side effects are most severe with vein stripping and ligation. Rarely, this procedure can cause severe pain, infections, blood clots, and scarring.

Sclerotherapy

Sclerotherapy uses a liquid chemical to close off a varicose vein. The chemical is injected into the vein to cause irritation and scarring inside the vein. The irritation and scarring cause the vein to close off, and it fades away.

This procedure often is used to treat smaller varicose veins and spider veins. It can be done in your doctor's office, while you stand. You may need several treatments to completely close off a vein.

Treatments typically are done every 4 to 6 weeks. Following treatments, your legs will be wrapped in elastic bandaging to help with healing and decrease swelling.

Microsclerotherapy

Microsclerotherapy is used to treat spider veins and other very small varicose veins.

A small amount of liquid chemical is injected into a vein using a very fine needle. The chemical scars the inner lining of the vein, causing it to close off.

Laser Surgery

This procedure applies light energy from a laser onto a varicose vein. The laser light makes the vein fade away.

Laser surgery mostly is used to treat smaller varicose veins. No cutting or injection of chemicals is involved.

Endovenous Ablation Therapy

Endovenous ablation therapy uses lasers or radiowaves to create heat to close off a varicose vein.

Your doctor makes a tiny cut in your skin near the varicose vein. He or she then inserts a small tube called a catheter into the vein. A device at the tip of the tube heats up the inside of the vein and closes it off.

You'll be awake during this procedure, but your doctor will numb the area around the vein. You usually can go home the same day as the procedure.

Endoscopic Vein Surgery

For endoscopic vein surgery, your doctor will make a small cut in your skin near a varicose vein. He or she then uses a tiny camera at the end of a thin tube to move through the vein. A surgical device at the end of the camera is used to close the vein.

Endoscopic vein surgery usually is used only in severe cases when varicose veins are causing skin ulcers (sores). After the procedure, you usually can return to your normal activities within a few weeks.

Ambulatory Phlebectomy

For ambulatory phlebectomy, your doctor will make small cuts in your skin to remove small varicose veins. This procedure usually is done to remove the varicose veins closest to the surface of your skin.

You'll be awake during the procedure, but your doctor will numb the area around the vein. Usually, you can go home the same day that the procedure is done.

Vein Stripping and Ligation

Vein stripping and ligation typically is done only for severe cases of varicose veins. The procedure involves tying shut and removing the veins through small cuts in your skin.

You'll be given medicine to temporarily put you to sleep so you don't feel any pain during the procedure.

Vein stripping and ligation usually is done as an outpatient procedure. The recovery time from the procedure is about 1 to 4 weeks.

Living with Varicose Veins

Varicose veins are a common condition. They often cause few signs and symptoms. If your signs and symptoms are minor, your doctor may simply suggest making lifestyle changes.

If your condition is more severe—for example, if you have pain, blood clots, or skin ulcers (sores)—your doctor may recommend one or more medical procedures. Many treatments for varicose veins are quick and easy and don't require a long recovery.

Chapter 29

Vasculitis

What Is Vasculitis?

Vasculitis is a condition that involves inflammation in the blood vessels. The condition occurs if your immune system attacks your blood vessels by mistake. This may happen as the result of an infection, a medicine, or another disease or condition.

"Inflammation" refers to the body's response to injury, including injury to the blood vessels. Inflammation may involve pain, redness, warmth, swelling, and loss of function in the affected tissues.

In vasculitis, inflammation can lead to serious problems. Complications depend on which blood vessels, organs, or other body systems are affected.

Types of Vasculitis

There are many types of vasculitis. Each type involves inflamed blood vessels. However, most types differ in whom they affect and the organs that are involved.

The types of vasculitis often are grouped based on the size of the blood vessels they affect.

This chapter includes text excerpted from "Vasculitis," National Heart, Lung, and Blood Institute (NHLBI), September 23, 2014.

Mostly Large Vessel Vasculitis

These types of vasculitis usually, but not always, affect the body's larger blood vessels.

Behçet's Disease

Behçet's disease can cause recurrent, painful ulcers (sores) in the mouth, ulcers on the genitals, acne-like skin lesions, and eye inflammation called uveitis.

The disease occurs most often in people aged 20 to 40. Men are more likely to get it, but it also can affect women. Behçet's disease is more common in people of Mediterranean, Middle Eastern, and Far Eastern descent, although it rarely affects Blacks.

Researchers believe that a gene called the HLA-B51 gene may play a role in Behçet's disease. However, not everyone who has the gene gets the disease.

Cogan's Syndrome

Cogan's syndrome can occur in people who have a systemic vasculitis that affects the large blood vessels, especially the aorta and aortic valve. The aorta is the main artery that carries oxygen-rich blood from the heart to the body.

A systemic vasculitis is a type of vasculitis that affects you in a general or overall way.

Cogan's syndrome can lead to eye inflammation called interstitial keratitis. The syndrome also can cause hearing changes, including sudden deafness.

Giant Cell Arteritis

Giant cell arteritis usually affects the temporal artery, an artery on the side of your head. This condition also is called temporal arteritis. Symptoms of this condition can include headaches, scalp tenderness, jaw pain, blurred vision, double vision, and acute (sudden) vision loss.

Giant cell arteritis is the most common form of vasculitis in adults older than 50. It's more likely to occur in people of Scandinavian origin, but it can affect people of any race.

Polymyalgia Rheumatica

Polymyalgia rheumatica, or PMR, commonly affects the large joints in the body, such as the shoulders and hips. PMR typically causes stiffness and pain in the muscles of the neck, shoulders, lower back, hips, and thighs.

PMR usually occurs by itself, but 10–20 percent of people who have PMR also develop giant cell arteritis. Also, about half of the people who have giant cell arteritis may develop PMR.

Takayasu's Arteritis

Takayasu's arteritis affects medium- and large-sized arteries, particularly the aorta and its branches. The condition sometimes is called aortic arch syndrome.

Though rare, Takayasu's arteritis mainly affects teenage girls and young women. The condition is most common in Asians, but it can affect people of all races.

Takayasu's arteritis is a systemic disease. A systemic disease is one that affects you in a general or overall way.

Symptoms of Takayasu's arteritis may include tiredness and a sense of feeling unwell, fever, night sweats, sore joints, loss of appetite, and weight loss. These symptoms usually occur before other signs develop that point to arteritis.

Mostly Medium Vessel Vasculitis

These types of vasculitis usually, but not always, affect the body's medium-sized blood vessels.

Buerger's Disease

Buerger's disease, also known as thromboangiitis obliterans, typically affects blood flow to the hands and feet. In this disease, the blood vessels in the hands and feet tighten or become blocked. As a result, less blood flows to the affected tissues, which can lead to pain and tissue damage.

Rarely, Buerger's disease also can affect blood vessels in the brain, abdomen, and heart. The disease usually affects men aged 20 to 40 of Asian or Eastern European descent. The disease is strongly linked to cigarette smoking.

Symptoms of Buerger's disease include pain in the calves or feet when walking or pain in the forearms and hands with activity. Other symptoms include blood clots in the surface veins of the limbs and Raynaud's phenomenon.

In severe cases, ulcers may develop on the fingers and toes, leading to gangrene. The term "gangrene" refers to the death or decay of body tissues.

Surgical bypass of the blood vessels may help restore blood flow to some areas. Medicines generally don't work well to treat Buerger's disease. The best treatment is to stop using tobacco of any kind.

Central Nervous System Vasculitis

Central nervous system (CNS) vasculitis usually occurs as a result of a systemic vasculitis. A systemic vasculitis is one that affects you in a general or overall way.

Very rarely, vasculitis affects only the brain and/or spinal cord. When it does, the condition is called isolated vasculitis of the central nervous system or primary angiitis of the central nervous system.

Symptoms of CNS vasculitis include headaches, problems thinking clearly, changes in mental function, or stroke-like symptoms, such as muscle weakness and paralysis (an inability to move).

Kawasaki Disease

Kawasaki disease is a rare childhood disease in which the walls of the blood vessels throughout the body become inflamed. The disease can affect any blood vessel in the body, including arteries, veins, and capillaries.

Kawasaki disease also is known as mucocutaneous lymph node syndrome. This is because the disease is associated with redness of the mucous membranes in the eyes and mouth, redness of the skin, and enlarged lymph nodes. (Mucous membranes are tissues that line some organs and body cavities.)

Sometimes the disease affects the coronary arteries, which carry oxygen-rich blood to the heart. As a result, a small number of children who have Kawasaki disease may have serious heart problems.

Polyarteritis Nodosa

Polyarteritis nodosa can affect many parts of the body. This disorder often affects the kidneys, the digestive tract, the nerves, and the skin.

Symptoms often include fever, a general feeling of being unwell, weight loss, and muscle and joint aches, including pain in the calf muscles that develops over weeks or months.

Other signs and symptoms include anemia (a low red blood cell count), a lace- or web-like rash, bumps under the skin, and stomach pain after eating.

Researchers believe that this type of vasculitis is very rare, although the symptoms can be similar to those of other types of vasculitis. Some cases of polyarteritis nodosa seem to be linked to hepatitis B or C infections.

Mostly Small Vessel Vasculitis

These types of vasculitis usually, but not always, affect the body's small blood vessels.

Eosinophilic Granulomatosis with Polyangiitis

Eosinophilic granulomatosis with polyangiitis, or EGPA is a very rare disorder that causes blood vessel inflammation. The disorder is also known as Churg-Strauss syndrome or allergic angiitis and granulomatosis.

EGPA can affect many organs, including the lungs, skin, kidneys, nervous system, and heart. Symptoms can vary widely. They may include asthma, higher than normal levels of white blood cells in the blood and tissues, and abnormal lumps known as granulomas.

Cryoglobulinemia Vasculitis

Cryoglobulinemic vasculitis occurs when abnormal immune proteins (cryoglobulins) thicken the blood and impair blood flow. This causes pain and damage to the skin, joints, peripheral nerves, kidneys, and liver.

Cryoglobulins are abnormal immune proteins in the blood that clump together and thicken the blood plasma. Cryoglobulins can be detected in the laboratory by exposing a sample of blood to cold temperature (below normal body temperature). In cold temperatures, the immune proteins form clumps; but when the blood is rewarmed, the clumps dissolve.

The cause of cryoglobulinemic vasculitis is not always known. In some cases, it is associated with other conditions such as lymphoma, multiple myeloma, connective tissue diseases, and infection (particularly hepatitis C infection).

IgA Vasculitis

In IgA (immunoglobulin A) vasculitis (also known as Henoch-Schonlein purpura), abnormal IgA deposits develop in small blood vessels in the skin, joints, intestines, and kidneys. IgA a type of antibody (a protein) that normally helps defend the body against infections.

Symptoms of IgA vasculitis include a bruise-like, reddish-purple rash, most often seen on the buttocks, legs, and feet (but can be anywhere on the body); abdominal pain; swollen and painful joints; and blood in the urine. People with IgA vasculitis do not necessarily have all of the symptoms, but nearly all will have the characteristic rash.

IgA vasculitis is most often seen in children between 2 and 11 years of age, but it can affect people of all ages. More than 75 percent of the cases of IgA vasculitis follow an upper respiratory tract infection, a throat infection, or a gastrointestinal infection.

Most people with IgA vasculitis are well within 1 to 2 months and do not have any lasting problems. In rare cases symptoms can last longer or come back. All IgA vasculitis patients should have a full evaluation by a medical professional.

Hypersensitivity Vasculitis

Hypersensitivity vasculitis affects the skin. This condition also is known as allergic vasculitis, cutaneous vasculitis, or leukocytoclastic vasculitis.

A common symptom is red spots on the skin, usually on the lower legs. For people who are bedridden, the rash appears on the lower back.

An allergic reaction to a medicine or infection often causes this type of vasculitis. Stopping the medicine or treating the infection usually clears up the vasculitis. However, some people may need to take anti-inflammatory medicines, such as corticosteroids, for a short time. These medicines help reduce inflammation.

Microscopic Polyangiitis

Microscopic polyangiitis affects small blood vessels, particularly those in the kidneys and lungs. The disease mainly occurs in middle-aged people; it affects men slightly more often than women.

The symptoms often aren't specific, and they can begin gradually with fever, weight loss, and muscle aches. Sometimes the symptoms come on suddenly and progress quickly, leading to kidney failure.

If the lungs are affected, coughing up blood may be the first symptom. Sometimes microscopic polyangiitis occurs with a vasculitis that affects the intestinal tract, the skin, and the nervous system.

The signs and symptoms of microscopic polyangiitis are similar to those of Wegener's granulomatosis (another type of vasculitis). However, microscopic polyangiitis usually doesn't affect the nose and sinuses or cause abnormal tissue formations in the lungs and kidneys.

The results of certain blood tests can suggest inflammation. These results include a higher than normal erythrocyte sedimentation rate (ESR); lower than normal hemoglobin and hematocrit levels (which suggest anemia); and higher than normal white blood cell and platelet counts.

Also, more than half of the people who have microscopic polyangiitis have certain antibodies (proteins) in their blood. These antibodies are called antineutrophil cytoplasmic autoantibodies (ANCA). ANCA also occur in people who have Wegener's granulomatosis.

Testing for ANCA can't be used to diagnose either of these two types of vasculitis. However, testing can help evaluate people who have vasculitis-like symptoms.

Other Names for Vasculitis

- Angiitis

- Arteritis

What Causes Vasculitis?

Vasculitis occurs if your immune system attacks your blood vessels by mistake. What causes this to happen isn't fully known.

A recent or chronic (ongoing) infection may prompt the attack. Your body also may attack its own blood vessels in reaction to a medicine.

Sometimes an autoimmune disorder triggers vasculitis. Autoimmune disorders occur if the immune system makes antibodies (proteins) that attack and damage the body's own tissues or cells. Examples of these disorders include lupus, rheumatoid arthritis, and scleroderma. You can have these disorders for years before developing vasculitis.

Vasculitis also may be linked to certain blood cancers, such as leukemia and lymphoma.

Who Is at Risk for Vasculitis?

Vasculitis can affect people of all ages and races and both sexes. Some types of vasculitis seem to occur more often in people who:

- Have certain medical conditions, such as chronic hepatitis B or C infection

- Have certain autoimmune diseases, such a lupus, rheumatoid arthritis, and scleroderma

- Smoke

What Are the Signs and Symptoms of Vasculitis?

The signs and symptoms of vasculitis vary. They depend on the type of vasculitis you have, the organs involved, and the severity of the condition. Some people may have few signs and symptoms. Other people may become very sick.

Sometimes the signs and symptoms develop slowly, over months. Other times, the signs and symptoms develop quickly, over days or weeks.

Systemic Signs and Symptoms

Systemic signs and symptoms are those that affect you in a general or overall way. Common systemic signs and symptoms of vasculitis are:

- Fever

- Loss of appetite

- Weight loss

- Fatigue (tiredness)

- General aches and pains

Organ- or Body System-Specific Signs and Symptoms

Vasculitis can affect specific organs and body systems, causing a range of signs and symptoms.

Skin

If vasculitis affects your skin, you may notice skin changes. For example, you may have purple or red spots or bumps, clusters of small dots, splotches, bruises, or hives. Your skin also may itch.

Joints

If vasculitis affects your joints, you may ache or develop arthritis in one or more joints.

Lungs

If vasculitis affects your lungs, you may feel short of breath. You may even cough up blood. The results from a chest X-ray may show signs that suggest pneumonia, even though that may not be what you have.

Gastrointestinal Tract

If vasculitis affects your gastrointestinal tract, you may get ulcers (sores) in your mouth or have stomach pain.

In severe cases, blood flow to the intestines can be blocked. This can cause the wall of the intestines to weaken and possibly rupture (burst). A rupture can lead to serious problems or even death.

Sinuses, Nose, Throat, and Ears

If vasculitis affects your sinuses, nose, throat, and ears, you may have sinus or chronic (ongoing) middle ear infections. Other symptoms include ulcers in the nose and, in some cases, hearing loss.

Eyes

If vasculitis affects your eyes, you may develop red, itchy, burning eyes. Your eyes also may become sensitive to light, and your vision may blur. Rarely, certain types of vasculitis may cause blindness.

Brain

If vasculitis affects your brain, symptoms may include headaches, problems thinking clearly, changes in mental function, or stroke-like symptoms, such as muscle weakness and paralysis (an inability to move).

Nerves

If vasculitis affects your nerves, you may have numbness, tingling, and weakness in various parts of your body. You also may have a loss of feeling or strength in your hands and feet and shooting pains in your arms and legs.

How Is Vasculitis Diagnosed?

Your doctor will diagnose vasculitis based on your signs and symptoms, your medical history, a physical exam, and test results.

Specialists Involved

Depending on the type of vasculitis you have and the organs affected, your doctor may refer you to various specialists, including:

- A rheumatologist (joint and muscle specialist)

- An infectious disease specialist
- A dermatologist (skin specialist)
- A pulmonologist (lung specialist)
- A nephrologist (kidney specialist)
- A neurologist (nervous system specialist)
- A cardiologist (heart specialist)
- An ophthalmologist (eye specialist)
- A urologist (urinary tract and urogenital system specialist)

Diagnostic Tests and Procedures

Many tests are used to diagnose vasculitis.

- Blood Tests
- Biopsy
- Blood Pressure
- Urinalysis
- EKG (Electrocardiogram)
- Echocardiography
- Chest X-Ray
- Lung Function Tests
- Abdominal Ultrasound
- Computed Tomography Scan
- Magnetic Resonance Imaging

Other Advanced Imaging Techniques

Several new imaging techniques are now being used to help diagnose vasculitis. Duplex ultrasonography combines an image of the structure of the blood vessel with a color image of the blood flow through that vein or artery. 18F-fluorodeoxyglucose positron emission tomography (FDG-PET) identifies areas that show higher glucose metabolism leading to problems in the blood vessels.

Angiography

Angiography is a test that uses dye and special X-rays to show blood flowing through your blood vessels.

The dye is injected into your bloodstream. Special X-ray pictures are taken while the dye flows through your blood vessels. The dye helps highlight the vessels on the X-ray pictures.

How Is Vasculitis Treated?

Treatment for vasculitis will depend on the type of vasculitis you have, which organs are affected, and the severity of the condition.

People who have severe vasculitis are treated with prescription medicines. Rarely, surgery may be done. People who have mild vasculitis may find relief with over-the-counter pain medicines, such as acetaminophen, aspirin, ibuprofen, or naproxen.

The main goal of treating vasculitis is to reduce inflammation in the affected blood vessels. This usually is done by reducing or stopping the immune response that caused the inflammation.

Types of Treatment

Common prescription medicines used to treat vasculitis include corticosteroids and cytotoxic medicines.

Corticosteroids help reduce inflammation in your blood vessels. Examples of corticosteroids are prednisone, prednisolone, and methylprednisolone.

Doctors may prescribe **cytotoxic medicines** if vasculitis is severe or if corticosteroids don't work well. Cytotoxic medicines kill the cells that are causing the inflammation. Examples of these medicines are azathioprine, methotrexate, and cyclophosphamide.

Your doctor may prescribe both corticosteroids and cytotoxic medicines.

Other treatments may be used for certain types of vasculitis. For example, the standard treatment for Kawasaki disease is high-dose aspirin and immune globulin. Immune globulin is a medicine that's injected into a vein.

Certain types of vasculitis may require surgery to remove aneurysms that have formed as a result of the condition. (An aneurysm is an abnormal bulge in the wall of a blood vessel.)

Can Vasculitis Be Prevented?

No, you can't prevent vasculitis. However, treatment can help prevent or delay the complications of vasculitis.

People who have severe vasculitis are treated with prescription medicines. Rarely, surgery may be done. People who have mild vasculitis may find relief with over-the-counter pain medicines, such as acetaminophen, aspirin, ibuprofen, or naproxen.

Part Four

Cardiovascular Disorders in Specific Populations

Chapter 30

Cardiovascular Disease in Children

Chapter Contents

Section 30.1

Basic Facts about Congenital Heart Defects

This section contains text excerpted from the following sources: Text
beginning with the heading "What are Congenital Heart Defects
(CHDs)?" is excerpted from "Congenital Heart Defects (CHDs),"
Centers for Disease Control and Prevention (CDC), December 22,
2015; Text beginning with the heading "Common Heart Defects"
is excerpted from "Congenital Heart Defects," © 1995–2016. The
Nemours Foundation/KidsHealth®. Reprinted with permission;
Text beginning with the heading "Living with a Congenital Heart
Defect" is excerpted from "Congenital Heart Defects (CHDs),"
Centers for Disease Control and Prevention (CDC), May 18, 2016.

What are Congenital Heart Defects (CHDs)?

CHDs are present at birth and can affect the structure of a baby's
heart and the way it works. They can affect how blood flows through
the heart and out to the rest of the body. CHDs can vary from mild
(such as a small hole in the heart) to severe (such as missing or poorly
formed parts of the heart).

About 1 in 4 babies born with a heart defect has a critical CHD (also
known as critical congenital heart disease). Babies with a critical CHD
need surgery or other procedures in the first year of life.

Signs and Symptoms

Signs and symptoms for CHDs depend on the type and severity
of the particular defect. Some defects might have few or no signs
or symptoms. Others might cause a baby to have the following
symptoms:

- Blue-tinted nails or lips

- Fast or troubled breathing

- Tiredness when feeding

- Sleepiness

Diagnosis

Some CHDs may be diagnosed during pregnancy using a special type of ultrasound called a fetal echocardiogram, which creates ultrasound pictures of the heart of the developing baby. However, some CHDs are not detected until after birth or later in life, during childhood or adulthood. If a healthcare provider suspects a CHD may be present, the baby can get several tests (such as an echocardiogram) to confirm the diagnosis.

Treatment

Treatment for CHDs depends on the type and severity of the defect present. Some affected infants and children might need one or more surgeries to repair the heart or blood vessels. Some can be treated without surgery using a procedure called cardiac catheterization. A long tube, called a catheter, is threaded through the blood vessels into the heart, where a doctor can take measurements and pictures, do tests, or repair the problem. Sometimes the heart defect can't be fully repaired, but these procedures can improve blood flow and the way the heart works.

Causes

The causes of CHDs among most babies are unknown. Some babies have heart defects because of changes in their individual genes or chromosomes. CHDs also are thought to be caused by a combination of genes and other factors, such as things in the environment, the mother's diet, the mother's health conditions, or the mother's medication use during pregnancy. For example, certain conditions a mother has, like pre-existing diabetes or obesity, have been linked to heart defects in the baby. In addition, smoking during pregnancy as well as taking certain medications have also been linked to heart defects.

Common Heart Defects

Common types of congenital heart defects, which can affect any part of the heart or its surrounding structures, include:

Aortic Stenosis

In aortic stenosis, the aortic valve is stiffened and has a narrowed opening (a condition called stenosis). It does not open properly, which increases strain on the heart because the left ventricle has to pump harder to send blood out to the body. Sometimes the aortic valve also does not close properly, causing it to leak, a condition called aortic regurgitation.

Atrial Septal Defect (ASD)

ASD is a hole in the wall (called the septum) that separates the left atrium and the right atrium. This wall is called the atrial septum. When this hole is present, it allows extra blood flow to travel from the left atrium into the right heart and out to the lungs.

Atrioventricular Canal Defect

This defect—also known as endocardial cushion defect or atrioventricular septal defect—is caused by a poorly formed central area of the heart. Typically, there is a large hole between the upper chambers of the heart (the atria) and, often, an additional hole between the lower chambers of the heart (the ventricles). Instead of two separate valves allowing flow into the heart (tricuspid on the right and mitral valve on the left), there is one large common valve, which may be quite malformed. Atrioventricular canal defect is commonly seen in children with Down syndrome.

Coarctation of the Aorta

Coarctation of the aorta is a narrowing of a portion of the aorta, and often seriously decreases the blood flow from the heart out to the lower portion of the body.

Hypoplastic Left Heart Syndrome

When the structures of the left side of the heart (the left ventricle, the mitral valve, and the aortic valve) are underdeveloped, they're unable to pump blood adequately to the entire body. This condition is usually diagnosed within the first few days of life, at which point the baby may be critically ill.

Fortunately, many of these infants are recognized to have serious heart disease even before birth on ultrasound tests. A fetal echocardiogram is a specialized ultrasound that allows doctors to see the baby's heart in great detail and plan the best care for the baby while still in utero.

Patent Ductus Arteriosus (PDA)

The ductus arteriosus is a normal blood vessel in the developing fetus that diverts blood away from the lungs and sends it directly to the body. (The lungs are not used while the unborn fetus is in amniotic fluid—the fetus gets oxygen directly from the mother's placenta.) The ductus usually closes on its own shortly after birth; it is no longer needed once a newborn breathes independently. Patent ductus arteriosus (PDA) occurs when the ductus doesn't close, which can result in too much blood flow to a newborn's lungs. PDA is common in premature babies.

Patent Foramen Ovale (PFO)

The patent foramen ovale is a normal hole between the upper chambers of the heart. It is present in the unborn fetus and usually seals up in the first few months of life. In approximately 25% of people, this hole never fully closes. Usually, it does not cause problems and does not require treatment.

Pulmonary Atresia

In this defect, the pulmonic valve does not open at all and may indeed be completely absent, so that no blood can flow from the right ventricle to the lungs. The pulmonary artery, the main blood vessel that runs between the right ventricle and the lungs, also might be malformed, and the right ventricle may be too small. These babies usually appear blue (cyanotic) after birth and need immediate specialized care.

Pulmonary Stenosis

In pulmonary stenosis, the pulmonic valve is stiffened and has a narrowed opening (called stenosis). It does not open properly, which may increase strain on the right side of the heart because the right ventricle has to pump harder to send blood out to the lungs. If mild, pulmonary stenosis may never require any treatment.

Tetralogy of Fallot (TOF)

Tetralogy of Fallot is actually a combination of four heart defects: pulmonary stenosis; a thickened right ventricle (ventricular hypertrophy); a hole between the lower chambers (ventricular septal defect); and an aorta that can receive blood from both the left and right ventricles, instead of draining just the left. Because oxygen-poor (blue) blood can flow out to the body, children with this defect often appear bluish.

Total Anomalous Pulmonary Venous Connection

The pulmonary veins normally are the blood vessels that deliver oxygen-rich blood from the lungs to the left atrium. Sometimes these vessels don't join the left atrium during development. Instead they deliver blood to the heart by other pathways, which may be narrowed. Pressure builds up in this pathway and in the pulmonary veins, pushing fluid into the lungs, which decreases the amount of oxygen-rich blood that reaches the body. These infants often have trouble breathing and appear blue.

Transposition of the Great Arteries

In this condition, the pulmonary artery and the aorta (the major blood vessels leaving the heart) are switched so that the aorta arises from the right side of the heart and receives blue blood, which is sent right back out to the body without becoming oxygen-rich. The pulmonary artery arises from the left side of the heart, receives red blood and sends it back to the lungs again. As a result, babies with this condition often appear very blue and have low oxygen levels in the bloodstream. They usually come to medical attention within the first days after birth.

Tricuspid Atresia

Blood normally flows from the right atrium to the right ventricle through the tricuspid valve. In tricuspid atresia, the valve is replaced by a plate or membrane that does not open. The right ventricle therefore does not receive blood normally and is often small. Babies with this defect often appear bluish after birth and may need specialized care early in life.

Truncus Arteriosus

In an embryo, the aorta and the pulmonary artery are initially a single vessel. During normal development, that vessel splits to form the two major arteries, the aorta and the pulmonary artery. If that split does not occur, the child is born with a single common great blood vessel called the truncus arteriosus. There usually is a hole between the ventricles associated with this defect. The valve leading into the truncus arteriosus may be very abnormal.

Ventricular Septal Defect (VSD)

One of the most common congenital heart defects, VSD is a hole in the wall (septum) between the heart's left and right ventricles. These can occur at different locations and vary in size from very small to very large. Some of the smaller defects may gradually close on their own.

Living with Congenital Heart Defect

As medical care and treatment have improved, babies and children with CHDs are living longer and healthier lives. Most are now living into adulthood. Ongoing, appropriate medical care can help children and adults with a CHD live as healthy as possible.

Healthcare

It is important for parents of children with a heart defect and adults living with a heart defect to talk with a heart doctor (cardiologist) regularly. Regular visits with a cardiologist are important, because they allow the parents of children with heart defects to make the best possible choices for the health of their child. These visits also allow adults living with a heart defect to make the best possible choices for their own health.

Children and adults with CHDs can help with their healthcare by knowing their medical history, including the:

- Type(s) of heart defect(s) they have.

- Procedures or surgeries they have had performed.

- Medicines and doses of these medicines that they are prescribed currently and were prescribed in the past.

- Type(s) of medical care they are receiving now.

As children transition to adult healthcare, it is important to notify any new healthcare provider(s) about the child's CHD. Ongoing appropriate medical care for their specific heart defect will help children and adults with a CHD to live as healthy a life as possible.

Care across the Lifespan

At this time, even with improved treatments, many people with a CHD are not cured, even if their heart defect has been repaired. As a person with a heart defect grows and gets older, further heart problems may occur. Additional medications, surgeries, or other procedures may be needed after the initial childhood surgeries. Some people with heart defects need lifelong care to stay as healthy as possible and address certain health issues:

Nutrition

Some babies with a CHD can become tired while feeding and might not eat enough to gain weight. Furthermore, because of the extra work that their heart may have to do to compensate for having a defect, some children with CHDs burn more calories. As they grow up, these children might be smaller and thinner than other children. After treatment for their heart defect, growth and weight gain often improve. It is important to talk with a healthcare provider about diet and nutrition.

Medications

Some children and adults with a CHD will need medicine to help with problems associated with their heart defect. For example, some medicines help make the heart stronger, and others help lower blood pressure. It is important for children and adults with a CHD to take medications as prescribed.

Physical activity

Physical activity is an important part of staying healthy, and it can help the heart become strong. Adults and parents of children with a CHD should discuss with their healthcare providers which physical activities are safe for them or their children, respectively, and if there are any physical activities that should be avoided.

Pregnancy

Women with CHDs who are considering having a baby should talk with a healthcare provider before becoming pregnant to discuss how the pregnancy might affect them or their baby, or both. Many women with a heart defect have healthy, uneventful pregnancies. However, having a CHD is the most common heart problem for pregnant women. Pregnancy can put stress on the heart of women with some types of heart defects. The woman might need to have procedures done related to her heart condition before becoming pregnant or take certain medications to help her heart during pregnancy. Her baby also might be at risk for having a heart defect, so talking with a genetic counselor could be helpful.

Other Potential Health Problems

Many people with a CHD live independent lives. Some people with a heart defect have little or no disability. For others, disability might increase or develop over time. People with a heart defect might also have genetic problems or other health conditions that increase the risk for disability. People with a CHD can develop other health problems related to their heart defect over time. These problems may depend on their specific heart defect, the number of heart defects they have, and the severity of their heart defect.

Some health problems that might need treatment include:

Infective Endocarditis

Infective endocarditis is an infection in the layers of the heart. If left untreated, it can lead to other problems, such as a blood clot, heart valve damage, or heart failure. It is recommend that individuals with certain heart defects take oral antibiotics before having certain procedures, such as dental or surgical procedures. However, these guidelines have been updated, and many people with a CHD, such as those with valve stenosis or an unrepaired ventricular septal defect, no longer need to take antibiotics before procedures. Each person should discuss his or her condition with the doctor to find out if antibiotics are recommended for him or her.

Arrhythmia

Arrhythmia is a problem with how the heart beats. The heart can beat too fast, too slow, or irregularly. This can lead to a problem with the heart not pumping enough blood out to the body and can increase the risk for blood clots. Some people with a heart defect can have an arrhythmia associated with their heart defect or as a result of past treatments or procedures for their heart defect. Some people can have an arrhythmia even in the absence of any heart defects.

Pulmonary Hypertension

Pulmonary hypertension is high blood pressure in the arteries (blood vessels) that lead from the heart to the lungs. Certain heart defects can cause pulmonary hypertension, which forces the heart and lungs to work harder. If the pulmonary hypertension is not treated, over time the right side of the heart can become enlarged, and heart failure can occur.

Liver Disease

People with single ventricle heart defects can develop liver disease associated with their heart defect or as a result of past treatments or procedures for their heart defect. It is important for people with this type of heart defect to see a healthcare provider regularly to stay as healthy as possible.

Section 30.2

Kawasaki Syndrome: A Disorder with Cardiovascular Implications

This section includes text excerpted from "Kawasaki Syndrome," Genetic and Rare Diseases Information Center (GARD), February 3, 2016.

Overview

Kawasaki syndrome is a condition that involves inflammation of the blood vessels. It is typically diagnosed in young children, but older children and adults can also develop this condition. Kawasaki syndrome often begins with a fever that lasts at least 5 days. Other classic symptoms may include red eyes, lips, and mouth; rash; swollen and red hands and feet; and swollen lymph nodes. Sometimes the condition affects the coronary arteries (which carry oxygen-rich blood to the heart). This can lead to serious heart problems. Kawasaki syndrome occurs most often in people of Asian and Pacific Island descent. The cause of Kawasaki disease is unknown. An infection along with genetic factors may be involved. Treatment includes intravenous gamma globulin and high doses of aspirin in a hospital setting.

Signs and Symptoms of Kawasaki Syndrome

- Cheilitis
- Glossitis
- Lymphadenopathy
- Inflammatory abnormality of the eye

- Proteinuria
- Recurrent pharyngitis
- Skin rash
- Vasculitis
- Abdominal pain
- Abnormality of nail color
- Abnormality of temperature regulation
- Abnormality of the heart valves
- Abnormality of the pericardium
- Arthritis
- Diarrhea
- Dry skin
- Edema
- Leukocytosis
- Abnormality of the myocardium
- Arrhythmia
- Arthralgia
- Aseptic leukocyturia
- Behavioral abnormality
- Biliary tract abnormality
- Congestive heart failure
- Coronary artery disease
- Cranial nerve paralysis
- Dilatation of the ascending aorta
- Meningitis
- Migraine
- Nausea and vomiting
- Ptosis
- Restrictive lung disease

What Genes Are Related to Kawasaki Syndrome?

A variation in the *ITPKC* gene has been associated with an increased risk of developing Kawasaki syndrome. This gene provides instructions for making an enzyme called inositol 1,4,5-triphosphate 3-kinase C. This enzyme helps limit the activity of immune system cells called T cells, which identify foreign substances and defend the body against infection. Reducing the activity of T cells when appropriate prevents the overproduction of immune proteins called cytokines that lead to inflammation and can, when present in large quantities, can cause tissue damage. Researchers believe that variations in the *ITPKC* gene may interfere with the body's ability to reduce T cell activity, leading to inflammation that damages blood vessels and results in the symptoms of this disease. It is likely that other factors, including changes in additional genes, also influence the development of this complex disorder.

What Causes Kawasaki Syndrome?

The cause of Kawasaki syndrome isn't known. The body's response to a virus or infection combined with genetic factors may cause the disease. However, no specific virus or infection has been found, and the role of genetics is not well understood. Kawasaki syndrome is not contagious; it can't be passed from one child to another.

Is Kawasaki Syndrome Inherited?

A predisposition to Kawasaki syndrome appears to be passed through generations in families, but the inheritance pattern is unknown.

How Might Kawasaki Disease Be Treated?

Intravenous gamma globulin is the standard treatment for Kawasaki disease and is administered in high doses. Children with Kawasaki disease usually greatly improve within 24 hours of treatment with IV gamma globulin. Aspirin is often given in combination with the IV gamma globulin as part of the treatment plan.

Section 30.3

Rheumatic Heart Disease in Children

"Rheumatic Heart Disease Is More Common in Children Than in Adults" © 2016 Omnigraphics. Reviewed June 2016.

Rheumatic Heart Disease

Rheumatic heart disease occurs when the heart sustains permanent damage from rheumatic fever. Rheumatic fever is a rare but serious illness caused by group A *streptococcus*, the bacterium responsible for strep throat infections. In rheumatic fever, the antibodies that the body produces to fight an untreated strep infection begin attacking the body's own tissues, causing a severe inflammatory response. Among other long-term effects, rheumatic fever can damage or scar the heart valves, reducing the heart's ability to pump blood through the body.

The use of antibiotics to treat strep throat has significantly reduced the incidence of rheumatic fever. The complication occurs in about 0.3% of people who contract strep throat, usually affecting children between the ages of 5 and 15. It is most common in lesser developed parts of the world, such as sub-Saharan Africa and south-central Asia, although it still occurs in poor, inner-city neighborhoods in the United States.

Symptoms

Rheumatic fever only occurs after a person has been infected by group A *streptococcus*. To prevent rheumatic fever, it is important to be aware of the symptoms of strep throat and treat the infection promptly with antibiotics. Experts recommend seeing a medical practitioner for a strep test if you notice the following symptoms:

- a sore throat, especially in the absence of cold symptoms
- swollen or tender lymph nodes
- a fever of 101°F or above
- inflamed tonsils, often with white patches
- a red rash
- small red spots on the roof of the mouth
- a thick, bloody discharge from the nose
- nausea or vomiting
- headache

The symptoms of rheumatic fever typically appear two to four weeks after the initial strep infection. The symptoms may persist for several weeks or even months. Although the symptoms vary widely, they may include the following:

- red, swollen, painful joints—especially the knees, ankles, elbows, and wrists
- nodules—or small, painless bumps—protruding under the skin of affected joints
- pain that migrates from one joint to another joint

- fever

- a red, raised rash on the chest, abdomen, or back

- weakness or shortness of breath

- lethargy, fatigue, or decreased attention span

- chest pain

- rapid fluttering or pounding heart palpitations

- nosebleeds

- stomach pain

- vomiting

- rapid, jerky, uncontrolled movements of the arms or legs, or twitching of the facial muscles (chorea)

- inappropriate emotional outbursts, such as laughing or crying

Diagnosis and Treatment

To diagnose rheumatic fever, doctors will first perform blood tests to check for the presence of strep bacteria. Next, they will look for inflammation in the joints, nodules beneath the skin, and a skin rash. They may also perform movement tests to detect chorea, or nervous system dysfunction.

In patients diagnosed with rheumatic fever, the most serious potential long-term complication is damage to the heart valves. Doctors will typically listen to the heart through a stethoscope to check for abnormalities. They may also perform additional tests, such as an electrocardiogram to measure the electrical activity in the heart muscle, or an echocardiogram to produce sound wave images of the heart.

In more than half of all cases of rheumatic fever, the patient develops rheumatic heart disease. Damage to the heart valves forces the heart muscle to work harder to circulate blood through the body. Eventually, the heart is unable to perform its vital function, leading to heart failure. Other heart conditions that may develop from rheumatic fever include valve stenosis, valve regurgitation, and atrial fibrillation.

The main treatment for rheumatic fever involves antibiotics to rid the body of group A *streptococcus*. Long-term antibiotic treatment may be prescribed to prevent the infection from taking hold again later. Other forms of treatment are generally used to control the symptoms of rheumatic fever and help patients feel more comfortable, including anti-inflammatory medications to reduce swelling and pain, anticon-vulsant medications to reduce involuntary movements, and bed rest or restricted activity to allow the heart to heal.

Prevention

The most effective methods of preventing rheumatic heart disease include avoiding strep infections, treating strep throat quickly and thoroughly with antibiotics, and being aware of risk factors for rheumatic fever.

Basic hygiene such as washing hands, covering the mouth when sneezing or coughing, and avoiding contact with people who are sick can help prevent strep infections. It is also important to recognize the symptoms of strep throat in children, seek medical attention promptly, and follow the recommended treatment—including completing the full course of antibiotics. It may also be a good idea to schedule a follow-up visit to ensure that patient is no longer producing antibodies to strep bacteria.

Although rheumatic fever is rare, certain factors may increase a person's risk of developing it. Some of the risk factors include a family history of the disease, the strain of strep bacteria that causes the initial infection, and poor sanitation and public health conditions often found in developing countries.

References

1. Johnson, Shannon. "Rheumatic Fever," Healthline, 2016.

2. "Understanding Rheumatic Fever—The Basics," WebMD, 2016.

Chapter 31

Cardiovascular Disease in Men

Chapter Contents

Section 31.1

Men and Cardiovascular Disease: A Statistical Overview

This section includes text excerpted from "Men and Heart Disease Fact Sheet," Centers for Disease Control and Prevention (CDC), November 30, 2015.

Heart Disease Facts in Men

- Heart disease is the leading cause of death for men in the United States, killing 307,225 men in 2009—that's **1 in every 4 male** deaths.

- Heart disease is the **leading cause** of death for men of most racial/ethnic groups in the United States, including African Americans, American Indians or Alaska Natives, Hispanics, and whites. For Asian American or Pacific Islander men, heart disease is second only to cancer.

- About 8.5% of all white men, 7.9% of black men, and 6.3% of Mexican American men have coronary heart disease.

- **Half** of the men who die suddenly of coronary heart disease have **no previous symptoms**. Even if you have no symptoms, you may still be at risk for heart disease.

- **Between 70% and 89%** of sudden cardiac events occur in men.

Risk Factors

High blood pressure, high LDL cholesterol, and smoking are key risk factors for heart disease. About **half of Americans** (49%) have at least one of these three risk factors.

Several other medical conditions and lifestyle choices can also put people at a higher risk for heart disease, including:

- Diabetes

- Overweight and obesity

- Poor diet

- Physical inactivity

- Excessive alcohol use

Section 31.2

Cardiovascular Implications of Erectile Dysfunction

"Cardiovascular Implications of Erectile Dysfunction," © 2016
Omnigraphics. Reviewed June 2016.

The inability to achieve or sustain an erection as needed for sexual intercourse is known as erectile dysfunction (ED) or impotence. It is believed to affect around 10 percent of adult men on a regular or long-term basis, while a much higher percentage of men experience occasional problems. Men who fail to achieve an erection more than half the time are considered to have a physical or psychological ailment that requires treatment.

A key reason to seek treatment for erectile dysfunction is that it is often linked to cardiovascular health. Studies have shown that ED is a major risk factor for heart disease. For men younger than 50, in fact, it carries a similar risk as smoking or a family history of coronary artery disease. In addition, obtaining treatment for current heart disease and related conditions can improve erectile dysfunction.

Causes and Treatment

The ability to achieve an erection depends on three factors: adequate blood circulation in the penis; proper nerve function in the penis; and stimulus from the brain. Erectile dysfunction can result from various diseases, conditions, and medications that interfere with one or more of these factors. Some common causes of ED include the following:

- Vascular diseases such as atherosclerosis (hardening of the arteries), hypertension (high blood pressure), and high cholesterol, which can restrict blood flow to the penis

- Diabetes, which can cause nerve and artery damage

- Kidney disease, which can affect circulation, nerve function, and libido (sex drive)

- Neurological diseases such as multiple sclerosis (MS), stroke, Parkinson disease, and Alzheimer disease, which can interfere with nerve impulses between the brain and penis

- Treatments for prostate, bladder, or colon cancer

- More than 200 different types of prescription medications

- Tobacco, alcohol, or drug use, which can damage blood vessels and restrict blood flow to the penis

- Injury to the penis, brain, or spinal cord

- Chronic illness

- Psychological conditions such as depression or performance anxiety

It is important to note that ED is not considered a normal part of the aging process. Although older men may require more stimulation to achieve an erection, they should be capable of sexual intercourse. There are several prescription drugs available to treat ED, including sildenafil (Viagra), vardenafil (Levitra), and tadalafil (Cialis). These drugs work by relaxing the cavernosal smooth muscle in order to increase the blood flow to the penis.

ED and Cardiovascular Health

Erectile dysfunction is a major predictor of heart disease. In fact, most men who experience ED will develop symptoms of cardiovascular illness within five years. One study found that 64 percent of men who were hospitalized for a heart attack and 57 percent of men who underwent heart bypass surgery had experienced ED. Although ED does not always point to an underlying heart problem, experts recommend that men with ED that does not have an obvious cause should undergo a complete cardiovascular health screening.

Doctors are uncertain about the exact nature of the link between erectile dysfunction and heart problems. One possible explanation is that the buildup of plaques in the arteries—which often occurs in people with heart disease—might also reduce blood flow to the penis. Many doctors attribute the link to dysfunction of the endothelium that lines the blood vessels, which impairs blood flow to the heart, penis, and other organs.

The link between erectile dysfunction and cardiovascular health also extends to risk factors that are shared between the two conditions, such as:

- Smoking

- Drinking alcohol

- Diabetes

- High blood pressure

- High cholesterol

- Obesity

- Low testosterone

For men who have both erectile dysfunction and heart disease, adopting healthy lifestyle changes can lead to improvements in both conditions. Some suggested changes include quitting smoking, drinking alcohol in moderation if at all, exercising regularly, maintaining a healthy weight, and choosing a healthy diet that is low in saturated fats. It is also important to note that some medications used to treat heart disease, including nitrates, are not safe to use in conjunction with the drugs used to treat erectile dysfunction.

References

1. "Erectile Dysfunction: A Sign of Heart Disease?" Mayo Clinic, 2016.

2. "Heart Disease and Erectile Dysfunction," Cleveland Clinic, 2012.

Section 31.3

HIV-Infected Men at Increased Risk for Heart Disease

This section includes text excerpted from "HIV-Infected Men at Increased Risk for Heart Disease, Large Study Finds," National Institutes of Health (NIH), March 31, 2014.

The buildup of soft plaque in arteries that nourish the heart is more common and extensive in HIV-infected men than HIV-uninfected men, independent of established cardiovascular disease risk factors, according to a new study by National Institutes of Health grantees. The findings suggest that HIV-infected men are at greater risk for a heart attack than their HIV-uninfected peers, the researchers write in Annals of Internal Medicine.

In addition, blockage in a coronary artery was most common among HIV-infected men whose immune health had declined the most over the course of their infection and who had taken anti-HIV drugs the longest, the scientists found, placing these men at even higher risk for a heart attack.

"These findings from the largest study of its kind tell us that men with HIV infection are at increased risk for the development of coronary artery disease and should discuss with a care provider the potential need for cardiovascular risk factor screening and appropriate risk reduction strategies," said Gary H. Gibbons, M.D., director of the National Heart, Lung, and Blood Institute (NHLBI), part of NIH.

"Thanks to effective treatments, many people with HIV infection are living into their 50s and well beyond and are dying of non-AIDS-related causes—frequently, heart disease," said Anthony S. Fauci, M.D., director of the National Institute of Allergy and Infectious Diseases (NIAID), also part of NIH. "Consequently, the prevention and treatment of non-infectious chronic diseases in people with HIV infection has become an increasingly important focus of our research."

Past studies of the association between heart disease and HIV infection have reached inconsistent conclusions. To help clarify whether an association exists, the current investigation drew participants from the Multicenter AIDS Cohort Study (MACS), a study of HIV/AIDS in gay and bisexual men established by NIAID nearly 30 years ago.

"One advantage of the MACS is that it includes HIV-uninfected men who are similar to the HIV-infected men in the study in their sexual orientation, lifestyle, socioeconomic status and risk behavior, which makes for a good comparison group," said Wendy S. Post, M.D., who led the study. Dr. Post is a professor of medicine and epidemiology at the Johns Hopkins School of Medicine and the Johns Hopkins Bloomberg School of Public Health in Baltimore.

Another advantage was the MACS' size, with nearly 7,000 men cumulatively enrolled, 1,001 of whom participated in the new study. The participants included 618 men who were HIV-infected and 383 who were not. All were 40 to 70 years of age, weighed less than 200 pounds, and had had no prior surgery to restore blood flow to the coronary arteries.

Dr. Post and colleagues investigated whether the prevalence and extent of plaque buildup in coronary arteries, a condition called coronary atherosclerosis, is greater in HIV-infected men than HIV-uninfected men and whether that plaque is soft or hard. Coronary atherosclerosis, especially soft plaque, is more likely to be a precursor of heart attack than hard plaque.

The scientists found coronary atherosclerosis due to soft plaque in 63 percent of the HIV-infected men and 53 percent of the HIV-uninfected men. After adjusting for cardiovascular disease risk factors, including high blood pressure, diabetes, high cholesterol, high body mass index and smoking, the presence of soft plaque and the cumulative size of individual soft plaques were significantly greater in men with HIV infection.

In addition, by examining a subgroup of HIV-infected men, the scientists discovered two predictors of advanced atherosclerosis in this population. The first predictor deals with white blood cells called CD4+ T cells, which are the primary target of HIV and whose level, or count, is a measure of immune health. The researchers found that for every 100 cells per cubic millimeter decrease in a man's lowest CD4+ T cell count, his risk of coronary artery blockage rose by 20 percent. The scientists also found that for every year a man had taken anti-HIV drugs, his risk of coronary artery blockage rose by 9 percent.

Because the investigators examined coronary artery plaque at a single point in time, further research is needed to determine whether coronary artery plaque in HIV-infected men is less likely to harden over time, or whether these men simply develop greater amounts of soft plaque, according to Dr. Post. In addition, she said, studies on therapies and behavioral changes to reduce risk for cardiovascular disease in men and women infected with HIV are needed to determine how best to prevent progression of atherosclerosis in this population.

Chapter 32

Cardiovascular Disease in Women

Chapter Contents

Section 32.1

Basic Facts about Heart Disease in Women

This section includes text excerpted from "Women and Heart Disease Fact Sheet," Centers for Disease Control and Prevention (CDC), November 30, 2015.

Facts on Women and Heart Disease

- Heart disease is the leading cause of death for women in the United States, killing 292,188 women in 2009—that's **1 in every 4** female deaths.

- Although heart disease is sometimes thought of as a "man's disease," around the same number of women and men die each year of heart disease in the United States. Despite increases in awareness over the past decade, only **54%** of women recognize that heart disease is their **number 1 killer**.

- Heart disease is the **leading cause** of death for African American and white women in the United States. Among Hispanic women, heart disease and cancer cause roughly the same number of deaths each year. For American Indian or Alaska Native and Asian or Pacific Islander women, heart disease is second only to cancer.

- About 5.8% of all white women, 7.6% of black women, and 5.6% of Mexican American women have coronary heart disease.

- Almost **two-thirds** (64%) of women who die suddenly of coronary heart disease have **no previous symptoms**. Even if you have no symptoms, you may still be at risk for heart disease.

Symptoms

While some women have no symptoms, others experience angina (dull, heavy to sharp chest pain or discomfort), pain in the neck/jaw/throat or pain in the upper abdomen or back. These may occur during rest, begin during physical activity, or be triggered by mental stress.

Women are more likely to describe chest pain that is sharp, burning and more frequently have pain in the neck, jaw, throat, abdomen or back.

Sometimes heart disease may be silent and not diagnosed until a woman experiences signs or symptoms of a heart attack, heart failure, an arrhythmia, or stroke.

These symptoms may include

- **Heart Attack**: Chest pain or discomfort, upper back pain, indigestion, heartburn, nausea/vomiting, extreme fatigue, upper body discomfort, and shortness of breath.

- **Arrhythmia:** Fluttering feelings in the chest (palpitations).

- **Heart Failure:** Shortness of breath, fatigue, swelling of the feet/ankles/legs/abdomen.

- **Stroke:** Sudden weakness, paralysis (inability to move) or numbness of the face/arms/legs, especially on one side of the body. Other symptoms may include: confusion, trouble speaking or understanding speech, difficulty seeing in one or both eyes, shortness of breath, dizziness, loss of balance or coordination, loss of consciousness, or sudden and severe headache.

Risk Factors

High blood pressure, high LDL cholesterol, and smoking are key risk factors for heart disease. About **half of Americans** (49%) have at least one of these three risk factors.

Several other medical conditions and lifestyle choices can also put people at a higher risk for heart disease, including:

- Diabetes
- Overweight and obesity
- Poor diet
- Physical inactivity
- Excessive alcohol use

Screening

To reduce your chances of getting heart disease it's important to

- Know your **blood pressure.** Having uncontrolled blood pressure can result in heart disease. High blood pressure has no symptoms so it's important to have your blood pressure checked regularly.

- Talk to your healthcare provider about whether you should be tested for diabetes. Having uncontrolled **diabetes** raises your chances of heart disease.

- **Quit smoking.**

- Discuss checking your **cholesterol and triglycerides** with your healthcare provider.

- Make **healthy food** choices. Being overweight and obese raises your risk of heart disease.

- **Limit alcohol** intake to one drink a day.

- **Lower your stress** level and find healthy ways to cope with stress.

Section 32.2

Women and Heart Disease: Some Gender Differences

This section includes text excerpted from "Heart Disease in Women," National Heart, Lung, and Blood Institute (NHLBI), April 21, 2014.

How Does Heart Disease Affect Women?

In the United States, 1 in 4 women dies from heart disease. In fact, coronary heart disease (CHD)—the most common type of heart disease—is the #1 killer of both men and women in the United States.

Other types of heart disease, such as coronary microvascular disease (MVD) and broken heart syndrome, also pose a risk for women. These disorders, which mainly affect women, are not as well understood as CHD.

Coronary Heart Disease

CHD is a disease in which plaque builds up on the inner walls of your coronary arteries. These arteries carry oxygen-rich blood to your heart. When plaque builds up in the arteries, the condition is called atherosclerosis.

Plaque is made up of fat, cholesterol, calcium, and other substances found in the blood. Over time, plaque can harden or rupture (break open).

Hardened plaque narrows the coronary arteries and reduces the flow of oxygen-rich blood to the heart. This can cause chest pain or discomfort called angina.

If the plaque ruptures, a blood clot can form on its surface. A large blood clot can mostly or completely block blood flow through a coronary artery. This is the most common cause of a heart attack. Over time, ruptured plaque also hardens and narrows the coronary arteries.

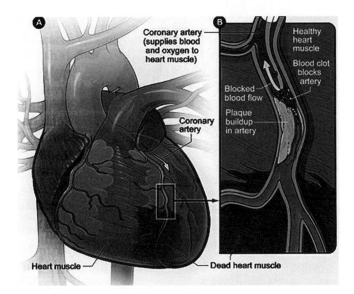

Figure 32.1. *Heart With Muscle Damage and a Blocked Artery*

(A) is an overview of a heart and coronary artery showing damage (dead heart muscle) caused by a heart attack. (B) is a cross-section of the coronary artery with plaque buildup and a blood clot resulting from plaque rupture.

Plaque also can develop within the walls of the coronary arteries. Tests that show the insides of the coronary arteries may look normal in people who have this pattern of plaque. Studies are under way to see whether this type of plaque buildup occurs more often in women than in men and why.

In addition to angina and heart attack, CHD can cause other serious heart problems. The disease may lead to heart failure, irregular heartbeats called arrhythmias, and sudden cardiac arrest (SCA).

Coronary Microvascular Disease

Coronary MVD is heart disease that affects the heart's tiny arteries. This disease is also called cardiac syndrome X or nonobstructive CHD. In coronary MVD, the walls of the heart's tiny arteries are damaged or diseased.

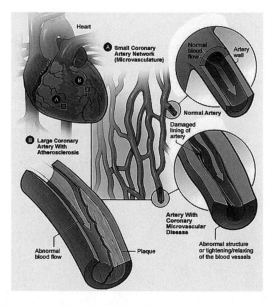

Figure 32.2. *Coronary Microvascular Disease*

(A) shows the small coronary artery network (microvasculature), containing a normal artery and an artery with coronary MVD. (B) shows a large coronary artery with plaque buildup.

Women are more likely than men to have coronary MVD. Many researchers think that a drop in estrogen levels during menopause combined with other heart disease risk factors causes coronary MVD.

Although death rates from heart disease have dropped in the last 30 years, they haven't dropped as much in women as in men. This may be the result of coronary MVD.

Standard tests for CHD are not designed to detect coronary MVD. Thus, test results for women who have coronary MVD may show that they are at low risk for heart disease.

Broken Heart Syndrome

Women are also more likely than men to have a condition called broken heart syndrome. In this recently recognized heart problem, extreme emotional stress can lead to severe (but often short-term) heart muscle failure.

Broken heart syndrome is also called stress-induced cardiomyopathy or takotsubo cardiomyopathy.

Doctors may misdiagnose broken heart syndrome as a heart attack because it has similar symptoms and test results. However, there's no evidence of blocked heart arteries in broken heart syndrome, and most people have a full and quick recovery.

Researchers are just starting to explore what causes this disorder and how to diagnose and treat it. Often, patients who have broken heart syndrome have previously been healthy.

Outlook

Women tend to have CHD about 10 years later than men. However, CHD remains the #1 killer of women in the United States.

The good news is that you can control many CHD risk factors. CHD risk factors are conditions or habits that raise your risk for CHD and heart attack. These risk factors also can increase the chance that existing CHD will worsen.

Lifestyle changes, medicines, and medical or surgical procedures can help women lower their risk for CHD. Thus, early and ongoing CHD prevention is important.

Other Names for Heart Disease

- Arrhythmia
- Broken heart syndrome, which also is called stress-induced cardiomyopathy or takotsubo cardiomyopathy
- Coronary heart disease, which also is called coronary artery disease
- Coronary microvascular disease, which also is called cardiac syndrome X or nonobstructive coronary heart disease
- Heart failure
- Sudden cardiac arrest

What Causes Heart Disease?

Research suggests that coronary heart disease (CHD) begins with damage to the lining and inner layers of the coronary (heart) arteries. Several factors contribute to this damage. They include:

- Smoking, including secondhand smoke

- High amounts of certain fats and cholesterol in the blood

- High blood pressure

- High amounts of sugar in the blood due to insulin resistance or diabetes

- Blood vessel inflammation

Plaque may begin to build up where the arteries are damaged. The buildup of plaque in the coronary arteries may start in childhood.

Over time, plaque can harden or rupture (break open). Hardened plaque narrows the coronary arteries and reduces the flow of oxygen-rich blood to the heart. This can cause chest pain or discomfort called angina.

If the plaque ruptures, blood cell fragments called platelets stick to the site of the injury. They may clump together to form blood clots.

Blood clots can further narrow the coronary arteries and worsen angina. If a clot becomes large enough, it can mostly or completely block a coronary artery and cause a heart attack.

In addition to the factors above, low estrogen levels before or after menopause may play a role in causing coronary microvascular disease (MVD). Coronary MVD is heart disease that affects the heart's tiny arteries.

The cause of broken heart syndrome isn't yet known. However, a sudden release of stress hormones may play a role in causing the disorder. Most cases of broken heart syndrome occur in women who have gone through menopause.

Who Is at Risk for Heart Disease?

Certain traits, conditions, or habits may raise your risk for coronary heart disease (CHD). These conditions are known as risk factors. Risk factors also increase the chance that existing CHD will worsen.

Women generally have the same CHD risk factors as men. However, some risk factors may affect women differently than men. For example, diabetes raises the risk of CHD more in women. Also, some risk factors, such as birth control pills and menopause, only affect women.

There are many known CHD risk factors. Your risk for CHD and heart attack rises with the number of risk factors you have and their severity. Risk factors tend to "gang up" and worsen each other's effects.

Having just one risk factor doubles your risk for CHD. Having two risk factors increases your risk for CHD fourfold. Having three or more risk factors increases your risk for CHD more than tenfold.

Also, some risk factors, such as smoking and diabetes, put you at greater risk for CHD and heart attack than others.

More than 75 percent of women aged 40 to 60 have one or more risk factors for CHD. Many risk factors start during childhood; some even develop within the first 10 years of life. You can control most risk factors, but some you can't.

Risk Factors You Can Control

Smoking

Smoking is the most powerful risk factor that women can control. Smoking tobacco or long-term exposure to secondhand smoke raises your risk for CHD and heart attack.

Smoking exposes you to carbon monoxide. This chemical robs your blood of oxygen and triggers a buildup of plaque in your arteries.

Smoking also increases the risk of blood clots forming in your arteries. Blood clots can block plaque-narrowed arteries and cause a heart attack. The more you smoke, the greater your risk for a heart attack.

Even women who smoke fewer than two cigarettes a day are at increased risk for CHD.

High Blood Cholesterol and High Triglyceride Levels

Cholesterol travels in the bloodstream in small packages called lipoproteins. The two major kinds of lipoproteins are low-density lipoprotein (LDL) cholesterol and high-density lipoprotein (HDL) cholesterol.

LDL cholesterol is sometimes called "bad" cholesterol. This is because it carries cholesterol to tissues, including your heart arteries. HDL cholesterol is sometimes called "good" cholesterol. This is because it helps remove cholesterol from your arteries.

A blood test called a lipoprotein panel is used to measure cholesterol levels. This test gives information about your total cholesterol, LDL cholesterol, HDL cholesterol, and triglycerides (a type of fat found in the blood).

Cholesterol levels are measured in milligrams (mg) of cholesterol per deciliter (dL) of blood. A woman's risk for CHD increases if she has a total cholesterol level greater than 200 mg/dL, an LDL cholesterol level greater than 100 mg/dL, or an HDL cholesterol level less than 50 mg/dL.

A triglyceride level greater than 150 mg/dL also increases a woman's risk for CHD. A woman's HDL cholesterol and triglyceride levels predict her risk for CHD better than her total cholesterol or LDL cholesterol levels.

High Blood Pressure

Blood pressure is the force of blood pushing against the walls of the arteries as the heart pumps blood. If this pressure rises and stays high over time, it can damage the body in many ways.

Women who have blood pressure greater than 120/80 mmHg are at increased risk for CHD. (The mmHg is millimeters of mercury—the units used to measure blood pressure.)

High blood pressure is defined differently for people who have diabetes or chronic kidney disease. If you have one of these diseases, work with your doctor to set a healthy blood pressure goal.

Diabetes and Prediabetes

Diabetes is a disease in which the body's blood sugar level is too high. This is because the body doesn't make enough insulin or doesn't use its insulin properly.

Insulin is a hormone that helps move blood sugar into cells, where it's used for energy. Over time, a high blood sugar level can lead to increased plaque buildup in your arteries.

Prediabetes is a condition in which your blood sugar level is higher than normal, but not as high as it is in diabetes. Prediabetes puts you at higher risk for both diabetes and CHD.

Diabetes and prediabetes raise the risk of CHD more in women than in men. In fact, having diabetes doubles a woman's risk of developing CHD.

Before menopause, estrogen provides women some protection against CHD. However, in women who have diabetes, the disease counters the protective effects of estrogen.

Overweight and Obesity

The terms "overweight" and "obesity" refer to body weight that's greater than what is considered healthy for a certain height.

The most useful measure of overweight and obesity is body mass index (BMI). BMI is calculated from your height and weight. In adults, a BMI of 18.5 to 24.9 is considered normal. A BMI of 25 to 29.9 is considered overweight. A BMI of 30 or more is considered obese.

Studies suggest that where extra weight occurs on the body may predict CHD risk better than BMI. Women who carry much of their fat around the waist are at greatest risk for CHD. These women have "apple-shaped" figures.

Women who carry most of their fat on their hips and thighs— that is, those who have "pear-shaped" figures—are at lower risk for CHD.

To fully know how excess weight affects your CHD risk, you should know your BMI and waist measurement. If you have a BMI greater than 24.9 and a waist measurement greater than 35 inches, you're at increased risk for CHD.

If your waist measurement divided by your hip measurement is greater than 0.9, you're also at increased risk for CHD.

Studies also suggest that women whose weight goes up and down dramatically (typically due to unhealthy dieting) are at increased risk for CHD. These swings in weight can lower HDL cholesterol levels.

Metabolic Syndrome

Metabolic syndrome is the name for a group of risk factors that raises your risk for CHD and other health problems, such as diabetes and stroke. A diagnosis of metabolic syndrome is made if you have at least three of the following risk factors:

- A large waistline. Having extra fat in the waist area is a greater risk factor for CHD than having extra fat in other parts of the body, such as on the hips.

- A higher than normal triglyceride level (or you're on medicine to treat high triglycerides).

- A lower than normal HDL cholesterol level (or you're on medicine to treat low HDL cholesterol).

- Higher than normal blood pressure (or you're on medicine to treat high blood pressure).

- Higher than normal fasting blood sugar (or you're on medicine to treat diabetes)

Metabolic syndrome is more common in African American women and Mexican American women than in men of the same racial groups. The condition affects White women and men about equally.

Birth Control Pills

Women who smoke and take birth control pills are at very high risk for CHD, especially if they're older than 35. For women who take birth control pills but don't smoke, the risk of CHD isn't fully known.

Lack of Physical Activity

Inactive people are nearly twice as likely to develop CHD as those who are physically active. A lack of physical activity can worsen other CHD risk factors, such as high blood cholesterol and triglyceride levels, high blood pressure, diabetes and prediabetes, and overweight and obesity.

Unhealthy Diet

An unhealthy diet can raise your risk for CHD. For example, foods that are high in saturated and trans fats and cholesterol raise your LDL cholesterol level. A high-sodium (salt) diet can raise your risk for high blood pressure.

Foods with added sugars will give you extra calories without nutrients, such as vitamins and minerals. This can cause you to gain weight, which raises your risk for CHD.

Too much alcohol also can cause you to gain weight, and it will raise your blood pressure.

Stress or Depression

Stress may play a role in causing CHD. Stress can trigger your arteries to narrow. This can raise your blood pressure and your risk for a heart attack.

Getting upset or angry also can trigger a heart attack. Stress also may indirectly raise your risk for CHD if it makes you more likely to smoke or overeat foods high in fat and sugar.

People who are depressed are two to three times more likely to develop CHD than people who are not. Depression is twice as common in women as in men.

Anemia

Anemia is a condition in which your blood has a lower than normal number of red blood cells.

The condition also can occur if your red blood cells don't contain enough hemoglobin. Hemoglobin is an iron-rich protein that carries oxygen from your lungs to the rest of your organs.

If you have anemia, your organs don't get enough oxygen-rich blood. This causes your heart to work harder, which may raise your risk for CHD.

Anemia has many causes.

Sleep Apnea

Sleep apnea is a common disorder that causes pauses in breathing or shallow breaths while you sleep. Breathing pauses can last from a few seconds to minutes. They often occur 5 to 30 times or more an hour.

Typically, normal breathing starts again after the pause, sometimes with a loud snort or choking sound. Major signs of sleep apnea are snoring and daytime sleepiness.

When you stop breathing, the lack of oxygen triggers your body's stress hormones. This causes blood pressure to rise and makes the blood more likely to clot.

Untreated sleep apnea can raise your risk for high blood pressure, diabetes, and even a heart attack or stroke.

Women are more likely to develop sleep apnea after menopause.

Risk Factors You Can't Control

Age and Menopause

As you get older, your risk for CHD and heart attack rises. This is due in part to the slow buildup of plaque inside your heart arteries, which can start during childhood.

Before age 55, women have a lower risk for CHD than men. Estrogen provides women with some protection against CHD before menopause. After age 55, however, the risk of CHD increases in both women and men.

You may have gone through early menopause, either naturally or because you had your ovaries removed. If so, you're twice as likely to develop CHD as women of the same age who aren't yet menopausal.

Another reason why women are at increased risk for CHD after age 55 is that middle age is when you tend to develop other CHD risk factors.

Women who have gone through menopause also are at increased risk for broken heart syndrome.

Family History

Family history plays a role in CHD risk. Your risk increases if your father or a brother was diagnosed with CHD before 55 years of age, or if your mother or a sister was diagnosed with CHD before 65 years of age.

Also, a family history of stroke—especially a mother's stroke history—can help predict the risk of heart attack in women.

Having a family history of CHD or stroke doesn't mean that you'll develop heart disease. This is especially true if your affected family member smoked or had other risk factors that were not well treated.

Making lifestyle changes and taking medicines to treat risk factors often can lessen genetic influences and prevent or delay heart problems.

Preeclampsia

Preeclampsia is a condition that develops during pregnancy. The two main signs of preeclampsia are a rise in blood pressure and excess protein in the urine.

These signs usually occur during the second half of pregnancy and go away after delivery. However, your risk of developing high blood pressure later in life increases after having preeclampsia.

Preeclampsia also is linked to an increased lifetime risk of heart disease, including CHD, heart attack, and heart failure. (Likewise, having heart disease risk factors, such as diabetes or obesity, increases your risk for preeclampsia.)

If you had preeclampsia during pregnancy, you're twice as likely to develop heart disease as women who haven't had the condition. You're also more likely to develop heart disease earlier in life.

Preeclampsia is a heart disease risk factor that you can't control. However, if you've had the condition, you should take extra care to try and control other heart disease risk factors.

The more severe your preeclampsia was, the greater your risk for heart disease. Let your doctor know that you had preeclampsia so he or she can assess your heart disease risk and how to reduce it.

Emerging Risk Factors

Research suggests that inflammation plays a role in causing CHD. Inflammation is the body's response to injury or infection. Damage to the arteries' inner walls seems to trigger inflammation and help plaque grow.

High blood levels of a protein called C-reactive protein (CRP) are a sign of inflammation in the body. Research suggests that women who have high blood levels of CRP are at increased risk for heart attack.

Also, some inflammatory diseases, such as lupus and rheumatoid arthritis, may increase the risk for CHD.

Some studies suggest that women who have migraine headaches may be at greater risk for CHD. This is especially true for women who have migraines with auras (visual disturbances), such as flashes of light or zig-zag lines.

Low bone density and low intake of folate and vitamin B6 also may raise a woman's risk for CHD.

More research is needed to find out whether calcium supplements with or without vitamin D affect CHD risk. You may want to talk with your doctor to find out whether these types of supplements are right for you.

Researchers are just starting to learn about broken heart syndrome risk factors. Most women who have this disorder are White and have gone through menopause.

Many of these women have other heart disease risk factors, such as high blood pressure, high blood cholesterol, diabetes, and smoking. However, these risk factors tend to be less common in women who have broken heart syndrome than in women who have CHD.

How Is Heart Disease Diagnosed?

Your doctor will diagnose coronary heart disease (CHD) based on your medical and family histories, your risk factors, a physical exam, and the results from tests and procedures.

No single test can diagnose CHD. If your doctor thinks you have CHD, he or she may recommend one or more of the following tests.

- EKG (Electrocardiogram)
- Stress Testing
- Echocardiography
- Chest X-Ray
- Blood Tests
- Coronary Angiography and Cardiac Catheterization

Tests Used to Diagnose Broken Heart Syndrome

If your doctor thinks you have broken heart syndrome, he or she may recommend coronary angiography. Other tests are also used to diagnose this disorder, including blood tests, EKG, echo, and cardiac MRI.

How Is Heart Disease Treated?

Treatment for coronary heart disease (CHD) usually is the same for both women and men. Treatment may include lifestyle changes, medicines, medical and surgical procedures, and cardiac rehabilitation (rehab).

The goals of treatment are to:

- Relieve symptoms.

- Reduce risk factors in an effort to slow, stop, or reverse the buildup of plaque.

- Lower the risk of blood clots forming. (Blood clots can cause a heart attack.)

- Widen or bypass plaque-clogged coronary (heart) arteries.

- Prevent CHD complications.

Lifestyle Changes

Making lifestyle changes can help prevent or treat CHD. These changes may be the only treatment that some people need.

Quit Smoking

If you smoke or use tobacco, try to quit. Smoking can raise your risk for CHD and heart attack and worsen other CHD risk factors. Talk with your doctor about programs and products that can help you quit. Also, try to avoid secondhand smoke.

If you find it hard to quit smoking on your own, consider joining a support group. Many hospitals, workplaces, and community groups offer classes to help people quit smoking.

Follow a Healthy Diet

A healthy diet is an important part of a healthy lifestyle. A healthy diet includes a variety of vegetables and fruits. These foods can be fresh, canned, frozen, or dried. A good rule is to try to fill half of your plate with vegetables and fruits.

A healthy diet also includes whole grains, fat-free or low-fat dairy products, and protein foods, such as lean meats, poultry without skin, seafood, processed soy products, nuts, seeds, beans, and peas.

Choose and prepare foods with little sodium (salt). Too much salt can raise your risk for high blood pressure. Studies show that following the Dietary Approaches to Stop Hypertension (DASH) eating plan can lower blood pressure.

Try to avoid foods and drinks that are high in added sugars. For example, drink water instead of sugary drinks, like soda.

Also, try to limit the amount of solid fats and refined grains that you eat. Solid fats are saturated fat and trans fatty acids. Refined grains come from processing whole grains, which results in a loss of nutrients (such as dietary fiber).

If you drink alcohol, do so in moderation. Research suggests that regularly drinking small to moderate amounts of alcohol may lower the risk of CHD. Women should have no more than one alcoholic drink a day.

One drink a day can lower your CHD risk by raising your HDL cholesterol level. One drink is a glass of wine, beer, or a small amount of hard liquor.

If you don't drink, this isn't a recommendation to start using alcohol. Also, you shouldn't drink if you're pregnant, if you're planning to become pregnant, or if you have another health condition that could make alcohol use harmful.

Too much alcohol can cause you to gain weight and raise your blood pressure and triglyceride level. In women, even one drink a day may raise the risk of certain types of cancer.

Be Physically Active

Regular physical activity can lower many CHD risk factors, including high LDL cholesterol, high blood pressure, and excess weight.

Physical activity also can lower your risk for diabetes and raise your HDL cholesterol level. (HDL cholesterol helps remove cholesterol from your arteries.)

Talk with your doctor before you start a new exercise plan. Ask him or her how much and what kinds of physical activity are safe for you.

People gain health benefits from as little as 60 minutes of moderate-intensity aerobic activity per week. Walking is an excellent heart healthy exercise. The more active you are, the more you will benefit.

Maintain a Healthy Weight

Overweight and obesity are risk factors for CHD. If you're overweight or obese, try to lose weight. Cut back your calorie intake and do more physical activity. Eat smaller portions and choose lower calorie foods. Your healthcare provider may refer you to a dietitian to help you manage your weight.

A BMI of less than 25 and a waist circumference of 35 inches or less is the goal for preventing and treating CHD. BMI measures your weight in relation to your height and gives an estimate of your total body fat. You can use the NHLBI's online BMI calculator to figure out your BMI, or your doctor can help you.

To measure your waist, stand and place a tape measure around your middle, just above your hipbones. Measure your waist just after you breathe out. Make sure the tape is snug but doesn't squeeze the flesh.

Stress and Depression

Research shows that getting upset or angry can trigger a heart attack. Also, some of the ways people cope with stress—such as drinking, smoking, or overeating—aren't heart healthy.

Learning how to manage stress, relax, and cope with problems can improve your emotional and physical health.

Having supportive people in your life with whom you can share your feelings or concerns can help relieve stress. Physical activity, yoga, and relaxation therapy also can help relieve stress. You may want to consider taking part in a stress management program.

Depression can double or triple your risk for CHD. Depression also makes it hard to maintain a heart healthy lifestyle.

Talk with your doctor if you have symptoms of depression, such as feeling hopeless or not taking interest in daily activities. He or she may recommend counseling or prescribe medicines to help you manage the condition.

Medicines

You may need medicines to treat CHD if lifestyle changes aren't enough. Medicines can help:

- Reduce your heart's workload and relieve CHD symptoms

- Decrease your chance of having a heart attack or dying suddenly

- Lower your LDL cholesterol, blood pressure, and other CHD risk factors

- Prevent blood clots

- Prevent or delay the need for a procedure or surgery, such as angioplasty or coronary artery bypass grafting (CABG)

Women who have coronary microvascular disease and anemia may benefit from taking medicine to treat the anemia.

Women who have broken heart syndrome also may need medicines. Doctors may prescribe medicines to relieve fluid buildup, treat blood pressure problems, prevent blood clots, and manage stress hormones. Most people who have broken heart syndrome make a full recovery within weeks.

Take all of your medicines as prescribed. If you have side effects or other problems related to your medicines, tell your doctor. He or she may be able to provide other options.

Menopausal Hormone Therapy

Recent studies have shown that menopausal hormone therapy (MHT) doesn't prevent CHD. Some studies have even shown that MHT increases women's risk for CHD, stroke, and breast cancer.

However, these studies tested MHT on women who had been postmenopausal for at least several years. During that time, they could have already developed CHD.

Research is ongoing to see whether MHT helps prevent CHD when taken right when menopause starts. While questions remain, current findings suggest MHT shouldn't routinely be used to prevent or treat CHD.

Ask your doctor about other ways to prevent or treat CHD, including lifestyle changes and medicines.

Procedures and Surgery

You may need a procedure or surgery to treat CHD. Both angioplasty and CABG are used as treatments. You and your doctor can discuss which treatment is right for you.

Percutaneous Coronary Intervention

Percutaneous coronary intervention (PCI), commonly known as angioplasty, is a nonsurgical procedure that opens blocked or narrowed coronary arteries.

A thin, flexible tube with a balloon or other device on the end is threaded through a blood vessel to the narrowed or blocked coronary artery. Once in place, the balloon is inflated to compress the plaque against the wall of the artery. This restores blood flow through the artery.

PCI can improve blood flow to your heart and relieve chest pain. A small mesh tube called a stent usually is placed in the artery to help keep it open after the procedure.

Coronary Artery Bypass Grafting

CABG is a type of surgery. During CABG, a surgeon removes arteries or veins from other areas in your body and uses them to bypass (that is, go around) narrowed or blocked coronary arteries.

CABG can improve blood flow to your heart, relieve chest pain, and possibly prevent a heart attack.

Cardiac Rehabilitation

Your doctor may prescribe cardiac rehab for angina or after angioplasty, CABG, or a heart attack. Almost everyone who has CHD can benefit from cardiac rehab.

Cardiac rehab is a medically supervised program that can improve the health and well-being of people who have heart problems.

The cardiac rehab team may include doctors, nurses, exercise specialists, physical and occupational therapists, dietitians or nutritionists, and psychologists or other mental health specialists.

Cardiac rehab has two parts:

1. **Exercise training.** This part of rehab helps you learn how to exercise safely, strengthen your muscles, and improve your stamina. Your exercise plan will be based on your personal abilities, needs, and interests.

2. **Education, counseling, and training.** This part of rehab helps you understand your heart condition and find ways to lower your risk for future heart problems. The rehab team will help you learn how to cope with the stress of adjusting to a new lifestyle and with your fears about the future.

How Can Heart Disease Be Prevented?

Taking action to control your risk factors can help prevent or delay coronary heart disease (CHD). Your risk for CHD increases with the number of CHD risk factors you have.

One step you can take is to adopt a heart healthy lifestyle. A heart healthy lifestyle should be part of a lifelong approach to healthy living.

For example, if you smoke, try to quit. Smoking can raise your risk for CHD and heart attack and worsen other CHD risk factors. Talk with your doctor about programs and products that can help you quit. Also, try to avoid secondhand smoke.

Following a healthy diet also is an important part of a healthy lifestyle. A healthy diet includes a variety of vegetables and fruits. It also includes whole grains, fat-free or low-fat dairy products, and protein foods, such as lean meats, poultry without skin, seafood, processed soy products, nuts, seeds, beans, and peas.

A healthy diet is low in sodium (salt), added sugars, solid fats, and refined grains. Solid fats are saturated fat and trans fatty acids. Refined grains come from processing whole grains, which results in a loss of nutrients (such as dietary fiber).

The NHLBI's Therapeutic Lifestyle Changes (TLC) and Dietary Approaches to Stop Hypertension (DASH) are two programs that promote healthy eating.

If you're overweight or obese, work with your doctor to create a reasonable weight-loss plan. Controlling your weight helps you control CHD risk factors.

Be as physically active as you can. Physical activity can improve your fitness level and your health. Talk with your doctor about what types of activity are safe for you.

Know your family history of CHD. If you or someone in your family has CHD, be sure to tell your doctor.

If lifestyle changes aren't enough, you also may need medicines to control your CHD risk factors. Take all of your medicines as prescribed.

Living with Heart Disease

If you have coronary heart disease (CHD), you can take steps to control its risk factors and prevent complications. Lifestyle changes and ongoing care can help you manage the disease.

Having CHD raises your risk for a heart attack. Thus, knowing the warning signs of a heart attack is important. If you think you're having a heart attack, call 9–1–1 right away.

Lifestyle Changes

Adopting a heart healthy lifestyle can help you control CHD risk factors. However, making lifestyle changes can be a challenge.

Try to take things one step at a time. Learn about the benefits of lifestyle changes, and make a plan with specific, realistic goals. Reward yourself for your progress.

The good news is that many lifestyle changes help control several CHD risk factors at the same time. For example, physical activity lowers your blood pressure and LDL cholesterol level, helps control diabetes and prediabetes, reduces stress, and helps control your weight.

Ongoing Care

Your CHD risk factors can change over time, so having ongoing care is important. Your doctor will track your blood pressure, blood cholesterol, and blood sugar levels with routine tests. These tests will show whether your doctor needs to adjust your treatment.

Ask your doctor how often you should schedule followup visits and blood tests. Between visits, call your doctor if you have any new symptoms or if your symptoms worsen.

You may feel depressed or anxious if you've been diagnosed with CHD. You may worry about heart problems or making lifestyle changes.

Your doctor may recommend medicine, professional counseling, or relaxation therapy if you have depression or anxiety. It's important to treat these conditions because they raise your risk for CHD and heart attack. Depression and anxiety also can make it harder for you to make lifestyle changes.

Heart Attack Warning Signs

If you have CHD, learn the warning signs of a heart attack. Heart attack signs and symptoms include:

- Chest pain or discomfort. This involves uncomfortable pressure, squeezing, fullness, or pain in the center or left side of the chest that can be mild or strong. This pain or discomfort often lasts more than a few minutes or goes away and comes back.

- Upper body discomfort in one or both arms, the back, neck, jaw, or upper part of the stomach.

- Shortness of breath, which may occur with or before chest discomfort.

- Nausea (feeling sick to your stomach), vomiting, light-headedness or fainting, or breaking out in a cold sweat.

- Sleep problems, fatigue (tiredness), and lack of energy.

If you think you're having a heart attack, call 9–1–1 at once. Early treatment can prevent or limit damage to your heart muscle.

If you think you're having a heart attack, do not drive to the hospital or let someone else drive you. Call an ambulance so that medical personnel can begin life-saving treatment on the way to the emergency room.

Let the people you see regularly know you're at risk for a heart attack. They can seek emergency care if you suddenly faint, collapse, or have other severe symptoms.

Living with Broken Heart Syndrome

Most people who have broken heart syndrome make a full recovery within weeks. The risk is low for a repeat episode of this disorder.

To check your heart health, your doctor may recommend echocardiography about a month after you're diagnosed with the syndrome. Talk with your doctor about how often you should schedule followup visits.

Section 32.3

Menopause and Heart Disease

"Menopause and Heart Disease," © 2016 Omnigraphics.
Reviewed June 2016.

Menopause is the point in the female life cycle that marks the end of menstruation and fertility. It is a natural part of the aging process that begins around age 50 for most women. Menopause involves a number of physical changes, such as declining production of estrogen—the hormones that are primarily responsible for female sexual and reproductive development.

Research has shown that some of the changes associated with menopause can increase a woman's risk of developing heart disease. In fact, cardiovascular disease accounts for nearly half of the deaths of American women over the age of 50. For women who have experienced menopause, therefore, it is particularly important to make healthy diet and lifestyle choices to reduce the risk of heart disease.

Menopause and Heart Health

Researchers attribute at least some of the increase in heart disease risk after menopause to declining levels of estrogen in the bloodstream. Estrogen impacts the arteries by strengthening their walls and helping them to remain flexible. When estrogen levels decline, it may accelerate the process of atherosclerosis (hardening of the arteries), which is associated with coronary artery disease.

In addition to drops in estrogen levels, however, several other menopausal changes may increase heart disease risk. Women's blood pressure levels tend to rise during menopause, for instance, as do levels of triglycerides and LDL (bad) cholesterol in the bloodstream. The negative effects of menopausal changes are compounded in women who have other heart disease risk factors, such as obesity, diabetes, smoking, an inactive lifestyle, or a family history of cardiovascular illness.

To reduce the risk of heart disease during and after menopause, doctors recommend that women redouble their efforts to adopt a healthy lifestyle. Some tips for promoting heart health include the following:

- Quit smoking and avoid secondhand smoke.

- Get routine medical checkups that include heart health screenings, such as cholesterol, blood glucose, blood pressure, body mass index, and waist circumference.

- Obtain treatment as needed to control such medical conditions as high cholesterol, high blood pressure, and diabetes.

- Maintain a healthy body weight.

- Follow a regular exercise routine that includes at least 150 minutes of activity per week.

- Eat a healthy diet that is low in saturated fat and high in whole grains, fiber, legumes, vegetables, fruits, and lean proteins.

- Pay attention to mood and mental health, as depression can occur after menopause and affect cardiovascular health.

Hormone Replacement Therapy and Heart Health

Hormone replacement therapy (HRT) was once used extensively to relieve the symptoms of menopause, such as hot flashes, vaginal dryness, loss of sex drive, insomnia, and mood swings. Doctors also believed that HRT would help reduce the risk of chronic health conditions related to decreasing estrogen levels, such as osteoporosis and heart disease. In the early 2000s, however, studies showed that HRT actually led to an increased the risk of breast cancer, stroke, blood clots, and heart disease. The negative effects of HRT appeared most strongly in women over age 60.

The U.S. Food and Drug Administration (FDA) responded by changing its guidelines regarding hormone replacement therapy. Doctors are now encouraged to prescribe estrogen at the lowest possible dose over the shortest possible length of time to achieve treatment goals. Experts saw a significant drop in cases of heart disease and breast cancer in postmenopausal women over age 50 as soon as the new guidelines went into effect. As of 2016, only about 10 percent of women take HRT to treat severe menopausal symptoms, and it is no longer recommended as a method of reducing a woman's risk of heart disease.

References

1. "Menopause and Heart Disease," American Heart Association, 2016.
2. "Menopause and Heart Disease," WebMD, 2016.

Chapter 33

Cardiovascular Disease in Minority Populations

Chapter Contents

Section 33.1

Cardiovascular Disease among U.S. Racial and Ethnic Minorities: Some Statistics

This section contains text excerpted from the following sources: Text beginning with the heading "Heart Disease in the United States" is excerpted from "Heart Disease Facts," Centers for Disease Control and Prevention (CDC), August 10, 2015; Text beginning with the heading "Heart Disease in Minorities" is excerpted from "Heart Disease in Minorities," U.S. Food and Drug Administration (FDA), November 16, 2015.

Heart Disease in the United States

- About **610,000 people** die of heart disease in the United States every year—that's **1 in every 4 deaths.**

- Heart disease is the leading cause of death for both men and women. **More than half** of the deaths due to heart disease in 2009 were in men.

- Coronary heart disease (CHD) is the most common type of heart disease, killing over **370,000 people** annually.

- Every year about **735,000 Americans** have a heart attack. Of these, 525,000 are a first heart attack and 210,000 happen in people who have already had a heart attack.

Heart Disease Deaths Vary by Race and Ethnicity

Heart disease is the leading cause of death for people of most ethnicities in the United States, including African Americans, Hispanics, and whites. For American Indians or Alaska Natives and Asians or Pacific Islanders, heart disease is second only to cancer. Below are the percentages of all deaths caused by heart disease in 2008, listed by ethnicity.

Early Action Is Important for Heart Attack

Know the warning signs and symptoms of a heart attack so that you can act fast if you or someone you know might be having a heart

Table 33.1. Heart Disease Deaths Vary by Race and Ethnicity

Race of Ethnic Group	% of Deaths
American Indians or Alaska Natives	18.4
Asians or Pacific Islanders	22.2
Non-Hispanic Blacks	23.8
Non-Hispanic Whites	23.8
All	23.5

attack. The chances of survival are greater when emergency treatment begins quickly.

- In a 2005 survey, most respondents—92%—recognized chest pain as a symptom of a heart attack. **Only 27%** were aware of all major symptoms and knew to call 9-1-1 when someone was having a heart attack.

- **About 47%** of sudden cardiac deaths occur outside a hospital. This suggests that many people with heart disease don't act on early warning signs.

Heart attacks have several **major warning signs** and symptoms:

- Chest pain or discomfort.
- Upper body pain or discomfort in the arms, back, neck, jaw, or upper stomach.
- Shortness of breath.
- Nausea, lightheadedness, or cold sweats.

Americans at Risk for Heart Disease

High blood pressure, high cholesterol, and smoking are key risk factors for heart disease. About **half of Americans** (47%) have at least one of these three risk factors.

Several other medical conditions and lifestyle choices can also put people at a higher risk for heart disease, including:

- Diabetes
- Overweight and obesity
- Poor diet
- Physical inactivity
- Excessive alcohol use

Heart Disease in Minorities

Although heart disease is the leading cause of death for all Americans, some minority groups experience an unequal burden of the disease.

For example, African Americans have the highest rate of high blood pressure, the leading cause of heart disease and stroke. African Americans also tend to develop the disease earlier in life.

Other Health Disparities Increase Your Risk

African Americans, Latinos, and American Indians experience a higher burden of related health conditions as well. American Indians use tobacco products more than any other ethnic group, and all groups are affected by diabetes and obesity more than white Americans. All three conditions are major risk factors for heart disease.

Follow the ABCS to Reduce Your Risk:

A Appropriate aspirin therapy
B Blood pressure control
C Cholesterol management
S Smoking cessation

You can also find links to FDA-regulated medications and devices, which are among the most common methods used to manage cardiovascular disease.

Section 33.2

African Americans and Cardiovascular Disease

This section includes text excerpted from "Heart Disease and African Americans," Office of Minority Health (OMH), U.S. Department of Health and Human Services (HHS), January 28, 2016.

Heart Disease and African Americans

Although African American adults are 40 percent more likely to have high blood pressure, they are less as likely than their non-Hispanic White counterparts to have their blood pressure under control.

- In 2010, African Americans were 30 percent more likely to die from heart disease than non-Hispanic whites.

- African American women are 1.6 times more likely (60 percent more likely) than non-Hispanic white women to have high blood pressure.

At a Glance—Diagnosed Cases of Coronary Heart Disease

Table 33.2. Age-Adjusted Percentages of Coronary Heart Disease among Persons 18 Years of Age and over, 2012

Non- Hispanic Black	Non-Hispanic White	Non-Hispanic Black/Non-Hispanic White Ratio
6.5	6.2	1

Source: CDC 2014. Summary Health Statistics for U.S. Adults: 2012.

At a Glance—Death Rate

Table 33.3. Age-Adjusted Heart Disease Death Rates per 100,000 (2013)

	Non-Hispanic Black	Non-Hispanic White	Non-Hispanic Black/Non-Hispanic White Ratio
Men	289.1	217.9	1.2
Women	176.4	134.6	1.3
Total	215.5	171.8	1.3

Source: CDC, 2014. National Vital Statistics Report. Vol. 64, Num 2

At a Glance—Risk Factors

There are several risk factors related to heart disease. Some of these risk factors are:

Obesity and Overweight

Hypertension

Table 33.4. Age-Adjusted Percentage of Persons 20 Years of Age and over Who Have High Blood Pressure, 2009-2012.

	Non-Hispanic Black	Non-Hispanic White	Non-Hispanic Black/Non-Hispanic White Ratio
Men	42.5	29.6	1.4
Women	44.2	27.5	1.6

Source: CDC 2015 Health United States, 2014.

Table 33.5. Age-Adjusted Percentage of Persons 18 Years of Age and over Who Have High Blood Pressure, 2012.

Non-Hispanic Black	Non-Hispanic White	Non-Hispanic Black / Non-Hispanic White Ratio
33.2	23.4	1.4

Source: CDC 2014. Summary Health Statistics for U.S. Adults: 2012.

Table 33.6. Percent of Adults with Hypertension Whose Blood Pressure Is under Control, 2011-2012

Non-Hispanic Black	Non-Hispanic White	Non-Hispanic Black/Non-Hispanic White Ratio
48.7	53.9	0.9

Source: CDC 2015. Health Indicators Warehouse.

High Cholesterol

Table 33.7. Age-Adjusted Percentage of Persons 20 Years of Age and over Who Have High Cholesterol, 2009-2012.

	Non-Hispanic Black	Non-Hispanic White	Non-Hispanic Black/Non-Hispanic White Ratio
Men	25.6	28.1	0.9
Women	26.3	28.2	0.9

Source: CDC 2015. Health United States, 2014.

Table 33.8. Adults Who Received a Blood Cholesterol Measurement in the Last 5 Years, 2008

Non-Hispanic Black	Non-Hispanic White	Non-Hispanic Black/Non-Hispanic White Ratio
76.9	74.1	1

Source: AHRQ 2015. National Healthcare Quality and Disparities Reports. Data Query. Table 7 _5_ 1_ 4_2.1.

Table 33.9. Heart Disease and African Americans

Age-adjusted percentage of adults aged 20 and over screened for cholesterol, 2011-2012			
	Non-Hispanic Black	Non-Hispanic White	Non-Hispanic Black / Non- Hispanic White Ratio
Men	66.8	70.6	0.9
Women	75.9	72.9	1
Total	71.9	71.8	1

Source: CDC 2013. NCHS Data Brief, No. 132,

Cigarette Smoking

Table 33.10. Age-Adjusted Percentage of Persons 18 Years of Age and over Who Are Current Cigarette Smokers, 2009-2011.

	Non-Hispanic Black	Non-Hispanic White	Non-Hispanic Black/Non-Hispanic White Ratio
Men	22.5	22.1	1
Women	14.9	19.2	0.8

Source: CDC, 2015. Health United States, 2014

Table 33.11. Percentage of Current Smokers Age 18 and over with a Checkup Who Reported Receiving Advice to Quit Smoking, 2009

	Non-Hispanic Black	Non-Hispanic White	Non-Hispanic Black/Non-Hispanic White Ratio
Men	59	66.3	0.9
Women	61.5	73.8	0.8
Total	60.5	70.5	0.9

Source: 2013 National Healthcare Quality Report. Table T2_10_1_1-1_2b.

At a Glance—Treatment

Table 33.12. Hospital Patients with Heart Attack Who Were Prescribed ACE Inhibitor or ARB at Discharge, United States, 2012

Black	White	Black/ White Ratio
97.5	96.1	1

Source: AHRQ 2015. National Healthcare Quality and Disparities Reports. Data Query. Table 6_2_3_1_1.1.

Section 33.3

Cardiovascular Disease in the Hispanic Population

This section contains text excerpted from the following sources: Text beginning with the heading "Hispanic Health" is excerpted from "Hispanic Health," Centers for Disease Control and Prevention (CDC), May 5, 2015; Text beginning with the heading "Cardiovascular Disease Is the Leading Cause of Death Among U.S. Hispanics" is excerpted from "Cardiovascular Disease Is the Leading Cause of Death Among U.S. Hispanics," Centers for Disease Control and Prevention (CDC), April 22, 2013.

Hispanic Health

- About 1 in 6 people living in the United States are Hispanic (almost 57 million). By 2035, this could be nearly 1 in 4.

- Hispanic death rate is 24% lower than whites ("non-Hispanic whites").

- Hispanics are about 50% more likely to die from diabetes or liver disease than whites.

Hispanics or Latinos are the largest racial/ethnic minority population in the United States. Heart disease and cancer in Hispanics are the two leading causes of death, accounting for about 2 of 5 deaths, which is about the same for whites. Hispanics have lower deaths than whites from most of the 10 leading causes of death with three exceptions—more deaths from diabetes and chronic liver disease, and similar numbers of deaths from kidney diseases. Health risk can vary by Hispanic subgroup—for example, 66% more Puerto Ricans smoke than Mexicans. Health risk also depends partly on whether you were born in the United States or another country. Hispanics are almost 3 times as likely to be uninsured as whites. Hispanics in the United States are on average nearly 15 years younger than whites, so steps Hispanics take now to prevent disease can go a long way.

Problem

Health Risks Differ among Hispanics

Hispanics have different degrees of illness or health risks than whites.

- 35% less heart disease and 49% less cancer;
- A lower death rate overall, but about a 50% higher death rate from diabetes;
- 24% more poorly controlled high blood pressure;
- 23% more obesity;
- 28% less colorectal screening.

Hispanic subgroups have different degrees of health risk and more need to receive preventive screenings as recommended.

- Mexicans and Puerto Ricans are about twice as likely to die from diabetes as whites. Mexicans also are nearly twice as likely to die from chronic liver disease and cirrhosis as whites.

- Smoking overall among Hispanics (14%) is less common than among whites (24%), but is high among Puerto Rican males (26%) and Cuban males (22%).*

- Colorectal cancer screening varies for Hispanics ages 50 to 75 years.

  - About 40% of Cubans get screened (29% of men and 49% of women);

  - About 58% of Puerto Ricans get screened (54% of men and 61% of women).

- Hispanics are as likely as whites to have high blood pressure. But Hispanic women with high blood pressure are twice as likely as Hispanic men to get it under control.

Whether Hispanics were born in the United States makes a difference.

- Cancers related to infections (cervical, stomach, and liver) are more common among Hispanics born in another country.

- Compared with U.S.-born Hispanics, foreign-born Hispanics have:

  - About half as much heart disease;

  - 48% less cancer;

  - 29% less high blood pressure;

  - 45% more high total cholesterol.

- Social factors may play a major role in Hispanic health. Among Hispanics living in the United States:

  - About 1 in 3 has not completed high school;

  - About 1 in 4 lives below the poverty line;

  - About 1 in 3 does not speak English well.

  * National Health Interview Survey data, 2009-2013 combined, for ages 18-64 years.

Differences in the 10 Leading Causes of Death, Non-Hispanic Whites vs Hispanics

Non-Hispanic Whites

- Heart Disease
- Cancer
- Chronic Lower Respiratory Diseases
- Unintentional Injuries
- Stroke
- Alzheimer Disease
- Diabetes
- Influenza and Pneumonia
- Suicide
- Kidney Diseases*

Hispanics

- Cancer
- Heart Disease

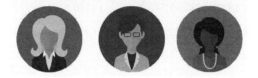

	Non-Hispanic Whites	Hispanics
Heart Disease	8%	5%
Cancer	4%	2%
High Blood Pressure	20%	17%
Poorly controlled High Blood Pressure	54%	68%

SOURCES: National Health Interview Survey, 2009-2013,
National Health and Nutrition Examination Survey, 2009-2012.

Figure 33.1. *Differences in Selected Chronic Disease Burden for Non-Hispanic Whites vs. Hispanics*

- Unintentional Injuries
- Stroke
- Diabetes
- Chronic Liver Disease and Cirrhosis
- Chronic Lower Respiratory Diseases
- Alzheimer Disease
- Influenza and Pneumonia
- Kidney Diseases*

* Types of kidney diseases–Nephritis, Nephrotic Syndrome and Nephrosis

Top Diseases and Risk Factors for Hispanics

Top Diseases

% of Hispanic population with disease

- Cancer: 2.7% U.S.-born, 1.4% Foreign-born.
- Heart Disease: 6.8% U.S.-born, 3.6% Foreign-born.

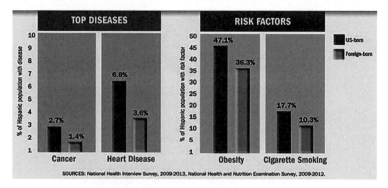

Figure 33.2. *Top Diseases and Risk Factors for Hispanics*

Risk Factors

% of Hispanic population with risk factor

- Obesity: 47.1% U.S.-born, 36.3% Foreign-born.
- Cigarette Smoking: 17.7% U.S.-born, 10.3% Foreign-born.

What Can Be Done?

Federal Government Is

- Helping eligible Hispanics get insurance coverage through the Affordable Care Act.

- Working to build capacity in communities to use community health workers (promotores de salud) to help improve the health of Hispanic communities.

- Leveraging existing programs to improve community health services and access to preventive care.

- Making efforts to better represent all Hispanics in national health surveillance data and research studies and use the data to help improve Hispanic health.

Doctors and Other Healthcare Professionals Can

- Work with interpreters to eliminate language barriers, when patient prefers to speak Spanish.

- Counsel patients on weight control and diet if they have or are at high risk for high blood pressure, diabetes, or cancer.

- Ask patients if they smoke and if they do, help them quit. www.espanol.smokefree.gov 1-800-QUIT-NOW (1-800-784-8669).

Engage community health workers (promotores de salud) to educate and link people to free or low-cost services.

Community Health Workers (Promotores De Salud) Can

Use resources that have been developed to educate the Hispanic community about health risks and preventive services.

Everyone Can

- Sign up for health insurance, if eligible, through the Affordable Care Act regardless of whether or not you have a pre-existing condition and find out if you are eligible for cost savings.

- Talk to your doctor or other healthcare professional about which cancer screening tests to get and how often, especially if you have a family history of cancer. Follow-up on any abnormal results.

- Make a strong effort to follow proven health tips such as quitting smoking, staying on medicine to control blood pressure and cholesterol, and maintaining a healthy weight by taking at least one brisk 10-minute walk, 3 times a day, 5 days a week.

- Learn about diabetes and how to prevent type 2 diabetes.

- Eat a healthy diet that is low in salt, low in total fat, saturated fat, and cholesterol, and rich in fresh fruits and vegetables.

Cardiovascular Disease Is the Leading Cause of Death among U.S. Hispanics

Just 40.7 percent of Hispanics said their blood pressure was under control. CDC and Million Hearts have developed educational resources to help Hispanics take control of their heart health.

A recent survey by the Centers for Disease Control and Prevention found that more than a quarter (26.1 percent) of Hispanics reported having high blood pressure, and nearly a third (30.4 percent) with high blood pressure weren't taking medication that could reduce their risk for heart attack and stroke. Educational resources to help Hispanics take control of their heart health is available from CDC and Million Hearts, a national public-private partnership that works to prevent 1 million heart attacks and strokes by 2017.

"Cardiovascular disease is the leading killer in every racial and ethnic group in America, and Million Hearts is committed to ensuring that everyone understands their risk," said Janet Wright, M.D., executive director of Million Hearts." These new resources will help Spanish-speaking Americans calculate their risk and, more importantly, take steps to reduce it."

A recent survey by the Centers for Disease Control and Prevention found that high blood pressure among Hispanic groups is a particular concern. More than a quarter (26.1 percent) of Hispanics reported having high blood pressure, and nearly a third (30.4 percent) with high blood pressure weren't taking medication that could reduce their risk for heart attack and stroke. Just 40.7 percent of Hispanics said their blood pressure was under control.

"If you have high blood pressure, work with your doctor to get it controlled and keep it controlled," said Thomas Frieden, MD, MPH, CDC director. "Take care of your heart for yourself, and for your family."

The new educational resources provide action steps and tips:

- The Four Steps for Heart Health fact sheet encourages individuals to work with their healthcare team to focus on the Million Hearts ABCS—**A**spirin for people at risk (people who have already experienced a heart attack or certain type of stroke and their doctor has advised them to take aspirin to prevent another), **B**lood pressure control, **C**holesterol management, and Smoking cessation—to help prevent heart attacks and strokes.

- How to Control Your Hypertension/Learning to Control Your Sodium Intake: a Fotonovela is an illustrated booklet that includes multi-generational advice on getting high blood pressure control by reducing sodium and is designed to be integrated into community health programs.

- The Million Hearts website offers guidance and tools for improving heart health, including a heart risk calculator, a journal to record blood pressure readings and track progress, and links to other resources.

The National Alliance for Hispanic Health, a non-profit science-based organization that focuses on improving the health and well-being of Hispanics, provided guidance on translation for cultural integrity during development of the materials. The Alliance will distribute the Four Steps for Heart Health fact sheet through its network of clinics and community health professionals.

"The Alliance is committed to the prevention of 1 million heart attacks and strokes by collaborating with Million Hearts to develop, promote, and distribute these new materials in the communities we serve," said Jane L. Delgado, Ph.D., M.S., president and CEO of the Alliance. "We consider this outreach a critical component of our ongoing efforts to improve the health of Hispanic communities and our work with others to secure health for all."

Section 33.4

Things to Know about Cardiovascular Disease in Asian Americans

This section includes text excerpted from "Heart Disease and Asians and Pacific Islanders," Office of Minority Health (OMH), U.S. Department of Health and Human Services (HHS), January 28, 2016.

Heart Disease and Asians and Pacific Islanders

Overall, Asian American adults are less likely than white adults to have heart disease and they are less likely to die from heart disease. In general, Asian American adults have lower rates of being overweight or obese, lower rates of hypertension, and they are less likely to be current cigarette smokers.

- Asian Americans are 50 percent less likely to die from heart disease than non-Hispanic whites.

At a Glance—Diagnosed Cases of Heart Disease

Table 33.13. Age-adjusted percentages of coronary heart disease among persons 18 years of age and over, 2012

	Non-Hispanic Whites	Hispanics
Heart Disease:	8.00%	5.00%
Cancer:	4.00%	2.00%
High Blood Pressure:	20.00%	17.00%
Poorly controlled High Blood Pressure:	54.00%	68.00%

Source: CDC 2014. Summary Health Statistics for U.S. Adults: 2012.

At a Glance—Death Rate

Table 33.14. Age-Adjusted Heart Disease Death Rates per 100,000 (2013)

Asians	Non-Hispanic White	Asian/Non-Hispanic White Ratio
4.5	6.2	0.7

Source: CDC, 2014. National Vital Statistics Report. Vol. 64, Num 2

At a Glance—Risk Factors

There are several risk factors related to diabetes. Some of these risk factors are:

Obesity and Overweight

Hypertension

Table 33.15. Age-Adjusted Percentage of Persons 18 Years of Age and over Who Have High Blood Pressure, 2012

	Asians/Pacific Islanders	Non-Hispanic White	Asians/Pacific Islanders /Non-Hispanic White Ratio
Men	118.4	217.9	0.5
Women	73.3	134.6	0.5
Total	92.8	171.8	0.5

Source: CDC 2014. Summary Health Statistics for U.S. Adults: 2012.
Percent of adults age 18 and over with hypertension whose blood pressure is under control not available.

High Cholesterol

Table 33.16. Age-Adjusted Percentage of Adults Aged 20 and over with High Total Cholesterol, 2011-2012

Asians	Non-Hispanic White	Asian/Non-Hispanic White Ratio
21.2	23.4	0.9

Source: CDC 2013. NCHS Data Brief, No. 132,

Table 33.17. Age-Adjusted Percentage of Adults Aged 20 and over Screened for Cholesterol, 2011-2012

Age-adjusted percentage of adults aged 20 and over with high total cholesterol, 2011-2012			
	Non-Hispanic Asian	Non-Hispanic White	Non-Hispanic Asian / Non- Hispanic White Ratio
Men	9.5	11.6	0.8
Women	10.9	15.2	0.7
Total	10.3	13.5	0.8

Source: CDC 2013. NCHS Data Brief, No. 132

Table 33.18. Age-Adjusted Percentage of Adults (Men and Women) with High Cholesterol, 2001-2002 (BRFSS, REACH 2010 Surveys)

Age-adjusted percentage of adults aged 20 and over screened for cholesterol, 2011-2012			
	Non-Hispanic Asian	Non-Hispanic White	Non-Hispanic Asian /Non-Hispanic White Ratio
Men	70.6	70.6	1
Women	70.9	72.9	1
Total	70.8	71.8	1

Source: CDC, 2004. Morbidity and Mortality Weekly Report: 53(33): 760-765

Table 33.19. Age-Adjusted Percentage of Adults (Men and Women) Who Had Their Blood Cholesterol Checked, 2001-2002 (BRFSS, REACH 2010 Surveys)

Population	% diagnosed with high cholesterol	Ratio vs. General Population
Asians	28.5	1
U.S. General Public	29.7	--
Cambodians (Lowell, MA)	24.5	0.8
Vietnamese (LA, Orange, and Santa Clara Counties, CA)	24.8	0.8

Source: CDC, 2004. Morbidity and Mortality Weekly Report: 53(33):760-765,

Table 33.20. Adults Who Received a Blood Cholesterol Measurement in the Last 5 Years, 2008

Population	% checked blood cholesterol	Ratio vs. General Population
Asians	70.1	0.9
U.S. General Public	77.4	--
Cambodians (Lowell, MA)	47.7	0.6
Vietnamese (LA, Orange, and Santa Clara Counties, CA)	68.3	0.9

Source: AHRQ 2015. National Healthcare Quality and Disparities Reports. Data Query.

Cigarette Smoking

Table 33.21. Age-adjusted percentage of persons 18 years of age and over who are current cigarette smokers, 2012

Asians	Non-Hispanic White	Asian/Non-Hispanic White Ratio
80.5	74.1	1.1

Source: CDC 2014. Summary Health Statistics for U.S. Adults: 2012. Percentage of current smokers age 18 and over with a checkup who reported receiving advice to quit smoking not available

Table 33.22. Age-Adjusted Percent of persons 18+ who currently smoke, 2011–2013.

Asian	Non-Hispanic White	Asian/White Ratio
10.4	20.6	0.5

Source: CDC 2015. Health United States, 2014.

At a Glance—Treatment

Table 33.23. Hospital Patients with Heart Attack Who Were Prescribed ACE Inhibitor or ARB at Discharge, United States, 2012

	Asians	Non-Hispanic White	Asians /Non-Hispanic White Ratio
Male	14.8	22.1	0.7
Female	5.2	19.2	0.3

Source: AHRQ 2015. National Healthcare Quality and Disparities Reports. Data Query

Section 33.5

Cardiovascular Disease among American Indians and Alaska Natives

This section contains text excerpted from the following sources:
Text in this section begins with excerpts from "American Indian
and Alaska Native Heart Disease and Stroke Fact Sheet," Centers
for Disease Control and Prevention (CDC), April 30, 2015; Text
beginning with the heading "Heart Disease and American Indians /
Alaska Natives" is excerpted from "Heart Disease and American
Indians / Alaska Natives," Office of Minority Health (OMH),
U.S. Department of Health and Human Services (HHS),
January 28, 2016.

Stroke is the fifth leading cause of death among American Indians
and Alaska Natives. In 2003, stroke caused 552 deaths among American Indians and Alaska Natives.

Heart disease and stroke are also major causes of disability and
can decrease a person's quality of life.

The American Indian and Alaska Native Population

- There are approximately 4.5 million American Indians and
  Alaska Natives in the United States, 1.5% of the population,
  including those of more than one race.

- The median age of American Indians and Alaska Natives is 30.7
  years, which is younger than the 36.2 years of the total U.S.
  population.

- California has the largest population of American Indians and
  Alaska Natives (696,600), followed by Oklahoma (401,100),
  and Arizona (334,700). Alaska has the highest proportion of
  American Indians and Alaska Natives in its populations (20%),
  followed by Oklahoma and New Mexico (11% each). Los Angeles County is the county with the most American Indians and
  Alaska Natives (154,000).

- A language other than English is spoken at home by 25% of
  American Indians and Alaska Natives aged 5 years and older.

- A high school diploma is held by 76% of American Indians and Alaska Natives over age 25; 14 percent have a bachelor's degree or higher. The poverty rate of people who report American Indian and Alaska Native race only is 25%.

- Approximately 177,000 American Indians and Alaska Natives are veterans.

American Indian and Alaska Native Heart Disease and Stroke Facts

- Heart Disease is the first and stroke the sixth leading cause of death Among American Indians and Alaska Natives.

- The heart disease death rate was 20 percent greater and the stroke death rate 14 percent greater among American Indians and Alaska Natives (1996–1998) than among all U.S. races (1997) after adjusting for misreporting of American Indian and Alaska Native race on state death certificates.

- The highest heart disease death rates are located primarily in South Dakota and North Dakota, Wisconsin, and Michigan.

- Counties with the highest stroke death rates are primarily in Alaska, Washington, Idaho, Montana, Wyoming, South Dakota, Wisconsin, and Minnesota.

- American Indians and Alaska Natives die from heart diseases at younger ages than other racial and ethnic groups in the United States. Thirty–six percent of those who die of heart disease die before age 65.

- Diabetes is an extremely important risk factor for cardiovascular disease among American Indians.

- Cigarette smoking, a risk factor for heart disease and stroke, is highest in the Northern Plains (44.1%) and Alaska (39.0%) and lowest in the Southwest (21.2%) among American Indians and Alaska Natives.

Preventing Heart Disease and Stroke among American Indians and Alaska Natives

Prevent and Control High Blood Cholesterol

High blood cholesterol is a major risk factor for heart disease. Preventing and treating high blood cholesterol includes eating a diet low in saturated fat and cholesterol and high in fiber, keeping a healthy weight, and getting regular exercise. All adults should have their cholesterol levels checked once every five years. If yours is high, your doctor may prescribe medicines to help lower it.

Prevent and Control High Blood Pressure

Lifestyle actions such as healthy diet, regular physical activity, not smoking, and healthy weight will help you to keep normal blood pressure levels. Blood pressure is easily checked, and all adults should have it checked on a regular basis. If your blood pressure is high, you can work with your doctor to treat it and bring it down to the normal range. A high blood pressure can usually be controlled with lifestyle changes and with medicines when needed.

Prevent and Control Diabetes

Diabetes has been shown to be a very important risk factor for heart disease among American Indians and Alaska Natives. People with diabetes have an increased risk for heart disease but can reduce their risk. Also, people can take steps to reduce their risk for diabetes in the first place, through weight loss and regular physical activity.

No Tobacco

Chewing, dipping, and cigarette smoking are non-traditional uses of tobacco among American Indians and Alaska Natives. Smoking increases the risk of high blood pressure, heart disease, and stroke. Never smoking is one of the best things a person can do to lower their risk. And, quitting smoking will also help lower a person's risk of heart disease. A person's risk of heart attack decreases soon after quitting. If you smoke, your doctor can suggest programs to help you quit smoking.

Moderate Alcohol Use

Excessive alcohol use increases the risk of high blood pressure, heart attack, and stroke. People who drink should do so only in moderation and always responsibly.

Maintain a Healthy Weight

Healthy weight status in adults is usually assessed by using weight and height to compute a number called the "body mass index" (BMI). BMI usually indicates the amount of body fat. An adult who has a BMI of 30 or higher is considered obese. Overweight is a BMI between 25 and 29.9. Normal weight is a BMI of 18 to 24.9. Proper diet and regular physical activity can help to maintain a healthy weight.

Regular Physical Activity

Adults should engage in moderate level physical activities for at least 30 minutes on most days of the week.

Diet and Nutrition

Along with healthy weight and regular physical activity, an overall healthy diet can help to lower blood pressure and cholesterol levels and prevent obesity, diabetes, heart disease, and stroke. This includes eating lots of fresh fruits and vegetables, lowering or cutting out added salt or sodium, and eating less saturated fat and cholesterol to lower these risks.

Treat Atrial Fibrillation

Atrial fibrillation is an irregular beating of the heart. It can cause clots that can lead to stroke. A doctor can prescribe medications to help reduce the chance of clots.

Genetic Risk Factors

Stroke can run in families. Genes play a role in stroke risk factors such as high blood pressure, heart disease, diabetes, and vascular conditions. It is also possible that an increased risk for stroke within a family is due to factors such as a common sedentary lifestyle or poor eating habits, rather than hereditary factors.

CDC Activities to Reduce the Burden of Heart Disease and Stroke among American Indians and Alaska Natives

Atlas of Heart Disease and Stroke Among American Indians and Alaska Natives is the first in a series of atlases to focus on a specific racial or ethnic group. It contains county level heart disease and stroke mortality maps (1995–1999) as well as state level surveillance data on heart disease and stroke risk factors (2001–2003). This information can help health professionals and concerned citizens tailor prevention policies and programs to communities with the greatest burden and risk.

Heart Disease and American Indians / Alaska Natives

American Indians / Alaska Natives, on average, are more likely to be diagnosed with heart disease than their white counterparts. In addition, American Indians / Alaska Native adults are more likely to be obese than white adults, more likely to have high blood pressure, and they are more likely to be current cigarette smokers than white adults-all risk factors for heart disease

- American Indian / Alaska Native men are 20 percent more likely than white men to be current cigarette smokers.

- American Indian / Alaska Native adults are 30 percent more likely than white adults to have high blood pressure.

At a Glance–Diagnosed Cases of Coronary Heart Disease:

Table 33.24. Age-Adjusted Percentages of Coronary Heart Disease among Persons 18 Years of Age and over, 2012

Asian	White	Asian / White Ratio
97.2	96.1	1

Source: CDC 2014. Summary Health Statistics for U.S. Adults: 2014

At a Glance–Death Rate:

Table 33.25. Age-Adjusted Heart Disease Death Rates per 100,000 (2013)

	American Indians / Alaska Natives	Non-Hispanic White	American Indians / Alaska Natives / Non-Hispanic White Ratio
Men	152.3	217.9	0.7
Women	93.9	134.6	0.7
Total	120.6	171.8	0.7

Source:CDC 2014. National Vital Statistics Report. Vol. 64, Num 2

At a Glance–Risk Factors:

There are several factors related to diabetes. Some of these risk factors are:

Obesity and Overweight

Hypertension

Table 33.26. Age-Adjusted Percentage of Persons 18 Years of Age and over Who Have High Blood Pressure, 2012.

American Indian / Alaska Native	Non-Hispanic White	American Indian / Alaska Native / Non-Hispanic White Ratio
24.8	23.4	1.1

Source: CDC 2014. Summary Health Statistics for U.S. Adults: 2012.

High Cholesterol

Age-adjusted percentage of persons 20 years of age and over who have high cholesterol
Not available at this time.

Table 33.27. Adults Who Received a Blood Cholesterol Measurement in the Last 5 Years, 2008

American Indian / Alaska Natives	Non-Hispanic White	American Indian / Alaska Native / Non-Hispanic White Ratio
66.5	74.1	0.9

Source: AHRQ 2015. National Healthcare Quality and Disparities Reports. Data Query. BRFSS

Table 33.28. Age-Adjusted Percentage of Persons 18 Years of Age and over Who Are Current Cigarette Smokers, 2012

American Indian / Alaska Natives	Non-Hispanic White	American Indian / Alaska Native / Non-Hispanic White Ratio
18.8	20.6	0.9

Source: CDC 2014. Summary Health Statistics for U.S. Adults 2012.

Table 33.29. Age-Adjusted Percent of Persons 18+ Who Currently Smoke, 2011-2013

	American Indian / Alaska Natives	Non-Hispanic White	American Indian / Alaska Natives / Non-Hispanic White Ratio
Male	25.6	22.1	1.2
Women	19.1	19.2	1

Source: CDC 2014. Health United States, 2013. Percentage of current smokers age 18 and over with a checkup who reported receiving advice to quit smoking Not available at this time.

At a Glance–Treatment:

Table 33.30. Hospital Patients with Heart Attack Who Were Prescribed ACE Inhibitor or ARB at Discharge, United States, 2012

American Indians / Alaska Natives	White	American Indians / Alaska Natives/White Ratio
96.6	96.1	1

Source: AHRQ 2015. National Healthcare Quality and Disparities Reports. Data Query.

Part Five

Diagnosing Cardiovascular Disorders

Chapter 34

Recognizing Signs and Symptoms of Heart Disease

The five major symptoms of a heart attack are

1. Pain or discomfort in the jaw, neck, or back.

2. Feeling weak, light-headed, or faint.

3. Chest pain or discomfort.

4. Pain or discomfort in arms or shoulder.

5. Shortness of breath.

Other symptoms of a heart attack could include unusual or unexplained tiredness and nausea or vomiting. Women are more likely to have these other symptoms.

What Are the Signs and Symptoms of Heart Disease?

The signs and symptoms of coronary heart disease (CHD) may differ between women and men. Some women who have CHD have no signs or symptoms. This is called silent CHD.

This chapter contains text excerpted from the following sources: Text in this chapter begins with excerpts from "Heart Attack Signs and Symptoms," Centers for Disease Control and Prevention (CDC), August 5, 2015; Text under the heading "What Are the Signs and Symptoms of Heart Disease?" is excerpted from "Heart Disease in Women," National Heart, Lung, and Blood Institute (NHLBI), April 21, 2014.

Silent CHD may not be diagnosed until a woman has signs and symptoms of a heart attack, heart failure, or an arrhythmia (irregular heartbeat). Other women who have CHD will have signs and symptoms of the disease.

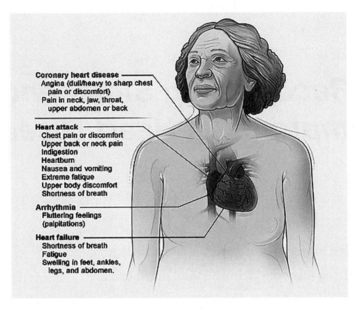

Figure 34.1. *Heart Disease Signs and Symptoms*

The illustration shows the major signs and symptoms of coronary heart disease.

A common symptom of CHD is angina. Angina is chest pain or discomfort that occurs when your heart muscle doesn't get enough oxygen-rich blood.

In men, angina often feels like pressure or squeezing in the chest. This feeling may extend to the arms. Women can also have these angina symptoms. But women also tend to describe a sharp, burning chest pain. Women are more likely to have pain in the neck, jaw, throat, abdomen, or back.

In men, angina tends to worsen with physical activity and go away with rest. Women are more likely than men to have angina while they're resting or sleeping.

In women who have coronary microvascular disease, angina often occurs during routine daily activities, such as shopping or cooking, rather than while exercising. Mental stress also is more likely to trigger angina pain in women than in men.

The severity of angina varies. The pain may get worse or occur more often as the buildup of plaque continues to narrow the coronary (heart) arteries.

Signs and Symptoms Coronary Heart Disease Complications

Heart Attack

The most common heart attack symptom in men and women is chest pain or discomfort. However, only half of women who have heart attacks have chest pain.

Women are more likely than men to report back or neck pain, indigestion, heartburn, nausea (feeling sick to the stomach), vomiting, extreme fatigue (tiredness), or problems breathing.

Heart attacks also can cause upper body discomfort in one or both arms, the back, neck, jaw, or upper part of the stomach. Other heart attack symptoms are light-headedness and dizziness, which occur more often in women than men.

Men are more likely than women to break out in a cold sweat and to report pain in the left arm during a heart attack.

Heart Failure

Heart failure is a condition in which your heart can't pump enough blood to meet your body's needs. Heart failure doesn't mean that your heart has stopped or is about to stop working. It means that your heart can't cope with the demands of everyday activities.

Heart failure causes shortness of breath and fatigue that tends to increase with physical exertion. Heart failure also can cause swelling in the feet, ankles, legs, abdomen, and veins in the neck.

Arrhythmia

An arrhythmia is a problem with the rate or rhythm of the heartbeat. During an arrhythmia, the heart can beat too fast, too slow, or with an irregular rhythm.

Some people describe arrhythmias as fluttering or thumping feelings or skipped beats in their chests. These feelings are called palpitations.

Some arrhythmias can cause your heart to suddenly stop beating. This condition is called sudden cardiac arrest (SCA). SCA causes loss of consciousness and death if it's not treated right away.

Signs and Symptoms of Broken Heart Syndrome

The most common signs and symptoms of broken heart syndrome are chest pain and shortness of breath. In this disorder, these symptoms tend to occur suddenly in people who have no history of heart disease.

Arrhythmias or cardiogenic shock also may occur. Cardiogenic shock is a condition in which a suddenly weakened heart isn't able to pump enough blood to meet the body's needs.

Some of the signs and symptoms of broken heart syndrome differ from those of heart attack. For example, in people who have broken heart syndrome:

- Symptoms occur suddenly after having extreme emotional or physical stress.

- EKG (electrocardiogram) results don't look the same as the EKG results for a person having a heart attack. (An EKG is a test that records the heart's electrical activity.)

- Blood tests show no signs or mild signs of heart damage.

- Tests show no signs of blockages in the coronary arteries.

- Tests show ballooning and unusual movement of the lower left heart chamber (left ventricle).

- Recovery time is quick, usually within days or weeks (compared with the recovery time of a month or more for a heart attack).

Chapter 35

Blood Tests Used to Diagnose Cardiovascular Disorders

Blood tests help doctors check for certain diseases and conditions. They also help check the function of your organs and show how well treatments are working.

Specifically, blood tests can help doctors:

- Evaluate how well organs—such as the kidneys, liver, thyroid, and heart—are working

- Diagnose diseases and conditions such as cancer, HIV/AIDS, diabetes, anemia, and coronary heart disease

- Find out whether you have risk factors for heart disease

- Check whether medicines you're taking are working

- Assess how well your blood is clotting

This chapter contains text from the following sources: Text in this chapter begins with excerpts from "Blood Tests," National Heart, Lung, and Blood Institute (NHLBI), January 6, 2012. Reviewed June 2016; Text under the heading "Other Blood Tests to Assess Heart Disease Risk," is © 2016 Omnigraphics. Reviewed June 2016.

What Are the Risks of Blood Tests?

The main risks of blood tests are discomfort and bruising at the site where the needle goes in. These complications usually are minor and go away shortly after the tests are done.

What Do Blood Tests Show?

Blood tests show whether the levels of different substances in your blood fall within a normal range.

For many blood substances, the normal range is the range of levels seen in 95 percent of healthy people in a certain group. For many tests, normal ranges vary depending on your age, gender, race, and other factors.

Your blood test results may fall outside the normal range for many reasons. Abnormal results might be a sign of a disorder or disease. Other factors—such as diet, menstrual cycle, physical activity level, alcohol intake, and medicines (both prescription and over the counter)—also can cause abnormal results.

Your doctor should discuss any unusual or abnormal blood test results with you. These results may or may not suggest a health problem.

Many diseases and medical problems can't be diagnosed with blood tests alone. However, blood tests can help you and your doctor learn more about your health. Blood tests also can help find potential problems early, when treatments or lifestyle changes may work best.

Types of Blood Tests

Some of the most common blood tests are:

- A complete blood count (CBC)
- Blood chemistry tests
- Blood enzyme tests
- Blood tests to assess heart disease risk

Complete Blood Count

The CBC is one of the most common blood tests. It's often done as part of a routine checkup.

The CBC can help detect blood diseases and disorders, such as anemia, infections, clotting problems, blood cancers, and immune system disorders. This test measures many different parts of your blood.

Blood Chemistry Tests / Basic Metabolic Panel

The basic metabolic panel (BMP) is a group of tests that measures different chemicals in the blood. These tests usually are done on the fluid (plasma) part of blood. The tests can give doctors information about your muscles (including the heart), bones, and organs, such as the kidneys and liver.

The BMP includes blood glucose, calcium, and electrolyte tests, as well as blood tests that measure kidney function. Some of these tests require you to fast (not eat any food) before the test, and others don't. Your doctor will tell you how to prepare for the test(s) you're having.

Blood Enzyme Tests

Enzymes are chemicals that help control chemical reactions in your body. There are many blood enzyme tests. These include troponin and creatine kinase (CK) tests.

Blood Tests to Assess Heart Disease Risk

A lipoprotein panel is a blood test that can help show whether you're at risk for coronary heart disease (CHD). This test looks at substances in your blood that carry cholesterol.

A lipoprotein panel gives information about your:

- Total cholesterol.

- LDL ("bad") cholesterol. This is the main source of cholesterol buildup and blockages in the arteries. (For more information about blockages in the arteries, go to the Diseases and Conditions Index Atherosclerosis article.)

- HDL ("good") cholesterol. This type of cholesterol helps decrease blockages in the arteries.

- Triglycerides. Triglycerides are a type of fat in your blood.

A lipoprotein panel measures the levels of LDL and HDL cholesterol and triglycerides in your blood. Abnormal cholesterol and triglyceride levels may be signs of increased risk for CHD.

Most people will need to fast for 9 to 12 hours before a lipoprotein panel.

Other Blood Tests to Assess Heart Disease Risk

Cardiac Biomarker Tests

Cardiac biomarkers are substances, such as hormones, enzymes, and proteins, that are released into the bloodstream when a heart is stressed or damaged. Testing the level of these biomarkers facilitates an evaluation of heart function and allows medical personnel to analyze conditions that may arise from improper blood flow to the heart, such as cardiac ischemia and acute coronary syndrome (ACS).

Some biomarkers that may be used to diagnose and monitor individuals suspected of having ACS include:

- **Troponin (I or T):** Troponin I and Troponin T are proteins that are released into the bloodstream when there is damage to the heart muscle. A troponin test is commonly used because it is the most specific of all biomarkers and is highly sensitive. It is released into the bloodstream within a few hours of heart attack or other heart injury and lasts longer than other biomarkers.

- **High-sensitivity (HS) troponin:** Though this test is not yet approved in the United States, it is even more sensitive than the standard test and can detect ACS much sooner and at much lower levels of the protein. The HS-troponin may also be used to detect stable angina, even when there are no symptoms. In such instances, it can also reveal the risk of future occurrence of heart damage, such as heart attacks.

- **Creatinine kinase (CK) and CK-MB:** CK is a biomarker that, although not specific to heart damage, will usually elevate after a heart attack and can be measured a number of times over a 24-hour period. A second heart attack that occurs immediately after the first can sometimes be identified with this enzyme. CK-MB is a sub-type of CK that is generally elevated when there is an instance of heart attack. Since it is short-lived, this test cannot be used for late diagnosis.

- **Myoglobin:** This protein is occasionally measured along with troponin to diagnose heart attack, although this is also not a test that is specific to diagnosing heart damage.

Some other biomarker tests include:

- **HS-CRP:** A high-sensitivity C-reactive protein test may be used to evaluate an individual's risk for future heart attacks.

- **BNP (or NT-proBNP):** A Brain Natriuretic Peptide test may be used to detect heart damage and severity of heart failure. An increased level in individuals with existing ACS will reveal higher risk of a recurring event.

Other tests frequently ordered in conjunction with cardiac biomarkers include those that measure blood gases and electrolytes, as well as a complete blood count (CBC), electrocardiogram (EKG/ECG), echocardiogram, nuclear scan, coronary angiogram, and chest X-ray.

C-Reactive Protein Test

The C-reactive protein (CRP) is produced in the liver and released into the bloodstream as a response to an infection or inflammation. CRP levels can be measured to detect inflammation caused by conditions such as fungal or bacterial infections or pelvic inflammatory disease (PID). CRP level in the blood is measured to detect damage to the heart. It is typically compared with various signs and symptoms, as well as results of other tests, to diagnose acute or chronic inflammation in an individual. Though a CRP test on its own cannot be used to diagnose a particular disease, it can be treated as a general marker that warns a practitioner about other infections and inflammations.

Homocysteine Test

Homocysteine (an amino acid), when found in high levels in the bloodstream, is typically associated with blood clots and atherosclerosis. When an individual is diagnosed with heart attack, stroke, or blood clots in the absence of other common risk factors—such as obesity, high blood pressure, or smoking—a physician might order a homocysteine test. It may also be ordered to screen individuals at elevated risks of heart attack or stroke, especially when there is a family history of coronary artery disease.

References

1. "Cardiac Biomarkers," American Association for Clinical Chemistry, June 12, 2015.

2. "Cardiac Biomarkers (Blood)," University of Rochester Medical Center, n.d.

3. "C-Reactive Protein," American Association for Clinical Chemistry, March 30, 2015.

4. "Homocysteine," American Association for Clinical Chemistry, April 30, 2014.

5. "Homocysteine," eMedicineHealth, February 22, 2016.

Chapter 36

Electrocardiogram (ECG)

What Is an Electrocardiogram?

An electrocardiogram, also called an EKG or ECG, is a simple, painless test that records the heart's electrical activity. To understand this test, it helps to understand how the heart works.

With each heartbeat, an electrical signal spreads from the top of the heart to the bottom. As it travels, the signal causes the heart to contract and pump blood. The process repeats with each new heartbeat.

The heart's electrical signals set the rhythm of the heartbeat.

An EKG shows:

- How fast your heart is beating

- Whether the rhythm of your heartbeat is steady or irregular

- The strength and timing of electrical signals as they pass through each part of your heart

Doctors use EKGs to detect and study many heart problems, such as heart attacks, arrhythmias, and heart failure. The test's results also can suggest other disorders that affect heart function.

Other Names for an Electrocardiogram

An electrocardiogram also is called an EKG or ECG. Sometimes the test is called a 12-lead EKG or 12-lead ECG. This is because the heart's

This chapter includes text excerpted from "Electrocardiogram," National Heart, Lung, and Blood Institute (NHLBI), October 1, 2010. Reviewed June 2016.

electrical activity most often is recorded from 12 different places on the body at the same time.

Who Needs an Electrocardiogram?

Your doctor may recommend an electrocardiogram (EKG) if you have signs or symptoms that suggest a heart problem. Examples of such signs and symptoms include:

- Chest pain

- Heart pounding, racing, or fluttering, or the sense that your heart is beating unevenly

- Breathing problems

- Tiredness and weakness

- Unusual heart sounds when your doctor listens to your heartbeat

You may need to have more than one EKG so your doctor can diagnose certain heart conditions.

An EKG also may be done as part of a routine health exam. The test can screen for early heart disease that has no symptoms. Your doctor is more likely to look for early heart disease if your mother, father, brother, or sister had heart disease—especially early in life.

You may have an EKG so your doctor can check how well heart medicine or a medical device, such as a pacemaker, is working. The test also may be used for routine screening before major surgery.

Your doctor also may use EKG results to help plan your treatment for a heart condition.

What to Expect before an Electrocardiogram

You don't need to take any special steps before having an electrocardiogram (EKG). However, tell your doctor or his or her staff about the medicines you're taking. Some medicines can affect EKG results.

What to Expect during an Electrocardiogram

An electrocardiogram (EKG) is painless and harmless. A nurse or technician will attach soft, sticky patches called electrodes to the skin of your chest, arms, and legs. The patches are about the size of a quarter.

Often, 12 patches are attached to your body. This helps detect your heart's electrical activity from many areas at the same time. The nurse may have to shave areas of your skin to help the patches stick.

After the patches are placed on your skin, you'll lie still on a table while the patches detect your heart's electrical signals. A machine will record these signals on graph paper or display them on a screen.

The entire test will take about 10 minutes.

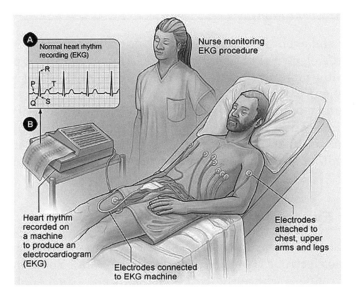

Figure 36.1. *EKG*

The image shows the standard setup for an EKG. (A), a normal heart rhythm recording shows the electrical pattern of a regular heartbeat. (B), a patient lies in a bed with EKG electrodes attached to his chest, upper arms, and legs. A nurse monitors the painless procedure.

Special Types of Electrocardiogram

The standard EKG described above, called a resting 12-lead EKG, only records seconds of heart activity at a time. It will show a heart problem only if the problem occurs during the test.

Many heart problems are present all the time, and a resting 12-lead EKG will detect them. But some heart problems, like those related to an irregular heartbeat, can come and go. They may occur only for a few minutes a day or only while you exercise.

Doctors use special EKGs, such as stress tests and Holter and event monitors, to help diagnose these kinds of problems.

Stress Test

Some heart problems are easier to diagnose when your heart is working hard and beating fast. During stress testing, you exercise to make your heart work hard and beat fast while an EKG is done. If you can't exercise, you'll be given medicine to make your heart work hard and beat fast.

Holter and Event Monitors

Holter and event monitors are small, portable devices. They record your heart's electrical activity while you do your normal daily activities. A Holter monitor records your heart's electrical activity for a full 24- or 48-hour period.

An event monitor records your heart's electrical activity only at certain times while you're wearing it. For many event monitors, you push a button to start the monitor when you feel symptoms. Other event monitors start automatically when they sense abnormal heart rhythms.

What to Expect after an Electrocardiogram

After an electrocardiogram (EKG), the nurse or technician will remove the electrodes (soft patches) from your skin. You may develop a rash or redness where the EKG patches were attached. This mild rash often goes away without treatment.

You usually can go back to your normal daily routine after an EKG.

What Does an Electrocardiogram Show?

Many heart problems change the heart's electrical activity in distinct ways. An electrocardiogram (EKG) can help detect these heart problems.

EKG recordings can help doctors diagnose heart attacks that are in progress or have happened in the past. This is especially true if doctors can compare a current EKG recording to an older one.

An EKG also can show:

- Lack of blood flow to the heart muscle (coronary heart disease)

- A heartbeat that's too fast, too slow, or irregular (arrhythmia)

- A heart that doesn't pump forcefully enough (heart failure)

- Heart muscle that's too thick or parts of the heart that are too big (cardiomyopathy)
- Birth defects in the heart (congenital heart defects)
- Problems with the heart valves (heart valve disease)
- Inflammation of the sac that surrounds the heart (pericarditis)

An EKG can reveal whether the heartbeat starts in the correct place in the heart. The test also shows how long it takes for electrical signals to travel through the heart. Delays in signal travel time may suggest heart block or long QT syndrome.

What Are the Risks of an Electrocardiogram?

An electrocardiogram (EKG) has no serious risks. It's a harmless, painless test that detects the heart's electrical activity. EKGs don't give off electrical charges, such as shocks.

You may develop a mild rash where the electrodes (soft patches) were attached. This rash often goes away without treatment.

Chapter 37

Echocardiography

What Is Echocardiography?

Echocardiography, or echo, is a painless test that uses sound waves to create moving pictures of your heart. The pictures show the size and shape of your heart. They also show how well your heart's chambers and valves are working.

Echo also can pinpoint areas of heart muscle that aren't contracting well because of poor blood flow or injury from a previous heart attack. A type of echo called Doppler ultrasound shows how well blood flows through your heart's chambers and valves.

Echo can detect possible blood clots inside the heart, fluid buildup in the pericardium (the sac around the heart), and problems with the aorta. The aorta is the main artery that carries oxygen-rich blood from your heart to your body.

Doctors also use echo to detect heart problems in infants and children.

Who Needs Echocardiography?

Your doctor may recommend echocardiography (echo) if you have signs or symptoms of heart problems.

For example, shortness of breath and swelling in the legs are possible signs of heart failure. Heart failure is a condition in which your

This chapter includes text excerpted from "Echocardiography," National Heart, Lung, and Blood Institute (NHLBI), October 31, 2011. Reviewed June 2016.

heart can't pump enough oxygen-rich blood to meet your body's needs. Echo can show how well your heart is pumping blood.

Echo also can help your doctor find the cause of abnormal heart sounds, such as heart murmurs. Heart murmurs are extra or unusual sounds heard during the heartbeat. Some heart murmurs are harmless, while others are signs of heart problems.

Your doctor also may use echo to learn about:

- The size of your heart. An enlarged heart might be the result of high blood pressure, leaky heart valves, or heart failure. Echo also can detect increased thickness of the ventricles (the heart's lower chambers). Increased thickness may be due to high blood pressure, heart valve disease, or congenital heart defects.

- Heart muscles that are weak and aren't pumping well. Damage from a heart attack may cause weak areas of heart muscle. Weakening also might mean that the area isn't getting enough blood supply, a sign of coronary heart disease.

- Heart valve problems. Echo can show whether any of your heart valves don't open normally or close tightly.

- Problems with your heart's structure. Echo can detect congenital heart defects, such as holes in the heart. Congenital heart defects are structural problems present at birth. Infants and children may have echo to detect these heart defects.

- Blood clots or tumors. If you've had a stroke, you may have echo to check for blood clots or tumors that could have caused the stroke.

Your doctor also might recommend echo to see how well your heart responds to certain heart treatments, such as those used for heart failure.

Types of Echocardiography

There are several types of echocardiography (echo)—all use sound waves to create moving pictures of your heart. This is the same technology that allows doctors to see an unborn baby inside a pregnant woman.

Unlike X-rays and some other tests, echo doesn't involve radiation.

Transthoracic Echocardiography

Transthoracic echo is the most common type of echocardiogram test. It's painless and noninvasive. "Noninvasive" means that no surgery is done and no instruments are inserted into your body.

This type of echo involves placing a device called a transducer on your chest. The device sends special sound waves, called ultrasound, through your chest wall to your heart. The human ear can't hear ultrasound waves.

As the ultrasound waves bounce off the structures of your heart, a computer in the echo machine converts them into pictures on a screen.

Stress Echocardiography

Stress echo is done as part of a stress test. During a stress test, you exercise or take medicine (given by your doctor) to make your heart work hard and beat fast. A technician will use echo to create pictures of your heart before you exercise and as soon as you finish.

Some heart problems, such as coronary heart disease, are easier to diagnose when the heart is working hard and beating fast.

Transesophageal Echocardiography

Your doctor may have a hard time seeing the aorta and other parts of your heart using a standard transthoracic echo. Thus, he or she may recommend transesophageal echo, or TEE.

During this test, the transducer is attached to the end of a flexible tube. The tube is guided down your throat and into your esophagus (the passage leading from your mouth to your stomach). This allows your doctor to get more detailed pictures of your heart.

Fetal Echocardiography

Fetal echo is used to look at an unborn baby's heart. A doctor may recommend this test to check a baby for heart problems. When recommended, the test is commonly done at about 18 to 22 weeks of pregnancy. For this test, the transducer is moved over the pregnant woman's belly.

Three-Dimensional Echocardiography

A three-dimensional (3D) echo creates 3D images of your heart. These detailed images show how your heart looks and works.

During transthoracic echo or TEE, 3D images can be taken as part of the process used to do these types of echo.

Doctors may use 3D echo to diagnose heart problems in children. They also may use 3D echo for planning and overseeing heart valve surgery.

Researchers continue to study new ways to use 3D echo.

Other Names for Echocardiography

- Echo

- Surface echo

- Ultrasound of the heart

What to Expect before Echocardiography

Echocardiography (echo) is done in a doctor's office or a hospital. No special preparations are needed for most types of echo. You usually can eat, drink, and take any medicines as you normally would.

The exception is if you're having a transesophageal echo. This test usually requires that you don't eat or drink for 8 hours prior to the test.

If you're having a stress echo, you may need to take steps to prepare for the stress test. Your doctor will let you know what steps you need to take.

What to Expect during Echocardiography

Echocardiography (echo) is painless; the test usually takes less than an hour to do. For some types of echo, your doctor will need to inject saline or a special dye into one of your veins. The substance makes your heart show up more clearly on the echo pictures.

The dye used for echo is different from the dye used during angiography (a test used to examine the body's blood vessels).

For most types of echo, you will remove your clothing from the waist up. Women will be given a gown to wear during the test. You'll lie on your back or left side on an exam table or stretcher.

Soft, sticky patches called electrodes will be attached to your chest to allow an EKG (electrocardiogram) to be done. An EKG is a test that records the heart's electrical activity.

A doctor or sonographer (a person specially trained to do ultrasounds) will apply gel to your chest. The gel helps the sound waves reach your heart. A wand-like device called a transducer will then be moved around on your chest.

The transducer transmits ultrasound waves into your chest. A computer will convert echoes from the sound waves into pictures of your heart on a screen. During the test, the lights in the room will be dimmed so the computer screen is easier to see.

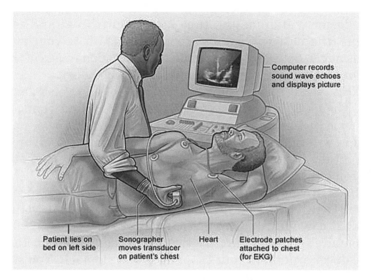

Figure 37.1. *Echocardiography*

The illustration shows a patient having echocardiography. The patient lies on his left side. A sonographer moves the transducer on the patient's chest, while viewing the echo pictures on a computer.

The sonographer will record pictures of various parts of your heart. He or she will put the recordings on a computer disc for a cardiologist (heart specialist) to review.

During the test, you may be asked to change positions or hold your breath for a short time. This allows the sonographer to get better pictures of your heart.

At times, the sonographer may apply a bit of pressure to your chest with the transducer. You may find this pressure a little uncomfortable, but it helps get the best picture of your heart. You should let the sonographer know if you feel too uncomfortable.

The process described above is similar to the process for fetal echo. For that test, however, the transducer is placed over the pregnant woman's belly at the location of the baby's heart.

Transesophageal Echocardiography

Transesophageal echo (TEE) is used if your doctor needs a more detailed view of your heart. For example, your doctor may use TEE to look for blood clots in your heart. A doctor, not a sonographer, will perform this type of echo.

TEE uses the same technology as transthoracic echo, but the transducer is attached to the end of a flexible tube.

Your doctor will guide the tube down your throat and into your esophagus (the passage leading from your mouth to your stomach). From this angle, your doctor can get a more detailed image of the heart and major blood vessels leading to and from the heart.

For TEE, you'll likely be given medicine to help you relax during the test. The medicine will be injected into one of your veins.

Your blood pressure, the oxygen content of your blood, and other vital signs will be checked during the test. You'll be given oxygen through a tube in your nose. If you wear dentures or partials, you'll have to remove them.

The back of your mouth will be numbed with gel or spray. Your doctor will gently place the tube with the transducer in your throat and guide it down until it's in place behind your heart.

The pictures of your heart are then recorded as your doctor moves the transducer around in your esophagus and stomach. You shouldn't feel any discomfort as this happens.

Although the imaging usually takes less than an hour, you may be watched for a few hours at the doctor's office or hospital after the test.

Stress Echocardiography

Stress echo is a transthoracic echo combined with either an exercise or pharmacological stress test.

For an exercise stress test, you'll walk or run on a treadmill or pedal a stationary bike to make your heart work hard and beat fast. For a pharmacological stress test, you'll be given medicine to increase your heart rate.

A technician will take pictures of your heart using echo before you exercise and as soon as you finish.

What You May See and Hear During Echocardiography

As the doctor or sonographer moves the transducer around, you will see different views of your heart on the screen of the echo machine.

The structures of your heart will appear as white objects, while any fluid or blood will appear black on the screen.

Doppler ultrasound often is used during echo tests. Doppler ultrasound is a special ultrasound that shows how blood is flowing through the blood vessels.

This test allows the sonographer to see blood flowing at different speeds and in different directions. The speed and direction of blood flow appear as different colors moving within the black and white images.

The human ear is unable to hear the sound waves used in echo. If you have a Doppler ultrasound, you may be able to hear "whooshing" sounds. Your doctor can use these sounds to learn about blood flow through your heart.

What to Expect after Echocardiography

You usually can go back to your normal activities right after having echocardiography (echo).

If you have a transesophageal echo (TEE), you may be watched for a few hours at the doctor's office or hospital after the test. Your throat might be sore for a few hours after the test.

You also may not be able to drive for a short time after having TEE. Your doctor will let you know whether you need to arrange for a ride home.

What Does Echocardiography Show?

Echocardiography (echo) shows the size, structure, and movement of various parts of your heart. These parts include the heart valves, the septum (the wall separating the right and left heart chambers), and the walls of the heart chambers. Doppler ultrasound shows the movement of blood through your heart.

Your doctor may use echo to:

• Diagnose heart problems

• Guide or determine next steps for treatment

• Monitor changes and improvement

• Determine the need for more tests

Echo can detect many heart problems. Some might be minor and pose no risk to you. Others can be signs of serious heart disease or other heart conditions.

Your doctor may use echo to learn about:

- The size of your heart. An enlarged heart might be the result of high blood pressure, leaky heart valves, or heart failure. Echo also can detect increased thickness of the ventricles (the heart's lower chambers). Increased thickness may be due to high blood pressure, heart valve disease, or congenital heart defects.

- Heart muscles that are weak and aren't pumping well. Damage from a heart attack may cause weak areas of heart muscle. Weakening also might mean that the area isn't getting enough blood supply, a sign of coronary heart disease.

- Heart valve problems. Echo can show whether any of your heart valves don't open normally or close tightly.

- Problems with your heart's structure. Echo can detect congenital heart defects, such as holes in the heart. Congenital heart defects are structural problems present at birth. Infants and children may have echo to detect these heart defects.

- Blood clots or tumors. If you've had a stroke, you may have echo to check for blood clots or tumors that could have caused the stroke.

What Are the Risks of Echocardiography?

Transthoracic and fetal echocardiography (echo) have no risks. These tests are safe for adults, children, and infants.

If you have a transesophageal echo (TEE), some risks are associated with the medicine given to help you relax. For example, you may have a bad reaction to the medicine, problems breathing, and nausea (feeling sick to your stomach).

Your throat also might be sore for a few hours after the test. Rarely, the tube used during TEE causes minor throat injuries.

Stress echo has some risks, but they're related to the exercise or medicine used to raise your heart rate, not the echo. Serious complications from stress tests are very uncommon.

Chapter 38

Carotid Ultrasound

What Is Carotid Ultrasound?

Carotid ultrasound is a painless and harmless test that uses high-frequency sound waves to create pictures of the insides of your carotid arteries.

You have two common carotid arteries, one on each side of your neck. They each divide into internal and external carotid arteries.

The internal carotid arteries supply oxygen-rich blood to your brain. The external carotid arteries supply oxygen-rich blood to your face, scalp, and neck.

Overview

Carotid ultrasound shows whether a waxy substance called plaque has built up in your carotid arteries. The buildup of plaque in the carotid arteries is called carotid artery disease.

Over time, plaque can harden or rupture (break open). Hardened plaque narrows the carotid arteries and reduces the flow of oxygen-rich blood to the brain.

If the plaque ruptures, a blood clot can form on its surface. A clot can mostly or completely block blood flow through a carotid artery, which can cause a stroke.

This chapter includes text excerpted from "Carotid Ultrasound," National Heart, Lung, and Blood Institute (NHLBI), February 3, 2012. Reviewed June 2016.

453

A piece of plaque or a blood clot also can break away from the wall of the carotid artery. The plaque or clot can travel through the bloodstream and get stuck in one of the brain's smaller arteries. This can block blood flow in the artery and cause a stroke.

A standard carotid ultrasound shows the structure of your carotid arteries. Your carotid ultrasound test might include a Doppler ultrasound. Doppler ultrasound is a special test that shows the movement of blood through your blood vessels.

Your doctor might need results from both types of ultrasound to fully assess whether you have a blood flow problem in your carotid arteries.

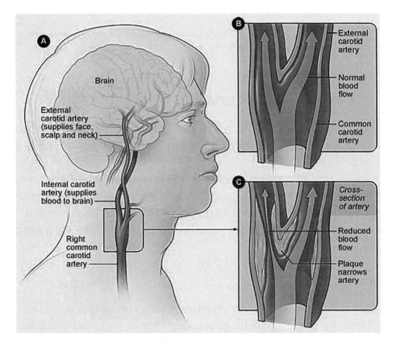

Figure 38.1. *Carotid Arteries*

(A) shows the location of the right carotid artery in the head and neck. (B) shows the inside of a normal carotid artery that has normal blood flow. (C) show the inside of a carotid artery that has plaque buildup and reduced blood flow.

Other Names for Carotid Ultrasound

- Doppler ultrasound
- Carotid duplex ultrasound

Who Needs Carotid Ultrasound?

A carotid ultrasound shows whether you have plaque buildup in your carotid arteries. Over time, plaque can harden or rupture (break open). This can reduce or block the flow of oxygen-rich blood to your brain and cause a stroke.

Your doctor may recommend a carotid ultrasound if you:

- Had a stroke or mini-stroke recently. During a mini-stroke, you may have some or all of the symptoms of a stroke. However, the symptoms usually go away on their own within 24 hours.

- Have an abnormal sound called a carotid bruit in one of your carotid arteries. Your doctor can hear a carotid bruit using a stethoscope. A bruit might suggest a partial blockage in your carotid artery, which could lead to a stroke.

Your doctor also may recommend a carotid ultrasound if he or she thinks you have:

- Blood clots in one of your carotid arteries

- A split between the layers of your carotid artery wall. The split can weaken the wall or reduce blood flow to your brain.

A carotid ultrasound also might be done to see whether carotid artery surgery, also called carotid endarterectomy, has restored normal blood flow through a carotid artery.

If you had a procedure called carotid stenting, your doctor might use carotid ultrasound afterward to check the position of the stent in your carotid artery. (The stent, a small mesh tube, supports the inner artery wall.)

Carotid ultrasound sometimes is used as a preventive screening test in people at increased risk of stroke, such as those who have high blood pressure and diabetes.

What to Expect before Carotid Ultrasound

Carotid ultrasound is a painless test, and typically there is little to do in advance. Your doctor will tell you how to prepare for your carotid ultrasound.

What to Expect during Carotid Ultrasound

Carotid ultrasound usually is done in a doctor's office or hospital. The test is painless and often doesn't take more than 30 minutes.

The ultrasound machine includes a computer, a screen, and a transducer. The transducer is a hand-held device that sends and receives ultrasound waves.

You will lie on your back on an exam table for the test. Your technician or doctor will put gel on your neck where your carotid arteries are located. The gel helps the ultrasound waves reach the arteries.

Your technician or doctor will put the transducer against different spots on your neck and move it back and forth. The transducer gives off ultrasound waves and detects their echoes as they bounce off the artery walls and blood cells. Ultrasound waves can't be heard by the human ear.

The computer uses the echoes to create and record pictures of the insides of the carotid arteries. These pictures usually appear in black and white. The screen displays these live images for your doctor to review.

Your carotid ultrasound test might include a Doppler ultrasound. Doppler ultrasound is a special test that shows the movement of blood through your arteries. Blood flow through the arteries usually appears in color on the ultrasound pictures.

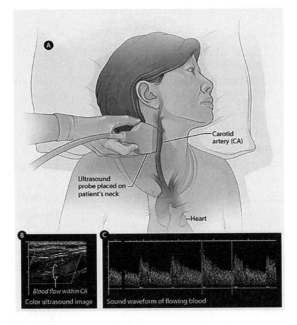

Figure 38.2. *Carotid Ultrasound*

(A) shows how the ultrasound probe (transducer) is placed over the carotid artery. (B) is a color ultrasound image showing blood flow (the red color in the image) in the carotid artery. (C) is a waveform image showing the sound of flowing blood in the carotid artery.

What to Expect after Carotid Ultrasound

You usually can return to your normal activities as soon as the carotid ultrasound is over. Your doctor will likely be able to tell you the results of the carotid ultrasound when it occurs or soon afterward.

What Does a Carotid Ultrasound Show?

A carotid ultrasound can show whether plaque buildup has narrowed one or both of your carotid arteries. If so, you might be at risk of having a stroke. The risk depends on the extent of the blockage and how much it has reduced blood flow to your brain.

To lower your risk of stroke, your doctor may recommend medical or surgical treatments to reduce or remove plaque from your carotid arteries.

What Are the Risks of Carotid Ultrasound?

Carotid ultrasound has no risks because the test uses harmless sound waves. They are the same type of sound waves that doctors use to record pictures of fetuses in pregnant women.

Chapter 39

Holter and Event Monitors

What Are Holter and Event Monitors?

Holter and event monitors are medical devices that record the heart's electrical activity. Doctors most often use these monitors to diagnose arrhythmias.

Arrhythmias are problems with the rate or rhythm of the heartbeat. During an arrhythmia, the heart can beat too fast, too slow, or with an irregular rhythm.

Holter and event monitors also are used to detect silent myocardial ischemia. In this condition, not enough oxygen-rich blood reaches the heart muscle. "Silent" means that no symptoms occur.

The monitors also can check whether treatments for an arrhythmia or silent myocardial ischemia are working.

This chapter focuses on using Holter and event monitors to diagnose problems with the heart's rate or rhythm.

Overview

Holter and event monitors are similar to an EKG (electrocardiogram). An EKG is a simple test that detects and records the heart's electrical activity. It's a common test for diagnosing heart rhythm problems.

This chapter includes text excerpted from "Holter and Event Monitors," National Heart, Lung, and Blood Institute (NHLBI), March 16, 2012. Reviewed June 2016.

However, a standard EKG only records the heartbeat for a few seconds. It won't detect heart rhythm problems that don't occur during the test.

Holter and event monitors are small, portable devices. You can wear one while you do your normal daily activities. This allows the monitor to record your heart for a longer time than an EKG.

Some people have heart rhythm problems that occur only during certain activities, such as sleeping or physical exertion. Using a Holter or event monitor increases the chance of recording these problems.

Although similar, Holter and event monitors aren't the same. A Holter monitor records your heart's electrical activity the entire time you're wearing it. An event monitor records your heart's electrical activity only at certain times while you're wearing it.

Types of Holter and Event Monitors

Holter Monitors

Holter monitors sometimes are called continuous EKGs (electrocardiograms). This is because Holter monitors record your heart rhythm continuously for 24 to 48 hours.

A Holter monitor is about the size of a large deck of cards. You can clip it to a belt or carry it in a pocket. Wires connect the device to sensors (called electrodes) that are stuck to your chest using sticky patches. These sensors detect your heart's electrical signals, and the monitor records your heart rhythm.

Wireless Holter Monitors

Wireless Holter monitors have a longer recording time than standard Holter monitors. Wireless monitors record your heart's electrical activity for a preset amount of time.

These monitors use wireless cellular technology to send the recorded data to your doctor's office or a company that checks the data. The device sends the data automatically at certain times. Wireless monitors still have wires that connect the device to the sensors on your chest.

You can use a wireless Holter monitor for days or even weeks, until signs or symptoms of a heart rhythm problem occur. These monitors usually are used to detect heart rhythm problems that don't occur often.

Although wireless Holter monitors work for longer periods, they have a down side. You must remember to write down the time of symptoms so your doctor can match it to the heart rhythm recording. Also, the batteries in the wireless monitor must be changed every 1–2 days.

Event Monitors

Event monitors are similar to Holter monitors. You wear one while you do your normal daily activities. Most event monitors have wires that connect the device to sensors. The sensors are stuck to your chest using sticky patches.

Unlike Holter monitors, event monitors don't continuously record your heart's electrical activity. They only record during symptoms. For many event monitors, you need to start the device when you feel symptoms. Some event monitors start automatically if they detect abnormal heart rhythms.

Event monitors tend to be smaller than Holter monitors because they don't need to store as much data.

Different types of event monitors work in slightly different ways. Your doctor will explain how to use the monitor before you start wearing it.

Postevent Recorders

Postevent recorders are among the smallest event monitors. You can wear a postevent recorder like a wristwatch or carry it in your pocket. The pocket version is about the size of a thick credit card. These monitors don't have wires that connect the device to chest sensors.

To start the recorder when you feel a symptom, you hold it to your chest. To start the wristwatch version, you touch a button on the side of the watch.

A postevent recorder only records what happens after you start it. It may miss a heart rhythm problem that occurs before and during the onset of symptoms. Also, it might be hard to start the monitor when a symptom is in progress.

In some cases, the missing data could have helped your doctor diagnose the heart rhythm problem.

Presymptom Memory Loop Recorders

Presymptom memory loop recorders are the size of a small cell phone. They're also called continuous loop event recorders.

You can clip this event monitor to your belt or carry it in your pocket. Wires connect the device to sensors on your chest.

These recorders are always recording and erasing data. When you feel a symptom, you push a button on the device. The normal erase process stops. The recording will show a few minutes of data from before, during, and after the symptom. This may make it possible for your doctor to see very brief changes in your heart rhythm.

Autodetect Recorders

Autodetect recorders are about the size of the palm of your hand. Wires connect the device to sensors on your chest.

You don't need to start an autodetect recorder during symptoms. These recorders detect abnormal heart rhythms and automatically record and send the data to your doctor's office.

Implantable Loop Recorders

You may need an implantable loop recorder if other event monitors can't provide enough data. Implantable loop recorders are about the size of a pack of gum. This type of event monitor is inserted under the skin on your chest. No wires or chest sensors are used.

Your doctor can program the device to record when you start it during symptoms or automatically if it detects an abnormal heart rhythm. Devices may differ, so your doctor will tell you how to use your recorder. Sometimes a special card is held close to the recorder to start it.

Other Names for Holter and Event Monitors

- Ambulatory EKG or ECG. (The terms "EKG" and "ECG" both stand for electrocardiogram.)

- Continuous EKG or ECG.

- EKG event monitors.

- Episodic monitors.

- Mobile cardiac outpatient telemetry systems. This is another name for autodetect recorders.

- Thirty-day event recorders.

- Transtelephonic event monitors. These monitors require the patient to send the collected data by telephone to a doctor's office or a company that checks the data.

462

Who Needs a Holter or Event Monitor?

Your doctor may recommend a Holter or event monitor if he or she thinks you have an arrhythmia. An arrhythmia is a problem with the rate or rhythm of the heartbeat.

Holter and event monitors most often are used to detect arrhythmias in people who have:

Issues with fainting or feeling dizzy. A monitor might be used if causes other than a heart rhythm problem have been ruled out.

Palpitations that recur with no known cause. Palpitations are feelings that your heart is skipping a beat, fluttering, or beating too hard or fast. You may have these feelings in your chest, throat, or neck.

People who are being treated for heart rhythm problems also may need to use Holter or event monitors. The monitors can show how well their treatments are working.

Heart rhythm problems may occur only during certain activities, such sleeping or physical exertion. Holter and event monitors record your heart rhythm while you do your normal daily routine. This allows your doctor to see how your heart responds to various activities.

What to Expect before Using a Holter or Event Monitor

Your doctor will do a physical exam before giving you a Holter or event monitor. He or she may:

- Check your pulse to find out how fast your heart is beating (your heart rate) and whether your heart rhythm is steady or irregular.

- Measure your blood pressure.

- Check for swelling in your legs or feet. Swelling could be a sign of an enlarged heart or heart failure, which may cause an arrhythmia. An arrhythmia is a problem with the rate or rhythm of the heartbeat.

- Look for signs of other diseases that might cause heart rhythm problems, such as thyroid disease.

You may have an EKG (electrocardiogram) test before your doctor sends you home with a Holter or event monitor.

An EKG is a simple test that records your heart's electrical activity for a few seconds. The test shows how fast your heart is beating and its rhythm (steady or irregular). An EKG also records the strength and timing of electrical signals as they pass through your heart.

A standard EKG won't detect heart rhythm problems that don't happen during the test. For this reason, your doctor may give you a Holter or event monitor. These monitors are portable. You can wear one while doing your normal daily activities. This increases the chance of recording symptoms that only occur once in a while.

Your doctor will explain how to wear and use the Holter or event monitor. Usually, you'll leave the office wearing it.

Each type of monitor is slightly different, but most have sensors (called electrodes) that attach to the skin on your chest using sticky patches. The sensors need good contact with your skin. Poor contact can cause poor results.

Oil, too much sweat, and hair can keep the patches from sticking to your skin. You may need to shave the area on your chest where your doctor will attach the patches. If you have to replace the patches, you'll need to clean the area with a special prep pad that the doctor will provide.

You may need to use a small amount of special paste or gel to help the patches stick to your skin. Some patches come with paste or gel on them.

What to Expect While Using a Holter or Event Monitor

Your experience while using a Holter or event monitor depends on the type of monitor you have. However, most monitors have some factors in common.

Recording the Heart's Electrical Activity

All monitors record the heart's electrical activity. Thus, maintaining a clear signal between the sensors (electrodes) and the recording device is important.

In most cases, the sensors are attached to your chest using sticky patches. Wires connect the sensors to the monitor. You usually can clip the monitor to your belt or carry it in your pocket. (Postevent recorders and implantable loop recorders don't have chest sensors.)

Holter or Event Monitor

A good stick between the patches and your skin helps provide a clear signal. Poor contact leads to a poor recording that's hard for your doctor to read.

Oil, too much sweat, and hair can keep the patches from sticking to your skin. You may need to shave the area where your doctor will attach the patches. If you have to replace the patches, you'll need to clean the area with a special prep pad that your doctor will provide.

You may need to use a small amount of special paste or gel to help the patches stick to your skin. Some patches come with paste or gel on them.

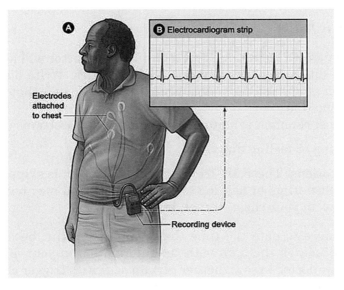

Figure 39.1. *Holter or Event Monitor*

(A) shows how a Holter or event monitor attaches to a patient. In this example, the monitor is clipped to the patient's belt and electrodes are attached to his chest. (B) shows an electrocardiogram strip, which maps the data from the Holter or event monitor.

Too much movement can pull the patches away from your skin or create "noise" on the EKG (electrocardiogram) strip. An EKG strip is a graph showing the pattern of the heartbeat. Noise looks like a lot of jagged lines; it makes it hard for your doctor to see the real rhythm of your heart.

When you have a symptom, stop what you're doing. This will ensure that the recording shows your heart's activity rather than your movement.

Your doctor will tell you whether you need to adjust your activity level during the testing period. If you exercise, choose a cool location to avoid sweating too much. This will help the patches stay sticky.

Other everyday items also can disrupt the signal between the sensors and the monitor. These items include magnets; metal detectors;

microwave ovens; and electric blankets, toothbrushes, and razors. Avoid using these items. Also avoid areas with high voltage.

Cell phones and MP3 players (such as iPods) may interfere with the signal between the sensors and the monitor if they're too close to the monitor. When using any electronic device, try to keep it at least 6 inches away from the monitor.

Keeping a Diary

While using a Holter or event monitor, your doctor will advise you to keep a diary of your symptoms and activities. Write down what type of symptoms you're having, when they occur, and what you were doing at the time.

The most common symptoms of heart rhythm problems include:

- Fainting or feeling dizzy.

- Palpitations. These are feelings that your heart is skipping a beat, fluttering, or beating too hard or fast. You may have these feelings in your chest, throat, or neck.

Make sure to note the time that symptoms occur, because your doctor will match the data with the information in your diary. This allows your doctor to see whether certain activities trigger changes in your heart rate and rhythm.

Also, include details in your diary about when you take any medicine or if you feel stress at certain times during the testing period.

What to Expect with Specific Monitors

Holter Monitors

Holter monitors are about the size of a large deck of cards. You'll wear one for 24 to 48 hours. You can't get your monitor wet, so you won't be able to bathe or shower. You can take a sponge bath if needed.

When the testing period is done, you'll return the device to your doctor's office. The results will be stored on the device.

The recording period for a standard Holter monitor might be too short to capture a heart rhythm problem. If this is the case, your doctor may recommend a wireless Holter monitor.

Wireless Holter Monitors

Wireless Holter monitors can record for a longer time than standard Holter monitors. You can use a wireless Holter monitor for days or even weeks, until signs or symptoms of a heart rhythm problem occur.

Wireless monitors record for a preset amount of time. Then they automatically send data to your doctor's office or a company that checks the data.

These monitors use wireless cellular technology to send data. However, they still have wires that connect the device to the sensors stuck to your chest.

The batteries in the wireless monitor must be changed every 1–2 days. You'll need to detach the sensors to shower or bathe and then reattach them.

Event Monitors

Event monitors are slightly smaller than Holter monitors. They can be worn for weeks or until symptoms occur. Most event monitors are worn like Holter monitors—clipped to a belt or carried in a pocket.

When you have symptoms, you simply push a button on your monitor to start recording. Some event monitors start automatically if they detect abnormal heart rhythms.

Postevent Recorders

Postevent recorders can be worn like a wristwatch or carried in a pocket. The pocket version is about the size of a thick credit card. These recorders don't have wires that connect the device to chest sensors.

To start the recorder when you feel a symptom, you hold it to your chest. To start the wristwatch version, you touch a button on the side of the watch.

You send the stored data to your doctor's office using a telephone. Your doctor will explain how to use the monitor before you leave his or her office.

Autodetect Recorders

Autodetect recorders are about the size of the palm of your hand. Wires connect the device to sensors on your chest.

You don't need to start an autodetect recorder. This type of monitor automatically starts recording if it detects abnormal heart rhythms. It then sends the data to your doctor's office.

Implantable Loop Recorders

Implantable loop recorders are about the size of a pack of gum. This type of event monitor is inserted under the skin on your chest. Your doctor will discuss the procedure with you. No chest sensors are used with implantable loop recorders.

Your doctor can program the device to record when you start it during symptoms or automatically if it detects an abnormal heart rhythm. Devices may differ, so your doctor will tell you how to use your recorder. Sometimes a special card is held close to the device to start it.

What to Expect after Using a Holter or Event Monitor

After you're finished using a Holter or event monitor, you'll return it to your doctor's office or the place where you picked it up.

If you were using an implantable loop recorder, your doctor will need to remove it from your chest. He or she will discuss the procedure with you.

Your doctor will tell you when to expect the results. Once your doctor has reviewed the recordings, he or she will discuss the results with you.

What Does a Holter or Event Monitor Show?

A Holter or event monitor may show what's causing symptoms of an arrhythmia. An arrhythmia is a problem with the rate or rhythm of the heartbeat.

A Holter or event monitor also can show whether a heart rhythm problem is harmless or requires treatment. The monitor might alert your doctor to medical conditions that can result in heart failure, stroke, or sudden cardiac arrest.

If the symptoms of a heart rhythm problem occur often, a Holter or event monitor has a good chance of recording them. You may not have symptoms while using a monitor. Even so, your doctor can learn more about your heart rhythm from the test results.

Sometimes Holter and event monitors can't help doctors diagnose heart rhythm problems. If this happens, talk with your doctor about other steps you can take.

One option might be to try a different type of monitor. Wireless Holter monitors and implantable loop recorders have longer recording periods. This may allow your doctor to get the data he or she needs to make a diagnosis.

What Are the Risks of Using a Holter or Event Monitor?

The sticky patches used to attach the sensors (electrodes) to your chest have a small risk of skin irritation. You also may have an allergic reaction to the paste or gel that's sometimes used to attach the patches. The irritation will go away once the patches are removed.

If you're using an implantable loop recorder, you may get an infection or have pain where the device is placed under the skin. Your doctor can prescribe medicine to treat these problems.

Chapter 40

Stress Testing

What Is Stress Testing?

Stress testing provides information about how your heart works during physical stress. Some heart problems are easier to diagnose when your heart is working hard and beating fast.

During stress testing, you exercise (walk or run on a treadmill or pedal a stationary bike) to make your heart work hard and beat fast. Tests are done on your heart while you exercise.

You might have arthritis or another medical problem that prevents you from exercising during a stress test. If so, your doctor may give you medicine to make your heart work hard, as it would during exercise. This is called a pharmacological stress test.

Overview

Doctors usually use stress testing to help diagnose coronary heart disease (CHD). They also use stress testing to find out the severity of CHD.

CHD is a disease in which a waxy substance called plaque builds up in the coronary arteries. These arteries supply oxygen-rich blood to your heart.

Plaque narrows the arteries and reduces blood flow to your heart muscle. The buildup of plaque also makes it more likely that blood clots will form in your arteries. Blood clots can mostly or completely

This chapter includes text excerpted from "Stress Testing," National Heart, Lung, and Blood Institute (NHLBI), December 14, 2011. Reviewed June 2016.

block blood flow through an artery. This can lead to chest pain called angina or a heart attack.

You may not have any signs or symptoms of CHD when your heart is at rest. But when your heart has to work harder during exercise, it needs more blood and oxygen. Narrow arteries can't supply enough blood for your heart to work well. As a result, signs and symptoms of CHD may occur only during exercise.

A stress test can detect the following problems, which may suggest that your heart isn't getting enough blood during exercise:

- Abnormal changes in your heart rate or blood pressure

- Symptoms such as shortness of breath or chest pain, especially if they occur at low levels of exercise

- Abnormal changes in your heart's rhythm or electrical activity

During a stress test, if you can't exercise for as long as what is considered normal for someone your age, it may be a sign that not enough blood is flowing to your heart. However, other factors besides CHD can prevent you from exercising long enough (for example, lung disease, anemia, or poor general fitness).

Doctors also may use stress testing to assess other problems, such as heart valve disease or heart failure.

Types of Stress Testing

The two main types of stress testing are a standard exercise stress test and an imaging stress test.

Standard Exercise Stress Test

A standard exercise stress test uses an EKG (electrocardiogram) to detect and record the heart's electrical activity.

An EKG shows how fast your heart is beating and the heart's rhythm (steady or irregular). It also records the strength and timing of electrical signals as they pass through your heart.

During a standard stress test, your blood pressure will be checked. You also may be asked to breathe into a special tube during the test. This allows your doctor to see how well you're breathing and measure the gases that you breathe out.

A standard stress test shows changes in your heart's electrical activity. It also can show whether your heart is getting enough blood during exercise.

Imaging Stress Test

As part of some stress tests, pictures are taken of your heart while you exercise and while you're at rest. These imaging stress tests can show how well blood is flowing in your heart and how well your heart pumps blood when it beats.

One type of imaging stress test involves echocardiography (echo). This test uses sound waves to create a moving picture of your heart. An exercise stress echo can show how well your heart's chambers and valves are working when your heart is under stress.

A stress echo also can show areas of poor blood flow to your heart, dead heart muscle tissue, and areas of the heart muscle wall that aren't contracting well. These areas may have been damaged during a heart attack, or they may not be getting enough blood.

Other imaging stress tests use radioactive dye to create pictures of blood flow to your heart. The dye is injected into your bloodstream before the pictures are taken. The pictures show how much of the dye has reached various parts of your heart during exercise and while you're at rest.

Tests that use radioactive dye include a thallium or sestamibi stress test and a positron emission tomography (PET) stress test. The amount of radiation in the dye is considered safe for you and those around you. However, if you're pregnant, you shouldn't have this test because of risks it might pose to your unborn child.

Imaging stress tests tend to detect CHD better than standard (non-imaging) stress tests. Imaging stress tests also can predict the risk of a future heart attack or premature death.

An imaging stress test might be done first (as opposed to a standard exercise stress test) if you:

- Can't exercise for enough time to get your heart working at its hardest. (Medical problems, such as arthritis or leg arteries clogged by plaque, might prevent you from exercising long enough.)

- Have abnormal heartbeats or other problems that prevent a standard exercise stress test from giving correct results.

- Had a heart procedure in the past, such as coronary artery bypass grafting or percutaneous coronary intervention, also known as coronary angioplasty, and stent placement.

Other Names for Stress Testing

- Exercise echocardiogram or exercise stress echo

473

- Exercise test

- Myocardial perfusion imaging

- Nuclear stress test

- PET stress test

- Pharmacological stress test

- Sestamibi stress test

- Stress EKG or ECG

- Treadmill test

Who Needs Stress Testing?

You may need stress testing if you've had chest pains, shortness of breath, or other symptoms of limited blood flow to your heart.

Imaging stress tests, especially, can show whether you have coronary heart disease (CHD) or a heart valve problem. (Heart valves are like doors; they open and shut to let blood flow between the heart's chambers and into the heart's arteries. So, like CHD, faulty heart valves can limit the amount of blood reaching your heart.)

If you've been diagnosed with CHD or recently had a heart attack, a stress test can show whether you can handle an exercise program. If you've had percutaneous coronary intervention, also known as coronary angioplasty, (with or without stent placement) or coronary artery bypass grafting, a stress test can show how well the treatment relieves your CHD symptoms.

You also may need a stress test if, during exercise, you feel faint, have a rapid heartbeat or a fluttering feeling in your chest, or have other symptoms of an arrhythmia (an irregular heartbeat).

If you don't have chest pain when you exercise but still get short of breath, your doctor may recommend a stress test. The test can help show whether a heart problem, rather than a lung problem or being out of shape, is causing your breathing problems.

For such testing, you breathe into a special tube. This allows a technician to measure the gases you breathe out. Breathing into the tube during stress testing also is done before a heart transplant to help assess whether you're a candidate for the surgery.

Stress testing shouldn't be used as a routine screening test for CHD. Usually, you have to have symptoms of CHD before a doctor will recommend stress testing.

However, your doctor may want to use a stress test to screen for CHD if you have diabetes. This disease increases your risk of CHD. Currently, though, no evidence shows that having a stress test will improve your outcome if you have diabetes.

What to Expect before Stress Testing

Stress testing is done in a doctor's office or at a medical center or hospital. You should wear shoes and clothes in which you can exercise comfortably. Sometimes you're given a gown to wear during the test.

Your doctor might ask you to fast (not eat or drink anything but water) for a short time before the test. If you're diabetic, ask your doctor whether you need to adjust your medicines on the day of the test.

For some stress tests, you can't drink coffee or other caffeinated drinks for a day before the test. Certain over-the-counter or prescription medicines also may interfere with some stress tests. Ask your doctor whether you need to avoid certain drinks or food or change how you take your medicine before the test.

If you use an inhaler for asthma or other breathing problems, bring it to the test. Make sure you let the doctor know that you use it.

What to Expect during Stress Testing

During all types of stress testing, a doctor, nurse, or technician will always be with you to closely check your health status.

Before you start the "stress" part of a stress test, the nurse will put sticky patches called electrodes on the skin of your chest, arms, and legs. To help an electrode stick to the skin, the nurse may have to shave a patch of hair where the electrode will be attached.

The electrodes will be connected to an EKG (electrocardiogram) machine. This machine records your heart's electrical activity. It shows how fast your heart is beating and the heart's rhythm (steady or irregular). An EKG also records the strength and timing of electrical signals as they pass through your heart.

The nurse will put a blood pressure cuff on your arm to check your blood pressure during the stress test. (The cuff will feel tight on your arm when it expands every few minutes.) Also, you might have to breathe into a special tube so the gases you breathe out can be measured.

Next, you'll exercise on a treadmill or stationary bike. If such exercise poses a problem for you, you might turn a crank with your arms instead. During the test, the exercise level will get harder. You can stop whenever you feel the exercise is too much for you.

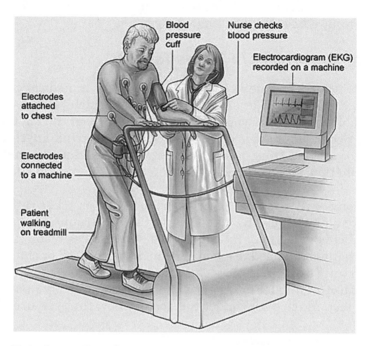

Figure 40.1. *Stress Testing*

The image shows a patient having a stress test. Electrodes are attached to the patient's chest and connected to an EKG (electrocardiogram) machine. The EKG records the heart's electrical activity. A blood pressure cuff is used to record the patient's blood pressure while he walks on a treadmill.

If you can't exercise, medicine might be injected into a vein in your arm or hand. The medicine will increase blood flow through your coronary arteries and make your heart beat fast, as it would during exercise. You can then have the stress test.

The medicine may make you flushed and anxious, but the effects go away as soon as the test is over. The medicine also may give you a headache.

While you're exercising or getting medicine to make your heart work harder, the nurse will ask you how you're feeling. You should tell him or her if you feel chest pain, short of breath, or dizzy.

The exercise or medicine infusion will continue until you reach a target heart rate, or until you:

- Feel moderate to severe chest pain

- Get too out of breath to continue
- Develop abnormally high or low blood pressure or an arrhythmia (an irregular heartbeat)
- Become dizzy

The nurse will continue to check your heart functions and blood pressure after the test until they return to normal levels.

The "stress" part of a stress test (when your heart is working hard) usually lasts about 15 minutes or less.

However, there's prep time before the test and monitoring time afterward. Both extend the total test time to about an hour for a standard stress test, and up to 3 hours or more for some imaging stress tests.

Exercise Stress Echocardiogram Test

For an exercise stress echocardiogram (echo) test, the nurse will take pictures of your heart using echocardiography before you exercise and as soon as you finish.

A sonographer (a person who specializes in using ultrasound techniques) will apply gel to your chest. Then, he or she will briefly put a transducer (a wand-like device) against your chest and move it around.

The transducer sends and receives high-pitched sounds that you probably won't hear. The echoes from the sound waves are converted into moving pictures of your heart on a screen.

You might be asked to lie on your side on an exam table for this test. Some stress echo tests also use dye to improve imaging. The dye is injected into your bloodstream while the test occurs.

Sestamibi or Other Imaging Stress Tests Involving Radioactive Dye

For a sestamibi stress test or other imaging stress test that uses radioactive dye, the nurse will inject a small amount of dye into your bloodstream. This is done through a needle placed in a vein in your arm or hand.

You'll get the dye about a half-hour before you start exercising or take medicine to make your heart work hard. The amount of radiation in the dye is considered safe for you and those around you. However, if you're pregnant, you shouldn't have this test because of risks it might pose to your unborn child.

Pictures will be taken of your heart at least two times: when it's at rest and when it's working its hardest. You'll lie down on a table, and a special camera or scanner that can detect the dye in your bloodstream will take pictures of your heart.

Some pictures may not be taken until you lie quietly for a few hours after the stress test. Some patients may even be asked to return in a day or so for more pictures.

What to Expect after Stress Testing

After stress testing, you'll be able to return to your normal activities. If you had a test that involved radioactive dye, your doctor may ask you to drink plenty of fluids to flush it out of your body. You shouldn't have certain other imaging tests until the dye is no longer in your body. Your doctor can advise you further.

What Does Stress Testing Show?

Stress testing shows how your heart works during physical stress (exercise) and how healthy your heart is.

A standard exercise stress test uses an EKG (electrocardiogram) to monitor changes in your heart's electrical activity. Imaging stress tests take pictures of blood flow throughout your heart. They also show your heart valves and the movement of your heart muscle.

Doctors use both types of stress tests to look for signs that your heart isn't getting enough blood flow during exercise. Abnormal test results may be due to coronary heart disease (CHD) or other factors, such as poor physical fitness.

If you have a standard exercise stress test and the results are normal, you may not need further testing or treatment. But if your test results are abnormal, or if you're physically unable to exercise, your doctor may want you to have an imaging stress test or other tests.

Even if your standard exercise stress test results are normal, your doctor may want you to have an imaging stress test if you continue having symptoms (such as shortness of breath or chest pain).

Imaging stress tests are more accurate than standard exercise stress tests, but they're much more expensive.

Imaging stress tests show how well blood is flowing in the heart muscle and reveal parts of the heart that aren't contracting strongly. They also can show the parts of the heart that aren't getting enough blood, as well as dead tissue in the heart, where no blood flows. (A heart attack can cause heart tissue to die.)

If your imaging stress test suggests significant CHD, your doctor may want you to have more testing and treatment.

What Are the Risks of Stress Testing?

Stress tests pose little risk of serious harm. The chance of these tests causing a heart attack or death is about 1 in 5,000. More common, but less serious side effects linked to stress testing include:

- An arrhythmia (irregular heartbeat). Often, an arrhythmia will go away quickly once you're at rest. But if it persists, you may need monitoring or treatment in a hospital.

- Low blood pressure, which can cause you to feel dizzy or faint. This problem may go away once your heart stops working hard; it usually doesn't require treatment.

- Jitteriness or discomfort while getting medicine to make your heart work hard and beat fast (you may be given medicine if you can't exercise). These side effects usually go away shortly after you stop getting the medicine. Sometimes the symptoms may last a few hours.

Also, some of the medicines used for pharmacological stress tests can cause wheezing, shortness of breath, and other asthma-like symptoms. Sometimes these symptoms are severe and require treatment.

Chapter 41

Tilt-Table Testing

Tilt-table testing is one of the many procedures that is used to assess syncope (fainting). The person undergoing the test lies on a special table, which when changed from a horizontal to a vertical position induces syncope and enables measurement of how the body reacts to the force of gravity. A nurse or technician keeps track of heart rate and blood pressure during the test to monitor response to the position changes.

Why Is It Needed?

A tilt-table test will be required if there are recurring episodes of fainting and when other causes of syncope have been eliminated through previous tests. A tilt-table test will analyze what makes you feel lightheaded or, in some instances, pass out completely. Typically, fainting may be caused by a number of factors, such as:

- abnormal heart rhythm (arrhythmia)

- a very slow heart rate (bradycardia)

- vasovagal syndrome (or, neurocardiogenic syncope), a sudden drop in blood pressure due to overstimulation of the vagus nerve

- changes in the structure of the heart muscle or valves causing the heart to malfunction

"Tilt-Table Testing," © 2016 Omnigraphics. Reviewed June 2016.

- damage to the heart muscle (or heart attack) caused by poor blood supply

- ventricular dysfunction, or complications in the functioning of ventricles

- reaction to certain medications

- severe dehydration

- low blood sugar (hypoglycemia)

- an extended period of bed-rest

Preparing for the Procedure

Before the test, the doctor will explain the procedure and will ask you to sign a consent form. It is important to let the doctor and technician know if:

- you have allergies

- you are sensitive to latex

- you are on medication (over-the-counter and prescription) or other supplements

- you are, or you think you may be, pregnant

- you have a pacemaker

The doctor will give instructions regarding fasting for this procedure. If you are diabetic, ask the doctor to adjust dosage of your regular medication for the day of the test. The doctor might request other specific preparation depending on your medical condition.

How Is It Performed?

The tilt-table test is performed by a trained nurse or a technician in a hospital or an electrophysiology (EP) lab. The test, which has two parts, is designed to trigger symptoms of syncope to analyze what causes it. The first part alone lasts for about 30 to 40 minutes, while both together take about 90 minutes.

The first part of the test is performed to analyze how the body reacts to position changes:

- You lie on your back on a special table. Straps at your knees and waist will help you stay in place.

- An IV line is started in your arm to administer medicine and IV fluids when needed, and electrocardiograph electrodes are attached to your chest to track heartbeat. A blood pressure cuff is placed on your arm and attached to a monitor.

- You will be asked to remain quiet and still until the end of the procedure, but you need to inform the nurse or technician if you feel uncomfortable.

- The table is tilted upward so that your head is slightly (30 degrees) above the rest of your body. Blood pressure and heart rate are checked by the nurse.

- A few minutes later, the table is further raised to almost vertical. Monitoring for symptoms, such as fainting, low blood pressure, low heart rate, and/or dizziness, will continue for up to 45 minutes.

- If there is a drop in blood pressure during this time, the table will be lowered and the test will be stopped. The second part of the test will not be required.

- If no symptoms occur, the table will be lowered and the second part of the test will be performed.

The second part of the tilt-table test measures the heart's response to a medication given to speed up the heart rate:

- You will be given a medicine, such as isoproterenol, through the IV tube to induce a faster heartbeat and thereby increase sensitivity to the tilt-table test.

- The table is tilted upward again, to an angle of 60 degrees, to determine whether any of the symptoms of syncope occur.

- If there is a drop in blood pressure within 15 minutes, the nurse will lower the table, stop the medicine, and end the test.

- If none of the symptoms occur, the test will be stopped once the nurse has all the necessary information. You will be allowed to rest for a while in flat position while heart rate and blood pressure continue to be monitored.

What Happens after the Test?

It is possible to feel a little tired or sick after the test. You may be asked to stay for 30 to 60 minutes in order for the nurse to keep track of your heart rate and blood pressure. Most people can drive home and get back to their normal routines right after the test, however those who lose consciousness during the test will need more testing and observation. It is advisable not to drive if you have fainted during the procedure.

What about the Results?

The result is either "negative" or "positive," and you are most likely to know the result right after the test. If there is no drop in blood pressure during the test, and if there are no other symptoms, the result is negative (normal). If there is a change in blood pressure, along with symptoms such as dizziness or feeling faint, the test is positive. In such a case, the doctor may prescribe further tests or a change in medication. If the fainting was induced by bradycardia, you may need a pacemaker.

What Are the Risks?

Some of the possible risks of a tilt-table test include:

- headache
- dizziness
- nausea
- episodes of fainting
- low or high blood pressure
- heart palpitations
- other risks, depending on already existing medical conditions

References

1. "Tilt-Table Test," American Heart Association, July 2015.
2. "Tilt Table Procedure," Johns Hopkins Medicine, n.d.

Chapter 42

Coronary Angiography

What Is Coronary Angiography?

Coronary angiography is a test that uses dye and special X-rays to show the insides of your coronary arteries. The coronary arteries supply oxygen-rich blood to your heart.

A waxy substance called plaque can build up inside the coronary arteries. The buildup of plaque in the coronary arteries is called coronary heart disease (CHD).

Over time, plaque can harden or rupture (break open). Hardened plaque narrows the coronary arteries and reduces the flow of oxygen-rich blood to the heart. This can cause chest pain or discomfort called angina.

If the plaque ruptures, a blood clot can form on its surface. A large blood clot can mostly or completely block blood flow through a coronary artery. This is the most common cause of a heart attack. Over time, ruptured plaque also hardens and narrows the coronary arteries.

Overview

During coronary angiography, special dye is released into the bloodstream. The dye makes the coronary arteries visible on X-ray pictures. This helps doctors see blockages in the arteries.

A procedure called cardiac catheterization is used to get the dye into the coronary arteries.

This chapter includes text excerpted from "Coronary Angiography," National Heart, Lung, and Blood Institute (NHLBI), March 2, 2012. Reviewed June 2016.

For this procedure, a thin, flexible tube called a catheter is put into a blood vessel in your arm, groin (upper thigh), or neck. The tube is threaded into your coronary arteries, and the dye is released into your bloodstream. X-ray pictures are taken while the dye is flowing through the coronary arteries.

Cardiologists (heart specialists) usually do cardiac catheterization in a hospital. You're awake during the procedure, and it causes little or no pain. However, you may feel some soreness in the blood vessel where the catheter was inserted.

Cardiac catheterization rarely causes serious complications.

Who Needs Coronary Angiography?

Your doctor may recommend coronary angiography if you have signs or symptoms of coronary heart disease (CHD). Signs and symptoms include:

- Angina. This is unexplained pain or pressure in your chest. You also may feel it in your shoulders, arms, neck, jaw, or back. The pain my even feel like indigestion. Angina may not only happen when you're active. Emotional stress also can trigger the pain associated with angina.

- Sudden cardiac arrest (SCA). This is a condition in which your heart suddenly and unexpectedly stops beating.

- Abnormal results from tests such as an EKG (electrocardiogram), exercise stress test, or other test.

Coronary angiography also might be done on an emergency basis, such as during a heart attack. If angiography shows blockages in your coronary arteries, your doctor may do a procedure called percutaneous coronary intervention, also known as angioplasty. This procedure can open blocked heart arteries and prevent further heart damage.

Coronary angiography also can help your doctor plan treatment after you've had a heart attack, especially if you have major heart damage or if you're still having chest pain.

What to Expect before Coronary Angiography

Before having coronary angiography, talk with your doctor about:

- How the test is done and how to prepare for it

- Any medicines you're taking, and whether you should stop taking them before the test

- Whether you have diseases or conditions that may require taking extra steps during or after the test to avoid complications. Examples of such conditions include diabetes and kidney disease.

Your doctor will tell you exactly which procedures will be done. For example, your doctor may recommend percutaneous coronary intervention, also known as coronary angioplasty, if the angiography shows a blocked artery.

You will have a chance to ask questions about the procedures. Also, you'll be asked to provide written informed consent to have the procedures.

It's not safe to drive after having cardiac catheterization, which is part of coronary angiography. You'll need to have someone drive you home after the procedure.

What to Expect during Coronary Angiography

During coronary angiography, you're kept on your back and awake. This allows you to follow your doctor's instructions during the test. You'll be given medicine to help you relax. The medicine might make you sleepy.

Your doctor will numb the area on the arm, groin (upper thigh), or neck where the catheter will enter your blood vessel. Then, he or she will use a needle to make a small hole in the blood vessel. The catheter will be inserted in the hole.

Next, your doctor will thread the catheter through the vessel and into the coronary arteries. Special X-ray movies are taken of the catheter as it's moved into the heart. The movies help your doctor see where to place the tip of the catheter.

Once the catheter is properly placed, your doctor will inject a special type of dye into the tube. The dye will flow through your coronary arteries, making them visible on an X-ray. This X-ray is called an angiogram.

If the angiogram reveals blocked arteries, your doctor may use percutaneous coronary intervention (PCI), commonly known as coronary angioplasty to restore blood flow to your heart.

After your doctor completes the procedure(s), he or she will remove the catheter from your body. The opening left in the blood vessel will then be closed up and bandaged.

A small sandbag or other type of weight might be placed on the bandage to apply pressure. This will help prevent major bleeding from the site.

What to Expect after Coronary Angiography

After coronary angiography, you'll be moved to a special care area in the hospital. You'll be carefully watched for several hours or overnight. During this time, you'll need to limit your movement to avoid bleeding from the site where the catheter was inserted.

While you recover in the special care area, nurses will check your heart rate and blood pressure regularly. They'll also watch for any bleeding at the catheter insertion site. You may develop a small bruise on your arm, groin (upper thigh), or neck at the catheter insertion site. That area may feel sore or tender for about a week.

Let your doctor know if you develop problems such as:

- A constant or large amount of blood at the catheter insertion site that can't be stopped with a small bandage

- Unusual pain, swelling, redness, or other signs of infection at or near the catheter insertion site

Your doctor will tell you whether you should avoid certain activities, such as heavy lifting, for a short time after the test.

What Are the Risks of Coronary Angiography?

Coronary angiography is a common medical test. It rarely causes serious problems. However, complications can include:

- Bleeding, infection, and pain at the catheter insertion site.

- Damage to blood vessels. Rarely, the catheter may scrape or poke a hole in a blood vessel as it's threaded to the heart.

- An allergic reaction to the dye that's used during the test.

Other, less common complications include:

- Arrhythmias (irregular heartbeats). These irregular heartbeats often go away on their own. However, your doctor may recommend treatment if they persist.

- Kidney damage caused by the dye that's used during the test.

- Blood clots that can trigger a stroke, heart attack, or other serious problems.

- Low blood pressure.

- A buildup of blood or fluid in the sac that surrounds the heart. This fluid can prevent the heart from beating properly.

As with any procedure involving the heart, complications can sometimes be fatal. However, this is rare with coronary angiography.

The risk of complications is higher in people who are older and in those who have certain diseases or conditions (such as chronic kidney disease and diabetes).

Chapter 43

Cardiac Computed Tomography (CT)

What Is Cardiac CT?

Cardiac computed tomography, or cardiac CT, is a painless test that uses an X-ray machine to take clear, detailed pictures of the heart. Doctors use this test to look for heart problems.

During a cardiac CT scan, an X-ray machine will move around your body in a circle. The machine will take a picture of each part of your heart. A computer will put the pictures together to make a three-dimensional (3D) picture of the whole heart.

Sometimes an iodine-based dye (contrast dye) is injected into one of your veins during the scan. The contrast dye highlights your coronary (heart) arteries on the X-ray pictures. This type of CT scan is called a coronary CT angiography, or CTA.

Overview

Doctors use cardiac CT to help detect or evaluate:

- Coronary heart disease (CHD). In CHD, a waxy substance called plaque narrows the coronary arteries and limits blood flow to the heart. A coronary CTA can show whether the coronary arteries are narrow or blocked.

This chapter includes text excerpted from "Cardiac CT," National Heart, Lung, and Blood Institute (NHLBI), February 29, 2012. Reviewed June 2016.

- Calcium buildup in the walls of the coronary arteries. This type of CT scan is called a coronary calcium scan. Calcium in the coronary arteries may be an early sign of CHD.

- Problems with the aorta. The aorta is the main artery that carries oxygen-rich blood from the heart to the body. Cardiac CT can detect two serious problems in the aorta:

    - Aneurysm. An aneurysm is a diseased area of a blood vessel wall that bulges out. An aneurysm can be life threatening if it bursts.

    - Dissection. A dissection is a split in one or more layers of the artery wall. The split causes bleeding into and along the layers of the artery wall. This condition can cause pain and may be life threatening.

- A pulmonary embolism (PE). A PE is a sudden blockage in a lung artery, usually due to a blood clot.

- Problems in the pulmonary veins. The pulmonary veins carry blood from the lungs to the heart. Problems with these veins may lead to an irregular heart rhythm called atrial fibrillation (AF). The pictures that cardiac CT creates of the pulmonary veins can help guide procedures used to treat AF.

- Problems with heart function and heart valves. In some cases, doctors may recommend cardiac CT instead of echocardiography or cardiac MRI (magnetic resonance imaging) to look for problems with heart function or heart valves.

- Pericardial disease. This is a disease that occurs in the pericardium, the sac around your heart. Cardiac CT can create clear, detailed pictures of the pericardium.

- Results of coronary artery bypass grafting (CABG). In CABG, arteries from other areas in your body are used to bypass (that is, go around) narrow coronary arteries. A CT scan can show whether the grafted arteries remain open after the surgery.

Different types of CT scans are used for different purposes. For example, multidetector computed tomography (MDCT) is a fast type of CT scanner. Because the heart is in motion, a fast scanner is able to produce high-quality pictures of the heart. MDCT also might be used to detect calcium in the coronary arteries.

Another type of CT scanner, called electron-beam computed tomography (EBCT), also is used to detect calcium in the coronary arteries.

Outlook

Because an X-ray machine is used, cardiac CT involves radiation. The amount of radiation used is considered small. Depending on the type of CT scan you have, the amount of radiation is similar to the amount you're naturally exposed to over 1–5 years.

There is a small chance that cardiac CT will cause cancer because of the radiation. The risk is higher in people younger than 40 years old. New cardiac CT methods are available that reduce the amount of radiation used during the test.

Researchers continue to study new and better ways to use cardiac CT.

Other Names for Cardiac CT

- CAT scan
- Coronary artery scan
- Coronary CT angiography
- CT angiography

What to Expect before Cardiac CT

Your doctor will tell you how to prepare for the cardiac CT scan. He or she may tell you to avoid caffeine and not eat anything for 4 hours before the scan. You're usually allowed to drink water before the test.

If you take medicine for diabetes, talk with your doctor about whether you'll need to change how you take it on the day of your cardiac CT scan.

Tell your doctor whether you:

- Are pregnant or might be pregnant. Even though cardiac CT uses a low radiation dose, the X-rays may harm your fetus.

- Have asthma or kidney problems or are allergic to any medicines, iodine, or shellfish. These problems can increase your chance of having an allergic reaction to the contrast dye that's sometimes used during cardiac CT.

A technician will ask you to remove your clothes above the waist and wear a hospital gown. You also will be asked to remove any jewelry from around your neck or chest.

If you don't have asthma, COPD (chronic obstructive pulmonary disease), or heart failure, your doctor may give you medicine to slow your heart rate. A slower heart rate will help produce better quality pictures. The medicine will be given by mouth or injected into a vein.

What to Expect during Cardiac CT

Cardiac CT is done in a hospital or outpatient office. A doctor who has experience with CT scanning will supervise the test.

The doctor may want to use an iodine-based dye (contrast dye) during the cardiac CT scan. If so, a needle connected to an intravenous (IV) line will be put in a vein in your hand or arm.

The doctor will inject the contrast dye through the IV line during the scan. You may have a warm feeling when this happens. The dye will make your blood vessels visible on the CT scan pictures.

The technician who runs the cardiac CT scanner will clean areas on your chest and apply sticky patches called electrodes. The patches are attached to an EKG (electrocardiogram) machine. The machine records your heart's electrical activity during the scan.

The CT scanner is a large machine that has a hollow, circular tube in the middle. You will lie on your back on a sliding table. The table can move up and down, and it goes inside the tunnel-like machine.

The table will slide slowly into the opening in the machine. Inside the scanner, an X-ray tube moves around your body to take pictures of different parts of your heart. A computer will put the pictures together to make a three-dimensional (3D) picture of the whole heart.

The technician controls the CT scanner from the next room. He or she can see you through a glass window and talk to you through a speaker.

Moving your body can cause the pictures to blur. You'll be asked to lie still and hold your breath for short moments, while each picture is taken.

A cardiac CT scan usually takes about 15 minutes to complete. However, it can take more than an hour to get ready for the test and for the medicine to slow your heart rate.

What to Expect after Cardiac CT

After the cardiac CT scan is done, you'll be able to return to your normal activities. A doctor who has experience with CT will provide your doctor with the results of your scan. Your doctor will discuss the findings with you.

What Does Cardiac CT Show?

Many X-ray pictures are taken during a cardiac CT scan. A computer puts the pictures together to make a three-dimensional (3D) picture of the whole heart. This picture shows the inside of the heart and the structures that surround the heart.

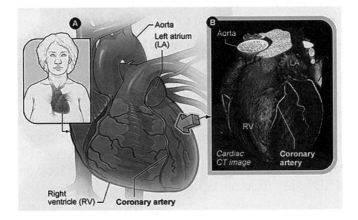

Figure 43.1. *Cardiac CT*

(A) is an illustration of the outside of the heart. The arrow shows the point of view of the cardiac CT image. The inset image shows the position of the heart in the body. (B) is a cardiac CT image showing the coronary arteries on the surface of the heart. This is a picture of the whole heart put together by a computer.

Doctors use cardiac CT to detect or evaluate:

- Coronary heart disease (CHD). In CHD, a waxy substance called plaque narrows the coronary arteries and limits blood flow to the heart. Contrast dye might be used during a cardiac CT scan to show whether the coronary arteries are narrow or blocked. When contrast dye is used, the test is called a coronary CT angiography, or CTA.

- Calcium buildup in the walls of the coronary arteries. This type of CT scan is called a coronary calcium scan. Calcium in the coronary arteries may be an early sign of CHD.

- Problems with the aorta. The aorta is the main artery that carries oxygen-rich blood from the heart to the body. Cardiac CT can detect two serious problems in the aorta:

  - Aneurysm. An aneurysm is a diseased area of a blood vessel wall that bulges out. An aneurysm can be life threatening if it bursts.

  - Dissection. A dissection is a split in one or more layers of the artery wall. The split causes bleeding into and along the layers of the artery wall. This condition can cause pain and may be life threatening.

- A pulmonary embolism (PE). A PE is a sudden blockage in a lung artery, usually due to a blood clot.

- Problems in the pulmonary veins. The pulmonary veins carry blood from the lungs to the heart. Problems with these veins may lead to an irregular heart rhythm called atrial fibrillation (AF). The pictures that cardiac CT creates of the pulmonary veins can help guide procedures used to treat AF.

- Problems with heart function and heart valves. In some cases, doctors may recommend cardiac CT instead of echocardiography or cardiac MRI (magnetic resonance imaging) to look for problems with heart function or heart valves.

- Pericardial disease. This is a disease that occurs in the pericardium, the sac around your heart. Cardiac CT can create clear, detailed pictures of the pericardium.

- Results of coronary artery bypass grafting (CABG). In CABG, arteries from other areas in your body are used to bypass (that is, go around) narrow coronary arteries. A CT scan can help determine whether the grafted arteries remain open after the surgery.

Doctors also might recommend cardiac CT scans before or after other heart procedures, such as cardiac resynchronization therapy. A CT scan can help your doctor pinpoint the areas of the heart or blood vessels where the procedure should be done. The scan also can help your doctor check your heart after the procedure.

Because the heart is in motion, a fast type of CT scanner, called multidetector computed tomography (MDCT), might be used to take high-quality pictures of the heart. MDCT also might be used to detect calcium in the coronary arteries.

Another type of CT scanner, called electron-beam computed tomography (EBCT), also is used to detect calcium in the coronary arteries.

What Are the Risks of Cardiac CT?

Cardiac CT involves radiation, although the amount used is considered small. Depending on the type of CT scan you have, the amount of radiation is similar to the amount you're naturally exposed to over 1–5 years.

There is a small chance that cardiac CT will cause cancer because of the radiation. The risk is higher for people younger than 40 years old. New cardiac CT methods are available that reduce the amount of radiation used during the test.

Cardiac CT scans are painless. Some people have side effects from the contrast dye that might be used during the scan. An itchy feeling or a rash may appear after the contrast dye is injected. Normally, neither side effect lasts for long, so medicine often isn't needed.

If you do want medicine to relieve the symptoms, your doctor may prescribe an antihistamine. This type of medicine is used to help stop allergic reactions.

Although rare, it is possible to have a serious allergic reaction to the contrast dye. This reaction may cause breathing problems. Doctors use medicine to treat serious allergic reactions.

People who have asthma, COPD (chronic obstructive pulmonary disease), or heart failure may have breathing problems during cardiac CT if they're given beta blockers to slow their heart rates.

Chapter 44

Cardiac Magnetic Resonance Imaging

What Is Cardiac MRI?

Magnetic resonance imaging (MRI) is a safe, noninvasive test that creates detailed pictures of your organs and tissues. "Noninvasive" means that no surgery is done and no instruments are inserted into your body.

MRI uses radio waves, magnets, and a computer to create pictures of your organs and tissues. Unlike other imaging tests, MRI doesn't use ionizing radiation or carry any risk of causing cancer.

Cardiac MRI creates both still and moving pictures of your heart and major blood vessels. Doctors use cardiac MRI to get pictures of the beating heart and to look at its structure and function. These pictures can help them decide the best way to treat people who have heart problems.

Cardiac MRI can help explain results from other tests, such as X-rays and computed tomography scans (also called CT scans).

Doctors sometimes use cardiac MRI instead of invasive procedures or tests that involve radiation (such as X-rays) or dyes containing iodine (these dyes may be harmful to people who have kidney problems).

A contrast agent, such as gadolinium, might be injected into a vein during cardiac MRI. The substance travels to the heart and highlights

This chapter includes text excerpted from "Cardiac MRI," National Heart, Lung, and Blood Institute (NHLBI), February 2, 2012. Reviewed June 2016.

the heart and blood vessels on the MRI pictures. This contrast agent often is used for people who are allergic to the dyes used in CT scanning.

People who have severe kidney or liver problems may not be able to have the contrast agent. As a result, they may have a noncontrast MRI (an MRI that does not involve contrast agent).

Other Names for Cardiac MRI

- Heart MRI

- Cardiovascular MRI

- Cardiac nuclear magnetic resonance (NMR)

What to Expect before Cardiac MRI

You'll be asked to fill out a screening form before having cardiac MRI. The form may ask whether you've had any previous surgeries. It also may ask whether you have any metal objects or medical devices (like a cardiac pacemaker) in your body. Some implanted medical devices, such as man-made heart valves and coronary stents, are safe around the MRI machine, but others are not. For example, the MRI machine can:

- Cause implanted cardiac pacemakers and defibrillators to malfunction.

- Damage cochlear (inner-ear) implants. Cochlear implants are small, electronic devices that help people who are deaf or who can't hear well understand speech and the sounds around them.

- Cause brain aneurysm clips to move as a result of the MRI's strong magnetic field. This can cause severe injury.

Talk to your doctor or the MRI technician if you have concerns about any implanted devices that may interfere with the MRI.

Your doctor will let you know if you shouldn't have a cardiac MRI because of a medical device. If so, consider wearing a medical ID bracelet or necklace or carrying a medical alert card that states that you shouldn't have an MRI.

If you're pregnant, make sure your doctor knows before you have an MRI. No harmful effects of MRI during pregnancy have been reported; however, more research on the safety of MRI during pregnancy is needed.

Your doctor or technician will tell you whether you need to change into a hospital gown for the test. Don't bring hearing aids, credit cards, jewelry and watches, eyeglasses, pens, removable dental work, or anything that's magnetic near the MRI machine.

Tell your doctor if being in a fairly tight or confined space causes you anxiety or fear. If so, your doctor might give you medicine to help you relax. Your doctor may ask you to fast (not eat) for 6 hours before you take this medicine on the day of the test.

Some newer cardiac MRI machines are open on all sides. If you're fearful in tight or confined spaces, ask your doctor to help you find a facility that has an open MRI machine.

Your doctor will let you know whether you need to arrange for a ride home after the test.

What to Expect during Cardiac MRI

Cardiac MRI takes place in a hospital or medical imaging facility. A radiologist or other doctor who has special training in medical imaging oversees MRI testing.

Cardiac MRI usually takes 30 to 90 minutes, depending on how many pictures are needed. The test may take less time with some newer MRI machines.

The MRI machine will be located in a special room that prevents radio waves from disrupting the machine. It also prevents the MRI machine's strong magnetic fields from disrupting other equipment.

Traditional MRI machines look like long, narrow tunnels. Newer MRI machines (called short-bore systems) are shorter, wider, and don't completely surround you. Some newer machines are open on all sides. Your doctor will help decide which type of machine is best for you.

Cardiac MRI is painless and harmless. You'll lie on your back on a sliding table that goes inside the tunnel-like machine.

The MRI technician will control the machine from the next room. He or she will be able to see you through a glass window and talk to you through a speaker. Tell the technician if you have a hearing problem.

The MRI machine makes loud humming, tapping, and buzzing noises. Some facilities let you wear earplugs or listen to music during the test.

You will need to remain very still during the MRI. Any movement can blur the pictures. If you're unable to lie still, you may be given medicine to help you relax.

The technician might ask you to hold your breath for 10 to 15 seconds at a time while he or she takes pictures of your heart. Researchers are studying ways that will allow someone having a cardiac MRI to breathe freely during the exam, while achieving the same image quality.

A contrast agent, such as gadolinium, might be used to highlight your blood vessels or heart in the pictures. The substance usually is injected into a vein in your arm using a needle.

You may feel a cool sensation during the injection and discomfort when the needle is inserted. Gadolinium doesn't contain iodine, so it won't cause problems for people who are allergic to iodine.

Your cardiac MRI might include a stress test to detect blockages in your coronary arteries. If so, you'll get other medicines to increase the blood flow in your heart or to increase your heart rate.

What to Expect after Cardiac MRI

You'll be able to return to your normal routine once the cardiac MRI is done.

If you took medicine to help you relax during the test, your doctor will tell you when you can return to your normal routine. The medicine will make you sleepy, so you'll need someone to drive you home.

What Does Cardiac MRI Show?

The doctor supervising your scan will provide your doctor with the results of your cardiac MRI. Your doctor will discuss the findings with you.

Cardiac MRI can reveal various heart diseases and conditions, such as:

- Coronary heart disease

- Damage caused by a heart attack

- Heart failure

- Heart valve problems

- Congenital heart defects (heart defects present at birth)

- Pericarditis (a condition in which the membrane, or sac, around your heart is inflamed)

- Cardiac tumors

Cardiac MRI is a fast, accurate tool that can help diagnose a heart attack. The test does this by detecting areas of the heart that don't move normally, have poor blood supply, or are scarred.

Cardiac MRI also can show whether any of the coronary arteries are blocked. A blockage prevents your heart muscle from getting enough oxygen-rich blood, which can lead to a heart attack.

Currently, coronary angiography is the most common procedure for looking at blockages in the coronary arteries. Coronary angiography is an invasive procedure that uses X-rays and iodine-based dye.

Researchers have found that cardiac MRI can sometimes replace coronary angiography, avoiding the need to use X-ray radiation and iodine-based dye. This use of MRI is called MR angiography (MRA).

Echocardiography (echo) is the main test for diagnosing heart valve disease. However, your doctor also might recommend cardiac MRI to assess the severity of valve disease.

A cardiac MRI can confirm information about valve defects or provide more detailed information about heart valve disease.

This information can help your doctor plan your treatment. An MRI also might be done before heart valve surgery to help your surgeon plan for the surgery.

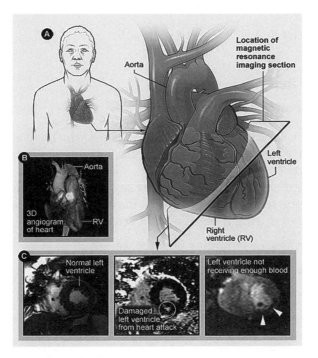

Figure 44.1. *Cardiac MRI*

(A) shows the heart's position in the body and the location and angle of the MRI pictures shown in (C). (B) is a magnetic resonance angiogram, which sometimes is used instead of a standard angiogram. (C) shows MRI pictures of a normal left ventricle (left image), a left ventricle damaged by a heart attack (middle image), and a left ventricle that isn't getting enough blood from the coronary arteries (right image).

Researchers are finding new ways to use cardiac MRI. In the future, cardiac MRI may replace X-rays as the main way to guide invasive procedures such as cardiac catheterization.

Also, improvements in cardiac MRI will likely lead to better methods for detecting heart disease in the future.

What Are the Risks of Cardiac MRI?

The magnetic fields and radio waves used in cardiac MRI have no side effects. This method of taking pictures of organs and tissues doesn't carry a risk of causing cancer or birth defects.

Serious reactions to the contrast agent used during some MRI tests are very rare. However, side effects are possible and include the following:

- Headache

- Nausea (feeling sick to your stomach)

- Dizziness

- Changes in taste

- Allergic reactions

Rarely, the contrast agent can harm people who have severe kidney or liver disease. The substance may cause a disease called nephrogenic systemic fibrosis.

If your cardiac MRI includes a stress test, more medicines will be used during the test. These medicines may have other side effects that aren't expected during a regular MRI scan, such as:

- Arrhythmias, or irregular heartbeats

- Chest pain

- Shortness of breath

- Palpitations (feelings that your heart is skipping a beat, fluttering, or beating too hard or fast)

Chapter 45

Coronary Calcium Scan

What Is a Coronary Calcium Scan?

A coronary calcium scan is a test that looks for specks of calcium in the walls of the coronary (heart) arteries. These specks of calcium are called calcifications.

Calcifications in the coronary arteries are an early sign of coronary heart disease (CHD). CHD is a disease in which a waxy substance called plaque builds up in the coronary arteries.

Over time, plaque can harden or rupture (break open). Hardened plaque narrows the coronary arteries and reduces the flow of oxygen-rich blood to the heart. This can cause chest pain or discomfort called angina.

If the plaque ruptures, a blood clot can form on its surface. A large blood clot can mostly or completely block blood flow through a coronary artery. This is the most common cause of a heart attack. Over time, ruptured plaque also hardens and narrows the coronary arteries.

CHD also can lead to heart failure and arrhythmias. Heart failure is a condition in which your heart can't pump enough blood to meet your body's needs. Arrhythmias are problems with the rate or rhythm of your heartbeat.

This chapter includes text excerpted from "Coronary Calcium Scan," National Heart, Lung, and Blood Institute (NHLBI), March 30, 2012. Reviewed June 2016.

Overview

Two machines can show calcium in the coronary arteries—electron beam computed tomography (EBCT) and multidetector computed tomography (MDCT).

Both use X-rays to create detailed pictures of your heart. Your doctor will study the pictures to see whether you're at risk for future heart problems.

A coronary calcium scan is a fairly simple test. You'll lie quietly in the scanner machine for about 10 minutes while it takes pictures of your heart. The pictures will show whether you have calcifications in your coronary arteries.

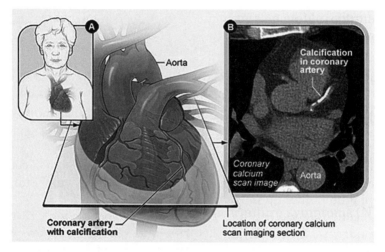

Figure 45.1. *Coronary Calcium Scan*

(A) shows the position of the heart in the body and the location and angle of the coronary calcium scan image. (B) is a coronary calcium scan image showing calcifications in a coronary artery.

Because calcifications are an early sign of CHD, a coronary calcium scan can show whether you're at risk for a heart attack or other heart problems before other signs and symptoms occur.

Outlook

A coronary calcium scan is most useful for people who are at moderate risk for heart attacks. You or your doctor can calculate your 10-year risk using the Risk Assessment Tool from the National Cholesterol Education Program.

People who are at moderate risk have a 10–20 percent chance of having a heart attack within the next 10 years. The coronary calcium scan may help doctors decide who within this group needs treatment.

Other Names for a Coronary Calcium Scan

• Calcium scan test

• Cardiac CT for calcium scoring

Some people refer to coronary calcium scans by the name of the machine used to take pictures of the heart:

• Electron beam computed tomography (EBCT) or electron beam tomography (EBT)

• Multidetector computed tomography (MDCT)

What to Expect before a Coronary Calcium Scan

You don't need to take any special steps before having a coronary calcium scan. However, your doctor may ask you to avoid caffeine and smoking for 4 hours before the test.

For the scan, you'll remove your clothes above the waist and wear a hospital gown. You also will remove any jewelry from around your neck or chest.

What to Expect during a Coronary Calcium Scan

A coronary calcium scan is done in a hospital or outpatient office. The X-ray machine that's used for the scan is called a computed tomography (CT) scanner.

The technician who runs the scanner will clean areas of your chest and apply sticky patches with sensors called electrodes. The patches are connected to an EKG (electrocardiogram) machine.

The EKG will record your heart's electrical activity during the scan. This makes it possible to take pictures of your heart when it's relaxed between beats.

The CT scanner is a large machine that has a hollow, circular tube in the center. You'll lie on your back on a sliding table. The table can move up and down, and it goes inside the tunnel-like machine.

The table will slowly slide into the opening in the machine. Inside the scanner, an X-ray tube will move around your body to take pictures of your heart. The technician will control the CT scanner from the next room. He or she will be able to see you through a glass window and talk to you through a speaker.

The technician will ask you to lie still and hold your breath for short periods while each picture is taken. You may be given medicine to slow your heart rate. This helps the machine take clearer pictures of your heart. The medicine will be given by mouth or injected into a vein.

The coronary calcium scan will take about 10–15 minutes, although the actual scanning will take only a few seconds. During the test, the machine will make clicking and whirring sounds as it takes pictures. The scan causes no discomfort, but the exam room might be chilly to keep the machine working properly.

If you get nervous in enclosed or tight spaces, you might receive medicine to help you stay calm. Your head will remain outside the opening in the machine during the test.

What to Expect after a Coronary Calcium Scan

You'll be able to return to your normal activities after the coronary calcium scan is done. Your doctor will discuss the results of the test with you.

What Does a Coronary Calcium Scan Show?

After a coronary calcium scan, you'll get a calcium score called an Agatston score. The score is based on the amount of calcium found in your coronary (heart) arteries. You may get an Agatston score for each major artery and a total score.

The test is negative if no calcifications are found in your arteries. This means your chance of having a heart attack in the next 2–5 years is low.

The test is positive if calcifications are found in your arteries. Calcifications are a sign of atherosclerosis and coronary heart disease (CHD). (Atherosclerosis is a condition in which plaque builds up in the arteries.) The higher your Agatston score is, the more severe the atherosclerosis.

An Agatston score of 0 is normal. In general, the higher your score, the more likely you are to have CHD. If your score is high, your doctor may recommend more tests.

What Are the Risks of a Coronary Calcium Scan?

Coronary calcium scans have very few risks. The test isn't invasive, which means that no surgery is done and no instruments are inserted into your body.

Unlike some CT scans, coronary calcium scans don't require an injection of contrast dye to make your heart or arteries visible on X-ray images.

Coronary calcium scans involve radiation, although the amount used is considered small. Electron beam computed tomography (EBCT) uses less radiation than multidetector computed tomography (MDCT).

In either case, the amount of radiation is about equal to the amount of radiation you're naturally exposed to in a single year.

Chapter 46

Nuclear Heart Scan

What Is a Nuclear Heart Scan?

A nuclear heart scan is a test that provides important information about the health of your heart.

For this test, a safe, radioactive substance called a tracer is injected into your bloodstream through a vein. The tracer travels to your heart and releases energy. Special cameras outside of your body detect the energy and use it to create pictures of your heart.

Nuclear heart scans are used for three main purposes:

- To check how blood is flowing to the heart muscle. If part of the heart muscle isn't getting blood, it may be a sign of coronary heart disease (CHD). CHD can lead to chest pain called angina, a heart attack, and other heart problems. When a nuclear heart scan is done for this purpose, it's called myocardial perfusion scanning.

- To look for damaged heart muscle. Damage might be the result of a previous heart attack, injury, infection, or medicine. When a nuclear heart scan is done for this purpose, it's called myocardial viability testing.

- To see how well your heart pumps blood to your body. When a nuclear heart scan is done for this purpose, it's called ventricular function scanning.

This chapter includes text excerpted from "Nuclear Heart Scan," National Heart, Lung, and Blood Institute (NHLBI), March 9, 2012. Reviewed June 2016.

Usually, two sets of pictures are taken during a nuclear heart scan. The first set is taken right after a stress test, while your heart is beating fast.

During a stress test, you exercise to make your heart work hard and beat fast. If you can't exercise, you might be given medicine to increase your heart rate. This is called a pharmacological stress test.

The second set of pictures is taken later, while your heart is at rest and beating at a normal rate.

Types of Nuclear Heart Scans

The two main types of nuclear heart scans are single photon emission computed tomography (SPECT) and cardiac positron emission tomography (PET).

Single Photon Emission Computed Tomography

Doctors use SPECT to help diagnose coronary heart disease (CHD). Combining SPECT with a stress test can show problems with blood flow to the heart. Sometimes doctors can detect these problems only when the heart is working hard and beating fast.

Doctors also use SPECT to look for areas of damaged or dead heart muscle tissue. These areas might be the result of a previous heart attack or other cause.

SPECT also can show how well the heart's lower left chamber (left ventricle) pumps blood to the body. Weak pumping ability might be the result of a heart attack, heart failure, and other causes.

Tracers commonly used during SPECT include thallium-201, technetium-99m sestamibi (Cardiolite®), and technetium-99m tetrofosmin (Myoview™).

Positron Emission Tomography

Doctors can use PET for the same purposes as SPECT—to diagnose CHD, check for damaged or dead heart muscle tissue, and check the heart's pumping strength.

Compared with SPECT, PET takes a clearer picture through thick layers of tissue (such as abdominal or breast tissue). PET also is better at showing whether CHD is affecting more than one of your heart's blood vessels.

Right now, however, there's no clear advantage of using one scan over the other in all situations. Research into advances in both SPECT and PET is ongoing.

PET uses different tracers than SPECT.

Other Names for a Nuclear Heart Scan

- Nuclear stress test

- SPECT scan

- PET scan

- Radionuclide scan

What to Expect before a Nuclear Heart Scan

A nuclear heart scan can take a lot of time. Most scans take between 2–5 hours, especially if your doctor needs two sets of pictures.

Discuss with your doctor how a nuclear heart scan is done. Talk with him or her about your overall health, including health problems such as asthma, COPD (chronic obstructive pulmonary disease), diabetes, and kidney disease.

If you have lung disease or diabetes, your doctor will give you special instructions before the nuclear heart scan.

If you're having a stress test as part of your nuclear heart scan, wear comfortable walking shoes and loose-fitting clothes for the test. You may be asked to wear a hospital gown during the test.

Let your doctor know about any medicines you take, including prescription and over-the-counter medicines, vitamins, minerals, and other supplements. Some medicines and supplements can interfere with the medicines that might be used during the stress test to raise your heart rate.

What to Expect during a Nuclear Heart Scan

Many nuclear medicine centers are located in hospitals. A doctor who has special training in nuclear heart scans—a cardiologist or radiologist—will oversee the test

Cardiologists are doctors who specialize in diagnosing and treating heart problems. Radiologists are doctors who have special training in medical imaging techniques.

Before the test begins, the doctor or a technician will use a needle to insert an intravenous (IV) line into a vein in your arm. Through this IV line, he or she will put radioactive tracer into your bloodstream at the right time.

You also will have EKG (electrocardiogram) patches attached to your body to check your heart rate during the test. (An EKG is a simple test that detects and records the heart's electrical activity.)

During the Stress Test

If you're having an exercise stress test as part of your nuclear scan, you'll walk on a treadmill or pedal a stationary bike. During this time, you'll be attached to EKG and blood pressure monitors.

Your doctor will ask you to exercise until you're too tired to continue, short of breath, or having chest or leg pain. You can expect that your heart will beat faster, you'll breathe faster, your blood pressure will increase, and you'll sweat.

Tell your doctor if you have any chest, arm, or jaw pain or discomfort. Also, report any dizziness, light-headedness, or other unusual symptoms.

If you're unable to exercise, your doctor may give you medicine to increase your heart rate. This is called a pharmacological stress test. The medicine might make you feel anxious, sick, dizzy, or shaky for a short time. If the side effects are severe, your doctor may give you other medicine to relieve the symptoms.

Before the exercise or pharmacological stress test ends, the tracer is injected through the IV line.

During the Nuclear Heart Scan

The nuclear heart scan will start shortly after the stress test. You'll lie very still on a padded table.

The nuclear heart scan camera, called a gamma camera, is enclosed in metal housing. The camera can be put in several positions around your body as you lie on the padded table.

For some nuclear heart scans, the metal housing is shaped like a doughnut (with a hole in the middle). You lie on a table that slowly moves through the hole. A computer nearby or in another room collects pictures of your heart.

Usually, two sets of pictures are taken. One will be taken right after the stress test and the other will be taken after a period of rest. The pictures might be taken all in 1 day or over 2 days. Each set of pictures takes about 15–30 minutes.

Some people find it hard to stay in one position during the test. Others may feel anxious while lying in the doughnut-shaped scanner. The table may feel hard, and the room may feel chilly because of the air conditioning needed to maintain the machines.

Let your doctor or technician know how you're feeling during the test so he or she can respond as needed.

What to Expect after a Nuclear Heart Scan

Your doctor may ask you to return to the nuclear medicine center on a second day for more pictures. Outpatients will be allowed to go home after the scan or leave the nuclear medicine center between the two scans.

Most people can go back to their daily routines after a nuclear heart scan. The radioactivity will naturally leave your body in your urine or stool. It's helpful to drink plenty of fluids after the test, as your doctor advises.

The cardiologist or radiologist will read and interpret the results of your test. He or she will report the results to your doctor, who will contact you to discuss them. Or, the cardiologist or radiologist may contact you directly to discuss the results.

What Does a Nuclear Heart Scan Show?

The results from a nuclear heart scan can help doctors:

- Diagnose heart conditions, such as coronary heart disease (CHD), and decide the best course of treatment.
- Manage certain heart diseases, such as CHD and heart failure, and predict short-term or long-term survival.
- Determine your risk for a heart attack.
- Decide whether other heart tests or procedures will help you. Examples of these tests and procedures include coronary angiography and cardiac catheterization.
- Decide whether procedures that increase blood flow to the coronary arteries will help you. Examples of these procedures include percutaneous coronary intervention, also known as coronary angioplasty, and coronary artery bypass grafting (CABG).
- Monitor procedures or surgeries that have been done, such as CABG or a heart transplant.

What Are the Risks of a Nuclear Heart Scan?

The radioactive tracer used during nuclear heart scanning exposes the body to a very small amount of radiation. No long-term effects have been reported from these doses.

515

Radiation dose might be a concern for people who need multiple scans. However, advances in hardware and software may greatly reduce the radiation dose people receive.

Some people are allergic to the radioactive tracer, but this is rare.

If you have coronary heart disease, you may have chest pain during the stress test while you're exercising or taking medicine to raise your heart rate. Medicine can relieve this symptom.

If you're pregnant, tell your doctor or technician before the scan. It might be postponed until after the pregnancy.

Chapter 47

Heart Biopsy

A biopsy is a procedure in which a small piece of tissue is removed from a body for examination. A heart biopsy, also known as a cardiac or myocardial biopsy, is performed to detect heart disease. A small catheter called a bioptome is used to collect a sample of the heart-muscle tissue, which is then sent to a laboratory for analysis.

Why Is It Needed?

A doctor will request a heart biopsy to diagnose:

- myocarditis or other heart disorders, such as cardiac amyloidosis or cardiomyopathy

- rejection of a transplanted heart by identifying tissue damage caused by the immune system

Preparing for the Procedure

A heart biopsy is conducted in a hospital as an outpatient procedure, although in rare circumstances you could be required to enter the hospital the night before the procedure. The doctor will give instructions on what food can be consumed before the biopsy. Generally, you should restrict intake of food and liquids six to eight hours before the test.

"Heart Biopsy," © 2016 Omnigraphics. Reviewed June 2016.

The doctor should be made aware of any current medication or supplements and their dosages, as well as allergies, if any. If you are diabetic, ask the doctor to adjust your medication dosage for the day of the test. Make sure that someone is available to drive you home after the test, since sedatives given during the procedure may make you feel groggy.

How Is It Performed?

A healthcare provider will first explain the procedure, including the risks involved. You will be given a hospital gown to wear for the procedure and will be asked to lie flat on your back on a special table with a large camera above it and several TV monitors nearby. An intravenous line will be started in your arm to transfer fluids to keep you hydrated during the procedure and administer medication to regulate heartbeat or blood pressure, if needed.

Depending on which region of the heart will be biopsied, as well as other factors, the doctor will make an incision in either on your neck, arm, or groin. It will most likely be the neck if you are not having another surgery at this time. You will be awake during the procedure, and a local anesthetic will be given to numb the incision site. A plastic introducer sheath (a short, hollow tube) will be inserted into the blood vessel to hold the incision open, which may cause some discomfort.

Once the tube in placed, a bioptome will be inserted into the blood vessel and threaded to the heart. Fluoroscopy, which is a special type of X-ray, will be used to guide the bioptome. When the device reaches the correct position, a jaw-like structure at its end will obtain a sample of the muscle tissue. Each sample is roughly the size of the head of a pin. The bioptome and the sheath are then removed and pressure is applied on the insertion site to stop bleeding. The whole procedure generally takes between 30 and 60 minutes and is constantly monitored by medical staff.

After the procedure, you will be instructed on how to care for the wound site and when you can go back to regular activities. The doctor will discuss the results of the test when they are available. If they are negative, it indicates that the analyzed tissues are normal.

A positive result may confirm a number of conditions, including:

- inflammation caused by an infection (myocarditis)
- disorders such as cardiac amyloidosis (a condition in which amyloid protein builds up in the heart

- different types of cardiomyopathy (diseased heart muscle)
- damage to the heart due to alcohol abuse
- the presence of rejection cells after heart transplant surgery

What Are the Risks?

Before the procedure, the possible risks involved will be explained, and you will be asked to sign a consent form. However, complications are rare when the biopsy is performed by an experienced doctor.

Some of the possible risks include:

- bleeding
- blood clots
- irregular heartbeat or aggravation of existing arrhythmia
- damage to the vein in which the bioptome is inserted
- damage to the recurrent laryngeal nerve, which controls speech
- infection
- collapsed lung
- in extremely rare cases, rupture of heart

References

1. Herndon, Jaime. "Myocardial Biopsy," Healthline, January 20, 2016.

2. Beckerman, James. "Heart Disease and the Heart Biopsy," WebMD, February 16, 2016.

Part Six

Treating Cardiovascular Disorders

Chapter 48

Medications for Treating Cardiovascular Disorders

Cardiovascular disease is the leading cause of death for Americans. A variety of medications have been developed to help alleviate symptoms of heart disease and extend patients' lives. Although medications can be very helpful when used as prescribed, lifestyle modifications are also important in avoiding the serious health consequences of heart disease, such as arrhythmias, heart attacks, and heart failure. The following are some of the medications most commonly prescribed to treat cardiovascular disorders:

Angiotensin-Converting Enzyme (ACE) Inhibitors

ACE inhibitors are typically prescribed to help lower blood pressure, which makes it easier for the heart to pump blood through the body. They work by reducing the levels of angiotensin, a hormone that constricts blood vessels. When the blood vessels dilate or expand, blood flows through them more easily and blood pressure decreases. ACE inhibitors such as benazepril (Lotensin), ramipril (Altacte), and captopril (Capoten) are usually prescribed for patients with high blood pressure, heart failure, or recent heart attacks to ease the workload on the heart muscle.

Angiotensin II Receptor Blockers (ARBs)

ARBs are similar to ACE inhibitors in that they reduce blood pressure and allow blood to flow more freely through the body. They work by completely blocking the effects of the hormone angiotensin II. ARBs such as losartan (Cozaar) and valsartan (Diovan) are commonly prescribed to treat high blood pressure, congestive heart failure, or a recent heart attack. The medication has also been shown to slow the progression of kidney disease in patients with type 2 diabetes.

Anticoagulants

Anticoagulants such as enoxaparin (Lovenox), heparin, and warfarin (Coumadin) help prevent blood clots from forming. Plaques in the arteries of people with coronary artery disease can rupture and create blood clots, which are associated with such serious health risks as heart attacks and strokes. Although anticoagulants cannot dissolve existing blood clots, they can help prevent new clots from forming.

Antiplatelet Agents

Antiplatelet medications are similar to anticoagulants because they help thin the blood and prevent blood clots from forming. Antiplatelet medications like aspirin, clopidogrel (Plavix), and prasurgel (Effient) are often prescribed to prevent heart attacks in people with coronary artery disease. They may also be prescribed for people who face an increased risk of blood clots due to abnormal heart rhythms, such as atrial fibrillation.

Beta Blockers

Beta blockers are a broad category of medications used to control and reduce the heart rate. They work by blocking the effects of adrenaline (epinephrine), a hormone produced in response to stress. Beta blockers such as metoprolol (Lopressor), labetalol (Trandate), and propanolol (Inderal) are often prescribed to treat arrhythmias, heart failure, chest pain, and high blood pressure. They may also help prevent heart attacks.

Calcium Channel Blockers

Since calcium triggers heart contractions, calcium channel blockers can slow the heart rate, relax the blood vessels, and increase the supply of oxygen to the heart. Medications such as amlodipine (Norvasc), dilti-azem (Cardizem), and nifedipine (Procardia) are commonly prescribed to treat high blood pressure, angina (chest pain), and arrhythmias.

Cholesterol-Lowering Medications

Cholesterol plays an important role in helping the body create new cells, lubricate nerves, and produce hormones. Yet cholesterol buildup in the blood vessels can create plaques that block arteries or rupture to form dangerous blood clots, increasing the risk of heart attack and stroke. Although adopting a healthier diet may help some patients lower their cholesterol levels, others may need medications to reduce their risk of coronary artery disease. Some of the main cholesterol-low-ering medications include statins like atorvastatin (Lipitor), pravasta-tin sodium (Pravachol), and simvastatin (Zocor); bile acid resins such as cholestyramine (Questran); cholesterol absorption inhibitors like ezetimibe (Zetia); fibric acid derivatives such as fenofibrate (Tricor); and niacin (Niacor, Nicolar). Patients whose high cholesterol levels do not respond to statins may benefit from proprotein convertase subtili-sin kexin type 9 (PCSK9) inhibitors, a new class of cholesterol-lowering drugs that block the action of a liver enzyme that prevents the removal of harmful cholesterol from the bloodstream.

Digitalis Medications

Digitalis medications like digoxin (Lanoxin) are used to increase the strength and efficiency of heart contractions. They are prescribed to treat patients with heart failure, irregular heartbeats, and poor circulation who may not experience benefits from ACE inhibitors and diuretics.

Diuretics

Diuretics trigger the kidneys to get rid of excess fluid from the tissues and bloodstream by excreting it as urine. Since excess fluid makes it more difficult for the heart to pump blood through the body, diuretics can help protect the heart. Commonly known as "water pills," they are used to treat high blood pressure and to reduce the swelling and water retention caused by heart failure. Aldosterone inhibitors are a type of diuretic that works by blocking aldosterone, a chemical in the body that causes fluid retention and salt buildup. Aldosterone inhibitors such as eplerenone (Inspra) and spironolactone (Aldoctone) may be prescribed for patients with severe heart failure that does not respond to other medications.

Inotropic Therapy

Inotropic therapy is another pharmacological approach for treating end-stage heart failure. It involves using intravenous medications to increase the force of the heart muscle's contractions and relax the blood vessels to allow blood to flow more smoothly. It is generally used to relieve symptoms of heart failure when other medications are no longer effective.

Potassium and Magnesium

Low levels of these minerals can cause abnormal heart rhythms, so potassium and magnesium are sometimes prescribed as supplements for patients with arrhythmias.

Vasodilators

Vasodilators relax the blood vessels to allow blood to flow more easily. They are generally prescribed to treat heart failure and control blood pressure in patients who cannot tolerate ACE inhibitors.

References

1. "Common Heart Disease Drugs," WebMD, 2016.
2. Donovan, Robin. "Drugs to Treat Heart Disease," Healthline, 2016.

Chapter 49

Procedures to Treat Narrowed or Blocked Arteries

Section 49.1

Cardiac Catheterization

This section includes excerpted from "Cardiac
Catheterization," National Heart, Lung, and Blood
Institute (NHLBI), January 30, 2012.
Reviewed June 2016.

What Is Cardiac Catheterization?

Cardiac catheterization is a medical procedure used to diagnose
and treat some heart conditions.

A long, thin, flexible tube called a catheter is put into a blood vessel
in your arm, groin (upper thigh), or neck and threaded to your heart.
Through the catheter, your doctor can do diagnostic tests and treatments on your heart.

For example, your doctor may put a special type of dye in the catheter. The dye will flow through your bloodstream to your heart. Then,
your doctor will take X-ray pictures of your heart. The dye will make
your coronary (heart) arteries visible on the pictures. This test is called
coronary angiography.

The dye can show whether a waxy substance called plaque has
built up inside your coronary arteries. Plaque can narrow or block the
arteries and restrict blood flow to your heart.

The buildup of plaque in the coronary arteries is called coronary
heart disease (CHD) or coronary artery disease.

Doctors also can use ultrasound during cardiac catheterization to
see blockages in the coronary arteries. Ultrasound uses sound waves
to create detailed pictures of the heart's blood vessels.

Doctors may take samples of blood and heart muscle during cardiac
catheterization or do minor heart surgery.

Cardiologists (heart specialists) usually do cardiac catheterization
in a hospital. You're awake during the procedure, and it causes little
or no pain. However, you may feel some soreness in the blood vessel
where the catheter was inserted.

Cardiac catheterization rarely causes serious complications.

Who Needs Cardiac Catheterization?

Doctors may recommend cardiac catheterization for various reasons. The most common reason is to evaluate chest pain.

Chest pain might be a symptom of coronary heart disease (CHD). Cardiac catheterization can show whether plaque is narrowing or blocking your coronary arteries.

Doctors also can treat CHD during cardiac catheterization using a procedure called percutaneous coronary intervention (PCI), also known as coronary angioplasty.

During PCI, a catheter with a balloon at its tip is threaded to the blocked coronary artery. Once in place, the balloon is inflated, pushing the plaque against the artery wall. This creates a wider path for blood to flow to the heart.

Sometimes a stent is placed in the artery during PCI. A stent is a small mesh tube that supports the inner artery wall.

Most people who have heart attacks have narrow or blocked coronary arteries. Thus, cardiac catheterization might be used as an emergency procedure to treat a heart attack. When used with PCI, the procedure allows your doctor to open up blocked arteries and prevent further heart damage.

Cardiac catheterization also can help your doctor figure out the best treatment plan for you if:

- You recently recovered from a heart attack, but are having chest pain

- You had a heart attack that caused major heart damage

- You had an EKG (electrocardiogram), stress test, or other test with results that suggested heart disease

Cardiac catheterization also might be used if your doctor thinks you have a heart defect or if you're about to have heart surgery. The procedure shows the overall shape of your heart and the four large spaces (heart chambers) inside it. This inside view of the heart will show certain heart defects and help your doctor plan your heart surgery.

Sometimes doctors use cardiac catheterization to see how well the heart valves work. Valves control blood flow in your heart. They open and shut to allow blood to flow between your heart chambers and into your arteries.

Your doctor can use cardiac catheterization to measure blood flow and oxygen levels in different parts of your heart. He or she also can check how well a man-made heart valve is working and how well your heart is pumping blood.

If your doctor thinks you have a heart infection or tumor, he or she may take samples of your heart muscle through the catheter. With the help of cardiac catheterization, doctors can even do minor heart surgery, such as repair certain heart defects.

What to Expect before Cardiac Catheterization

Before having cardiac catheterization, discuss with your doctor:

- How to prepare for the procedure

- Any medicines you're taking, and whether you should stop taking them before the procedure

- Whether you have any conditions (such as diabetes or kidney disease) that may require taking extra steps during or after the procedure to avoid problems

Your doctor will let you know whether you need to arrange for a ride home after the procedure.

What to Expect during Cardiac Catheterization

Cardiac catheterization is done in a hospital. During the procedure, you'll be kept on your back and awake. This allows you to follow your doctor's instructions during the procedure. You'll be given medicine to help you relax, which might make you sleepy.

Your doctor will numb the area on the arm, groin (upper thigh), or neck where the catheter will enter your blood vessel. Then, a needle will be used to make a small hole in the blood vessel. Your doctor will put a tapered tube called a sheath through the hole.

Next, your doctor will put a thin, flexible guide wire through the sheath and into your blood vessel. He or she will thread the wire through your blood vessel to your heart.

Your doctor will use the guide wire to correctly place the catheter. He or she will put the catheter through the sheath and slide it over the guide wire and into the coronary arteries.

Special X-ray movies will be taken of the guide wire and the catheter as they're moved into the heart. The movies will help your doctor see where to put the tip of the catheter.

When the catheter reaches the right spot, your doctor will use it to do tests or treatments on your heart. For example, your doctor may perform a percutaneous coronary intervention (PCI), also known as coronary angioplasty, and stenting.

During the procedure, your doctor may put a special type of dye in the catheter. The dye will flow through your bloodstream to your heart. Then, your doctor will take X-ray pictures of your heart. The dye will make your coronary (heart) arteries visible on the pictures. This test is called coronary angiography.

Coronary angiography can show how well the heart's lower chambers, called the ventricles, are pumping blood.

When the catheter is inside your heart, your doctor may use it to take blood and tissue samples or do minor heart surgery.

To get a more detailed view of a blocked coronary artery, your doctor may do intracoronary ultrasound. For this test, your doctor will thread a tiny ultrasound device through the catheter and into the artery. This device gives off sound waves that bounce off the artery wall (and its blockage). The sound waves create a picture of the inside of the artery.

If the angiogram or intracoronary ultrasound shows blockages in the coronary arteries, your doctor may use PCI to treat the blocked arteries.

After your doctor does all of the needed tests or treatments, he or she will pull back the catheter and take it out along with the sheath. The opening left in the blood vessel will be closed up and bandaged.

A small weight might be put on top of the bandage for a few hours to apply more pressure. This will help prevent major bleeding from the site.

What to Expect after Cardiac Catheterization

After cardiac catheterization, you will be moved to a special care area. You will rest there for several hours or overnight. During that time, you'll have to limit your movement to avoid bleeding from the site where the catheter was inserted.

While you recover in this area, nurses will check your heart rate and blood pressure regularly. They also will check for bleeding from the catheter insertion site.

A small bruise might form at the catheter insertion site, and the area may feel sore or tender for about a week. Let your doctor know if you have problems such as:

- A constant or large amount of bleeding at the insertion site that can't be stopped with a small bandage

- Unusual pain, swelling, redness, or other signs of infection at or near the insertion site

Talk to your doctor about whether you should avoid certain activities, such as heavy lifting, for a short time after the procedure.

What Are the Risks of Cardiac Catheterization?

Cardiac catheterization is a common medical procedure. It rarely causes serious problems. However, complications can include:

- Bleeding, infection, and pain at the catheter insertion site.
- Damage to blood vessels. Rarely, the catheter may scrape or poke a hole in a blood vessel as it's threaded to the heart.
- An allergic reaction to the dye that's used during coronary angiography.

Other, less common complications include:

- Arrhythmias (irregular heartbeats). These irregular heartbeats often go away on their own. However, your doctor may recommend treatment if they persist.
- Kidney damage caused by the dye used during coronary angiography.
- Blood clots that can trigger a stroke, heart attack, or other serious problems.
- Low blood pressure.
- A buildup of blood or fluid in the sac that surrounds the heart. This fluid can prevent the heart from beating properly.

As with any procedure involving the heart, complications sometimes can be fatal. However, this is rare with cardiac catheterization.

The risks of cardiac catheterization are higher in people who are older and in those who have certain diseases or conditions (such as chronic kidney disease and diabetes).

Section 49.2

Carotid Endarterectomy

This section includes text excerpted from "Questions and Answers about Carotid Endarterectomy," National Institute of Neurological Disorders and Stroke (NINDS), March 21, 2016.

What Is a Carotid Endarterectomy?

A carotid endarterectomy is a surgical procedure in which a doctor removes fatty deposits blocking one of the two carotid arteries, the main supply of blood for the brain. Carotid artery problems become more common as people age. The disease process that causes the buildup of fat and other material inside the artery walls is called atherosclerosis, popularly known as "hardening of the arteries." The fatty deposit is called plaque; the narrowing of the artery is called stenosis. The degree of stenosis is usually expressed as a percentage of the normal diameter of the opening.

Why Is Surgery Performed?

Carotid endarterectomy is performed to prevent stroke. Two large clinical trials supported by the National Institute of Neurological Disorders and Stroke (NINDS) have identified specific individuals for whom the surgery is beneficial when performed by surgeons and in institutions that can match the standards set in those studies. The surgery has been found highly beneficial for persons who have already had a stroke or experienced the symptoms of a stroke and have a severe stenosis of 70 to 99 percent. In this group, surgery reduces the estimated 2-year risk of stroke or death by more than 80 percent, from greater than 1 in 4 to less than 1 in 10.

For patients who have already had transient or mild stroke symptoms due to moderate carotid stenosis (50 to 69 percent), surgery reduces the 5-year risk of stroke or death by 6.5 percent. The failure rate for ipsilateral stroke or death for the medical group is 22.2 percent, and for the surgery group is 15.7 percent from greater than 1 in 4 to less than 1 in 7. Individuals who have already had stroke symptoms, and who have carotid stenosis greater than 50 percent, may wish to consider surgery to prevent future stroke. Based on findings of the North American Symptomatic Carotid Endarterectomy Trial (NASCET) trial, patients with moderate (50 to 69 percent) stenosis are now better able to make more informed decisions.

In another trial (Asymptomatic Carotid Atherosclerosis Study, or ACAS), the procedure has also been found highly beneficial for persons who are symptom-free but have a carotid stenosis of 60 to 99 percent. In this group, the surgery reduces the estimated 5-year risk of stroke by more than one-half, from about 1 in 10 to less than 1 in 20.

The Carotid Revascularization Endarterectomy vs. Stenting Trial (CREST) compared carotid endarterectomy surgery to carotid artery stenting and found no significance between the procedures regarding the 4-year rate of stroke or death in patients with or without a previous stroke. The pivotal differences were the lower rate of stroke following surgery and the lower rate of heart attack following stenting. The study also found that the age of the patient made a difference with a larger benefit for stenting, the younger the age of the patient. At age 69 and younger, stenting results were slightly better. Conversely, for patients older than 70, surgical benefits were slightly superior to stenting, with larger benefit for surgery, the older the patient.

How Important Is a Blockage as a Cause of Stroke

A blockage of a blood vessel is the most frequent cause of stroke and is responsible for about 80 percent of the approximately 700,000 strokes in the United States each year. With nearly 150,000 stroke deaths each year, stroke ranks as the fourth leading killer in the United States. Stroke is the leading cause of adult disability in the United States with 2 million of the 3 million Americans who have survived a stroke sustaining some permanent disability. The overall cost of stroke to the nation is $40 billion a year.

How Many Carotid Endarterectomies Are Performed Each Year?

An estimated 140,000 carotid endarterectomies were performed in the United States in 2009, according to the National Hospital Discharge Survey. The procedure was first described in the mid-1950s. It began to be used increasingly as a stroke prevention measure in the 1960s and 1970s. Its use peaked in the mid-1980s when more than 100,000 operations were performed each year. At that time, several authorities began to question the trend and the risk-benefit ratio for some groups, and the use of the procedure dropped precipitously. The NINDS-supported NASCET and ACAS trials were launched in the mid-1980s to identify the specific groups of people with carotid artery disease who would clearly benefit from the procedure.

What Are the Risk Factors and How Risky Is the Surgery?

Important risk factors in addition to the degree of stenosis include, gender, diabetes, the type of stroke symptoms, and blockage of the carotid artery on the opposite side. Without other complicating illnesses, age alone is not a worrisome risk factor. Risk factors can affect patients in two ways. They can, particularly in combination, greatly increase a person's risk of having a stroke. In addition, these risk factors can increase the likelihood of surgical complications.

How Is Carotid Artery Disease Diagnosed?

In some cases, the disease can be detected during a normal checkup by a physician. In other cases further testing is needed. Some of the tests a physician can use or order include ultrasound imaging, arteriography, and magnetic resonance angiography (MRA). Frequently these procedures are carried out in a stepwise fashion: from a doctor's evaluation of signs and symptoms to ultrasound, MRA, and arteriography for increasingly difficult cases.

- **History and physical exam.** A doctor will ask about symptoms of a stroke such as numbness or muscle weakness, speech or vision difficulties, or lightheadedness. Using a stethoscope, a doctor may hear a rushing sound, called a bruit, in the carotid artery. Unfortunately, dangerous levels of disease sometimes fail to make a sound, and some blockages with a low risk can make the same sound.

- **Ultrasound imaging**. This is a painless, noninvasive test in which sound waves above the range of human hearing are sent into the neck. Echoes bounce off the moving blood and the tissue in the artery and can be formed into an image. Ultrasound is fast, risk-free, relatively inexpensive, and painless compared to MRA and arteriography.

- **Arteriography.** This can be used to confirm the findings of ultrasound imaging which can be uncertain in some cases.

Arteriography is an X-ray of the carotid artery taken when a special dye is injected into the artery. A burning sensation may be felt when the dye is injected. An arteriogram is more expensive and carries its own small risk of causing a stroke.

- **Magnetic Resonance Angiography (MRA).** This is a new imaging technique that avoids most of the risks associated with arteriography. An MRA is a type of image that uses magnetism instead of X-rays to create an image of the carotid arteries.

What Is "Best Medical Therapy" for Stroke Prevention?

The mainstay of stroke prevention is risk factor management: smoking cessation, treatment of high blood pressure, and control of blood sugar levels among persons with diabetes. Additionally, physicians may prescribe aspirin, warfarin, or ticlopidine for some individuals.

Section 49.3

Coronary Angioplasty

This section includes text excerpted from "Percutaneous Coronary Intervention," National Heart, Lung, and Blood Institute (NHLBI), August 28, 2014.

What Is Percutaneous Coronary Intervention?

Percutaneous coronary intervention (PCI), commonly known as coronary angioplasty or simply angioplasty, is a non-surgical procedure used to open narrow or blocked coronary (heart) arteries. Percutaneous means "through the skin." The procedure is done by inserting a thin flexible tube (catheter) through the skin in the upper thigh or arm in the artery. The procedure restores blood flow to the heart muscle.

Overview

As you age, a waxy substance called plaque can build up inside your arteries. This condition is called atherosclerosis.

Atherosclerosis can affect any artery in the body. When atherosclerosis affects the coronary arteries, the condition is called coronary heart disease (CHD) or coronary artery disease.

Over time, plaque can harden or rupture (break open). Hardened plaque narrows the coronary arteries and reduces the flow of oxygen-rich blood to the heart. This can cause chest pain or discomfort called angina.

If the plaque ruptures, a blood clot can form on its surface. A large blood clot can mostly or completely block blood flow through a coronary artery. This is the most common cause of a heart attack. Over time, ruptured plaque also hardens and narrows the coronary arteries.

PCI can restore blood flow to the heart. During the procedure, a thin, flexible catheter (tube) with a balloon at its tip is threaded through a blood vessel to the affected artery. Once in place, the balloon is inflated to compress the plaque against the artery wall. This restores blood flow through the artery.

Doctors may use the procedure to improve symptoms of CHD, such as angina. The procedure also can reduce heart muscle damage caused by a heart attack.

Outlook

Serious complications from PCI don't occur often. However, they can happen no matter how careful your doctor is or how well he or she does the procedure. The most common complications are discomfort and bleeding at the catheter insertion site.

Other Names for Percutaneous Coronary Intervention

- Balloon angioplasty
- Coronary angioplasty
- Coronary artery angioplasty
- Percutaneous intervention
- Percutaneous transluminal angioplasty
- Percutaneous transluminal coronary angioplasty

Who Needs Percutaneous Coronary Intervention?

Your doctor may recommend percutaneous coronary intervention (PCI) if you have narrow or blocked coronary arteries as a result of coronary heart disease (CHD).

PCI is one treatment for CHD. Other treatments include medicines and coronary artery bypass grafting (CABG). CABG is a type of surgery in which a healthy artery or vein from the body is connected, or grafted, to a blocked coronary artery.

The grafted artery or vein bypasses (that is, goes around) the blocked portion of the coronary artery. This improves blood flow to the heart.

Compared with CABG, some advantages of PCI are that it:

- Doesn't require open-heart surgery

- Doesn't require general anesthesia (that is, you won't be given medicine to make you sleep during the procedure)

- Has a shorter recovery time

However, PCI isn't for everyone. For some people, CABG might be a better option. For example, CABG might be used to treat people who have severe CHD, narrowing of the left main coronary artery, or poor function in the lower left heart chamber.

In addition, recent studies show that people with CHD who also have diabetes may have greater benefit from CABG.

Your doctor will consider many factors when deciding which treatment(s) to recommend.

PCI also is used as an emergency treatment for heart attack. As plaque builds up in the coronary arteries, it can rupture. This can cause a blood clot to form on the surface of the plaque and block blood flow to the heart muscle.

Quickly opening the blockage restores blood flow and reduces heart muscle damage during a heart attack.

How Is Percutaneous Coronary Intervention Done?

Before you have percutaneous coronary intervention (PCI), your doctor will need to know the location and extent of the blockages in your coronary (heart) arteries. To find this information, your doctor will use coronary angiography. This test uses dye and special X-rays to show the insides of your arteries.

During angiography, a small tube (or tubes) called a catheter is inserted into an artery, usually in the groin (upper thigh). The catheter is threaded to the coronary arteries.

Special dye, which is visible on X-ray pictures, is injected through the catheter. The X-ray pictures are taken as the dye flows through your coronary arteries. The dye shows whether blockages are present and their location and severity.

During PCI, another catheter with a balloon at its tip (a balloon catheter) is inserted in the coronary artery and placed in the blockage. Then, the balloon is expanded. This pushes the plaque against the artery wall, relieving the blockage and improving blood flow.

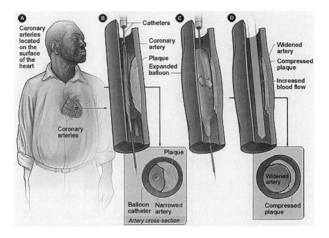

Figure 49.1. *Percutaneous Coronary Intervention*

(A) shows the location of the heart and coronary arteries. (B) shows a deflated balloon catheter inserted into a coronary artery narrowed by plaque. The inset image shows a cross-section of the artery with the inserted balloon catheter. In (C), the balloon is inflated, compressing the plaque against the artery wall. (D) shows the widened artery with increased blood flow. The inset image shows a cross-section of the widened artery and compressed plaque.

A small mesh tube called a stent usually is placed in the artery during the procedure. The stent is wrapped around the deflated balloon catheter before the catheter is inserted into the artery.

When the balloon is inflated to compress the plaque, the stent expands and attaches to the artery wall. The stent supports the inner artery wall and reduces the chance of the artery becoming narrow or blocked again.

Some stents are coated with medicine that is slowly and continuously released into the artery. They are called drug-eluting stents. The medicine helps prevent scar tissue from blocking the artery following PCI.

What to Expect before Percutaneous Coronary Intervention

Percutaneous coronary intervention (PCI) is done in a hospital. A cardiologist will perform the procedure. A cardiologist is a

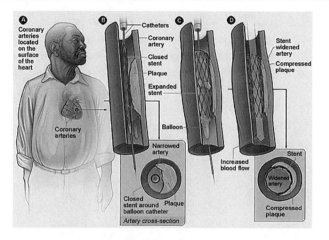

Figure 49.2. *Percutaneous Coronary Intervention with Stent Placement*

(A) shows the location of the heart and coronary arteries. (B) shows the deflated balloon catheter and closed stent inserted into the narrow coronary artery. The inset image shows a cross-section of the artery with the inserted balloon catheter and closed stent. In (C), the balloon is inflated, expanding the stent and compressing the plaque against the artery wall. (D) shows the stent-widened artery. The inset image shows a cross-section of the compressed plaque and stent-widened artery.

doctor who specializes in diagnosing and treating heart diseases and conditions.

If PCI isn't done as an emergency treatment, you'll meet with your cardiologist beforehand. He or she will go over your medical history (including the medicines you take), do a physical exam, and talk to you about the procedure.

Your doctor also may recommend tests, such as blood tests, an EKG (electrocardiogram), and a chest X-ray.

Once the procedure is scheduled, your doctor will advise you:

- When to begin fasting (not eating or drinking) before the procedure. Often, you have to stop eating and drinking 6–8 hours before the procedure.

- What medicines you should and shouldn't take on the day of the procedure.

- When to arrive at the hospital and where to go.

Even though PCI takes only 1–2 hours, you'll likely need to stay in the hospital overnight. Your doctor may advise you to not drive for a certain amount of time after the procedure. Thus, you'll probably need to arrange a ride home.

What to Expect during Percutaneous Coronary Intervention

Percutaneous coronary intervention (PCI) is done in a special part of the hospital called the cardiac catheterization laboratory. The "cath lab" has special video screens and X-ray machines.

Your doctor will use this equipment to see enlarged pictures of the blockages in your coronary arteries.

Preparation

In the cath lab, you'll lie down. An intravenous (IV) line will be placed in your arm to give you fluids and medicines. The medicines will relax you and help prevent blood clots from forming.

The area where your doctor will insert the catheter will be shaved. The catheter usually is inserted in your groin (upper thigh). The shaved area will be cleaned and then numbed. The numbing medicine may sting as it's going in.

The Procedure

During the PCI, you'll be awake but sleepy.

Your doctor will use a needle to make a small hole in an artery in your arm or groin. A thin, flexible guide wire will be inserted into the artery through the small hole. Then, your doctor will remove the needle and place a tapered tube called a sheath over the guide wire and into the artery.

Next, your doctor will put a long, thin, flexible tube called a guiding catheter through the sheath and slide it over the guide wire. The catheter is moved to the opening of a coronary artery, and the guide wire is removed.

Your doctor will inject special dye through the catheter. The dye will help show the inside of the coronary artery and any blockages on an X-ray picture called an angiogram.

Another guide wire is then put through the catheter into the coronary artery and threaded past the blockage. A thin catheter with a balloon at its tip (a balloon catheter) is threaded over the wire and through the guiding catheter.

The balloon catheter is positioned in the blockage. Then, the balloon is inflated. This pushes the plaque against the artery wall, relieving the blockage and improving blood flow through the artery. Sometimes the balloon is inflated and deflated more than once to widen the artery.

Your doctor may put a stent (small mesh tube) in your artery to help keep it open. If so, the stent will be wrapped around the balloon catheter.

When your doctor inflates the balloon, the stent will expand against the wall of the artery. When the balloon is deflated and pulled out of the artery with the catheter, the stent remains in place in the artery.

After the PCI is done, the sheath, guide wires, and catheters are removed from your artery. Pressure is applied to stop bleeding at the catheter insertion site. Sometimes a special device is used to seal the hole in the artery.

During the PCI, you'll receive strong antiplatelet medicines through your IV line. These medicines help prevent blood clots from forming in the artery or on the stent. Your doctor may start you on antiplatelet medicines before the procedure.

What to Expect after Percutaneous Coronary Intervention

After percutaneous coronary intervention (PCI), you'll be moved to a special care unit. You'll stay there for a few hours or overnight. You must lie still for a few hours to allow the blood vessel in your arm or groin (upper thigh) to seal completely.

While you recover, someone on your healthcare team will check your blood pressure, heart rate, oxygen level, and temperature. The site where the catheters were inserted also will be checked for bleeding. That area may feel sore or tender for a while.

Going Home

Most people go home the day after the procedure. When your doctor thinks you're ready to leave the hospital, you'll get instructions to follow at home, such as:

- How much activity or exercise you can do. (Most people are able to walk the day after the PCI procedure.)
- When you should follow up with your doctor.
- What medicines you should take.
- What you should look for daily when checking for signs of infection around the catheter insertion site. Signs of infection include redness, swelling, and drainage.

- When you should call your doctor. For example, you may need to call if you have shortness of breath; a fever; or signs of infection, pain, or bleeding.

- When you should call 9–1–1 (for example, if you have any chest pain).

Your doctor will prescribe medicine to help prevent blood clots from forming. Take all of your medicine as your doctor prescribes.

If you got a stent during the PCI, the medicine reduces the risk that blood clots will form in the stent. Blood clots in the stent can block blood flow and cause a heart attack.

Recovery and Recuperation

Most people recover from the PCI and return to work within a week of leaving the hospital.

Your doctor will want to check your progress after you leave the hospital. During the followup visit, your doctor will examine you, make changes to your medicines (if needed), do any necessary tests, and check your overall recovery.

Use this time to ask questions you may have about activities, medicines, or lifestyle changes, or to talk about any other issues that concern you.

Lifestyle Changes

Although PCI can reduce the symptoms of coronary heart disease (CHD), it isn't a cure for CHD or the risk factors that led to it. Making healthy lifestyle changes can help treat CHD and maintain the good results from PCI.

Talk with your doctor about your risk factors for CHD and the lifestyle changes you should make. Lifestyle changes might include changing your diet, quitting smoking, being physically active, losing weight or maintaining a healthy weight, and reducing stress.

Cardiac Rehabilitation

Your doctor may recommend cardiac rehabilitation (rehab). Cardiac rehab is a medically supervised program that helps improve the health and well-being of people who have heart problems.

Cardiac rehab includes exercise training, education on heart healthy living, and counseling to reduce stress and help you return to an active life. Your doctor can tell you where to find a cardiac rehab program near your home.

What Are the Risks of Percutaneous Coronary Intervention?

Percutaneous coronary intervention (PCI) is a common medical procedure. Serious complications don't occur often. However, they can happen no matter how careful your doctor is or how well he or she does the procedure.

PCI complications can include:

- Discomfort and bleeding at the catheter insertion site.

- Blood vessel damage from the catheters.

- An allergic reaction to the dye used during the procedure.

- An arrhythmia (irregular heartbeat).

- The need for emergency coronary artery bypass grafting during the procedure (less than 3 percent of people). This may occur if an artery closes down instead of opening up.

- Kidney damage caused by the dye used during the procedure.

- Heart attack (3–5 percent of people).

- Stroke (less than 1 percent of people).

Sometimes chest pain can occur during PCI because the balloon briefly blocks blood supply to the heart.

As with any procedure involving the heart, complications can sometimes be fatal. However, this is rare with PCI. Less than 2 percent of people die during the procedure.

The risk of complications is higher in:

- People aged 65 and older

- People who have chronic kidney disease

- People who are in shock

- People who have extensive heart disease and blockages in their coronary (heart) arteries

Research on PCI is ongoing to make it safer and more effective and to prevent treated arteries from narrowing again.

Complications from Stents

Restenosis

Another problem that can occur after PCI is too much tissue growth within the treated portion of the artery. This can cause the artery to become narrow or blocked again, often within 6 months. This complication is called restenosis.

When a stent (small mesh tube) isn't used during PCI, 30 percent of people have restenosis. When a stent is used, 15 percent of people have restenosis.

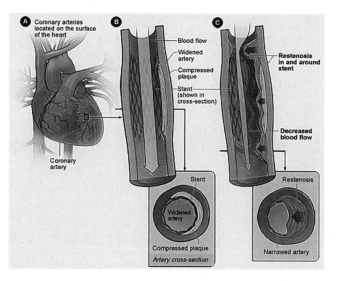

Figure 49.3. *Stent Restenosis*

(A) shows the coronary arteries located on the surface of the heart. (B) shows a stent-widened artery with normal blood flow. The inset image shows a cross-section of the stent-widened artery. In (C), tissue grows through and around the stent over time. This causes a partial blockage of the artery and abnormal blood flow. The inset image shows a cross-section of the tissue growth around the stent.

Stents coated with medicine (drug-eluting stents) reduce the growth of scar tissue around the stent. These stents further reduce the risk of restenosis. When these stents are used, about 10 percent of people have restenosis.

Other treatments, such as radiation, can help prevent tissue growth within a stent. For this procedure, a wire is put through a catheter to where the stent is placed. The wire releases radiation to stop any tissue growth that may block the artery.

Blood Clots

Studies suggest that there's a higher risk of blood clots forming in medicine-coated stents compared with bare metal stents. However, no firm evidence shows that these stents increase the chance of having a heart attack or dying if used as recommended. Researchers continue to study medicine-coated stents.

Taking medicine as prescribed by your doctor can lower your risk of blood clots. People who have medicine-coated stents usually are advised to take antiplatelet medicines, such as clopidogrel and aspirin, for up to a year or longer.

Section 49.4

Coronary Artery Bypass Grafting

This section includes excerpted from "Coronary Artery Bypass Grafting," National Heart, Lung, and Blood Institute (NHLBI), February 23, 2012. Reviewed June 2016.

What Is Coronary Artery Bypass Grafting?

Coronary artery bypass grafting (CABG) is a type of surgery that improves blood flow to the heart. Surgeons use CABG to treat people who have severe coronary heart disease (CHD).

CHD is a disease in which a waxy substance called plaque builds up inside the coronary arteries. These arteries supply oxygen-rich blood to your heart.

Over time, plaque can harden or rupture (break open). Hardened plaque narrows the coronary arteries and reduces the flow of oxygen-rich blood to the heart. This can cause chest pain or discomfort called angina.

If the plaque ruptures, a blood clot can form on its surface. A large blood clot can mostly or completely block blood flow through a coronary artery. This is the most common cause of a heart attack. Over time, ruptured plaque also hardens and narrows the coronary arteries.

CABG is one treatment for CHD. During CABG, a healthy artery or vein from the body is connected, or grafted, to the blocked coronary artery. The grafted artery or vein bypasses (that is, goes around) the blocked portion of the coronary artery. This creates a new path for oxygen-rich blood to flow to the heart muscle.

Surgeons can bypass multiple coronary arteries during one surgery.

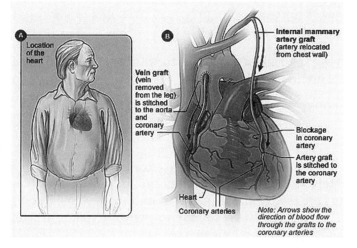

Figure 49.4. *Coronary Artery Bypass Grafting*

(A) shows the location of the heart. (B) shows how vein and artery bypass grafts are attached to the heart.

Overview

CABG is the most common type of open-heart surgery in the United States. Doctors called cardiothoracic surgeons do this surgery.

However, CABG isn't the only treatment for CHD. Other treatment options include lifestyle changes, medicines, and a procedure called percutaneous coronary intervention (PCI), also known as coronary angioplasty.

PCI is a nonsurgical procedure that opens blocked or narrow coronary arteries. During PCI, a stent might be placed in a coronary artery to help keep it open. A stent is a small mesh tube that supports the inner artery wall.

CABG or PCI may be options if you have severe blockages in your large coronary arteries, especially if your heart's pumping action has already grown weak.

CABG also may be an option if you have blockages in the heart that can't be treated with PCI. In this situation, CABG may work better than other types of treatment.

The goals of CABG may include:

- Improving your quality of life and reducing angina and other CHD symptoms

- Allowing you to resume a more active lifestyle

- Improving the pumping action of your heart if it has been damaged by a heart attack

- Lowering the risk of a heart attack (in some patients, such as those who have diabetes)

- Improving your chance of survival

Outlook

The results of CABG usually are excellent. The surgery improves or completely relieves angina symptoms in most patients. Although symptoms can recur, many people remain symptom-free for as long as 10 to 15 years. CABG also may lower your risk of having a heart attack and help you live longer.

You may need repeat surgery if blockages form in the grafted arteries or veins or in arteries that weren't blocked before. Taking medicines and making lifestyle changes as your doctor recommends can lower the risk of a graft becoming blocked.

Types of Coronary Artery Bypass Grafting

There are several types of coronary artery bypass grafting (CABG). Your doctor will recommend the best option for you based on your needs.

Traditional Coronary Artery Bypass Grafting

Traditional CABG is used when at least one major artery needs to be bypassed. During the surgery, the chest bone is opened to access the heart.

Medicines are given to stop the heart; a heart-lung bypass machine keeps blood and oxygen moving throughout the body during surgery. This allows the surgeon to operate on a still heart.

After surgery, blood flow to the heart is restored. Usually, the heart starts beating again on its own. Sometimes mild electric shocks are used to restart the heart.

Off-Pump Coronary Artery Bypass Grafting

This type of CABG is similar to traditional CABG because the chest bone is opened to access the heart. However, the heart isn't stopped, and a heart-lung bypass machine isn't used. Off-pump CABG sometimes is called beating heart bypass grafting.

Minimally Invasive Direct Coronary Artery Bypass Grafting

This type of surgery differs from traditional CABG because the chest bone isn't opened to reach the heart. Instead, several small cuts are made on the left side of the chest between the ribs. This type of surgery mainly is used to bypass blood vessels at the front of the heart.

Minimally invasive bypass grafting is a fairly new procedure. It isn't right for everyone, especially if more than one or two coronary arteries need to be bypassed.

Other Names for Coronary Artery Bypass Grafting

- Bypass surgery
- Coronary artery bypass surgery
- Heart bypass surgery

Who Needs Coronary Artery Bypass Grafting?

Coronary artery bypass grafting (CABG) is used to treat people who have severe coronary heart disease (CHD) that could lead to a heart attack. CABG also might be used during or after a heart attack to treat blocked arteries.

Your doctor may recommend CABG if other treatments, such as lifestyle changes or medicines, haven't worked. He or she also may recommend CABG if you have severe blockages in your large coronary (heart) arteries, especially if your heart's pumping action has already grown weak.

CABG also might be a treatment option if you have blockages in your coronary arteries that can't be treated with percutaneous coronary intervention (PCI), also known as coronary angioplasty.

Your doctor will decide whether you're a candidate for CABG based on factors such as:

- The presence and severity of CHD symptoms

- The severity and location of blockages in your coronary arteries
- Your response to other treatments
- Your quality of life
- Any other medical problems you have

Physical Exam and Diagnostic Tests

To find out whether you're a candidate for CABG, your doctor will give you a physical exam. He or she will check your heart, lungs, and pulse.

Your doctor also may ask you about any symptoms you have, such as chest pain or shortness of breath. He or she will want to know how often and for how long your symptoms occur, as well as how severe they are.

Your doctor will recommend tests to find out which arteries are clogged, how much they're clogged, and whether you have any heart damage.

EKG (Electrocardiogram)

An EKG is a simple test that detects and records your heart's electrical activity. The test shows how fast the heart is beating and its rhythm (steady or irregular). An EKG also records the strength and timing of electrical signals as they pass through each part of the heart.

An EKG can show signs of heart damage due to CHD and signs of a previous or current heart attack.

Echocardiography

Echocardiography (echo) uses sound waves to create a moving picture of your heart. The test shows the size and shape of your heart and how well your heart chambers and valves are working.

Echo also can show areas of poor blood flow to the heart, areas of heart muscle that aren't contracting normally, and previous injury to the heart muscle caused by poor blood flow.

There are several types of echo, including stress echo. This test is done both before and after a stress test. A stress echo usually is done to find out whether you have decreased blood flow to your heart, a sign of CHD.

Stress Test

Some heart problems are easier to diagnose when your heart is working hard and beating fast.

During stress testing, you exercise to make your heart work hard and beat fast while heart tests are done. If you can't exercise, you may be given medicine to raise your heart rate.

The heart tests done during stress testing may include nuclear heart scanning, echo, and positron emission tomography (PET) scanning of the heart.

Coronary Angiography and Cardiac Catheterization

Coronary angiography is a test that uses dye and special X-rays to show the insides of your coronary arteries.

To get the dye into your coronary arteries, your doctor will use a procedure called cardiac catheterization.

A thin, flexible tube called a catheter is put into a blood vessel in your arm, groin (upper thigh), or neck. The tube is threaded into your coronary arteries, and the dye is released into your bloodstream.

Special X-rays are taken while the dye is flowing through the coronary arteries. The dye lets your doctor study blood flow through the heart and blood vessels. This helps your doctor find blockages that can cause a heart attack.

Other Considerations

When deciding whether you're a candidate for CABG, your doctor also will consider your:

- History and past treatment of heart disease, including surgeries, procedures, and medicines

- History of other diseases and conditions

- Age and general health

- Family history of CHD, heart attack, or other heart diseases

Your doctor may recommend medicines and other medical procedures before CABG. For example, he or she may prescribe medicines to lower your cholesterol and blood pressure and improve blood flow through your coronary arteries.

PCI also might be tried. During this procedure, a thin, flexible tube with a balloon at its tip is threaded through a blood vessel to the narrow or blocked coronary artery.

Once in place, the balloon is inflated, pushing the plaque against the artery wall. This creates a wider path for blood to flow to the heart.

Sometimes a stent is placed in the artery during PCI. A stent is a small mesh tube that supports the inner artery wall.

What to Expect before Coronary Artery Bypass Grafting

You may have tests to prepare you for coronary artery bypass grafting (CABG). For example, you may have blood tests, an EKG (electrocardiogram), echocardiography, a chest X-ray, cardiac catheterization, and coronary angiography.

Your doctor will tell you how to prepare for CABG surgery. He or she will advise you about what you can eat or drink, which medicines to take, and which activities to stop (such as smoking). You'll likely be admitted to the hospital on the same day as the surgery.

If tests for coronary heart disease show that you have severe blockages in your coronary (heart) arteries, your doctor may admit you to the hospital right away. You may have CABG that day or the day after.

What to Expect during Coronary Artery Bypass Grafting

Coronary artery bypass grafting (CABG) requires a team of experts. A cardiothoracic surgeon will do the surgery with support from an anesthesiologist, perfusionist (heart-lung bypass machine specialist), other surgeons, and nurses.

There are several types of CABG. They range from traditional surgery to newer, less-invasive methods.

Traditional Coronary Artery Bypass Grafting

This type of surgery usually lasts 3–6 hours, depending on the number of arteries being bypassed. Many steps take place during traditional CABG.

You'll be under general anesthesia for the surgery. The term "anesthesia" refers to a loss of feeling and awareness. General anesthesia temporarily puts you to sleep.

During the surgery, the anesthesiologist will check your heartbeat, blood pressure, oxygen levels, and breathing. A breathing tube will be placed in your lungs through your throat. The tube will connect to a ventilator (a machine that supports breathing).

The surgeon will make an incision (cut) down the center of your chest. He or she will cut your chest bone and open your rib cage to reach your heart.

You'll receive medicines to stop your heart. This allows the surgeon to operate on your heart while it's not beating. You'll also receive medicines to protect your heart function during the time that it's not beating.

A heart-lung bypass machine will keep oxygen-rich blood moving throughout your body during the surgery.

The surgeon will take an artery or vein from your body—for example, from your chest or leg—to use as the bypass graft. For surgeries with several bypasses, both artery and vein grafts are commonly used.

- Artery grafts. These grafts are much less likely than vein grafts to become blocked over time. The left internal mammary artery most often is used for an artery graft. This artery is located inside the chest, close to the heart. Arteries from the arm or other places in the body also are used.

- Vein grafts. Although veins are commonly used as grafts, they're more likely than artery grafts to become blocked over time. The saphenous vein—a long vein running along the inner side of the leg—typically is used.

When the surgeon finishes the grafting, he or she will restore blood flow to your heart. Usually, the heart starts beating again on its own. Sometimes mild electric shocks are used to restart the heart.

You'll be disconnected from the heart-lung bypass machine. Then, tubes will be inserted into your chest to drain fluid.

The surgeon will use wire to close your chest bone (much like how a broken bone is repaired). The wire will stay in your body permanently. After your chest bone heals, it will be as strong as it was before the surgery.

Stitches or staples will be used to close the skin incision. The breathing tube will be removed when you're able to breathe without it.

Nontraditional Coronary Artery Bypass Grafting

Nontraditional CABG includes off-pump CABG and minimally invasive CABG.

Off-Pump Coronary Artery Bypass Grafting

Surgeons can use off-pump CABG to bypass any of the coronary (heart) arteries. Off-pump CABG is similar to traditional CABG because the chest bone is opened to access the heart.

However, the heart isn't stopped and a heart-lung-bypass machine isn't used. Instead, the surgeon steadies the heart with a mechanical device.

Off-pump CABG sometimes is called beating heart bypass grafting.

Minimally Invasive Direct Coronary Artery Bypass Grafting

There are several types of minimally invasive direct coronary artery bypass (MIDCAB) grafting. These types of surgery differ from traditional bypass surgery because the chest bone isn't opened to reach the heart. Also, a heart-lung bypass machine isn't always used for these procedures.

MIDCAB procedure. This type of surgery mainly is used to bypass blood vessels at the front of the heart. Small incisions are made between your ribs on the left side of your chest, directly over the artery that needs to be bypassed.

The incisions usually are about 3 inches long. (The incision made in traditional CABG is at least 6 to 8 inches long.) The left internal mammary artery most often is used for the graft in this procedure. A heart-lung bypass machine isn't used during MIDCAB grafting.

Port-access coronary artery bypass procedure. The surgeon does this procedure through small incisions (ports) made in your chest. Artery or vein grafts are used. A heart-lung bypass machine is used during this procedure.

Robot-assisted technique. This type of procedure allows for even smaller, keyhole-sized incisions. A small video camera is inserted in one incision to show the heart, while the surgeon uses remote-controlled surgical instruments to do the surgery. A heart-lung bypass machine sometimes is used during this procedure.

What to Expect after Coronary Artery Bypass Grafting

Recovery in the Hospital

After surgery, you'll typically spend 1 or 2 days in an intensive care unit (ICU). Your heart rate, blood pressure, and oxygen levels will be checked regularly during this time.

An intravenous line (IV) will likely be inserted into a vein in your arm. Through the IV line, you may get medicines to control blood circulation and blood pressure. You also will likely have a tube in your bladder to drain urine and a tube to drain fluid from your chest.

You may receive oxygen therapy (oxygen given through nasal prongs or a mask) and a temporary pacemaker while in the ICU. A pacemaker is a small device that's placed in the chest or abdomen to help control abnormal heart rhythms.

Your doctor may recommend that you wear compression stockings on your legs as well. These stockings are tight at the ankle and become looser as they go up the leg. This creates gentle pressure up the leg. The pressure keeps blood from pooling and clotting.

While in the ICU, you'll also have bandages on your chest incision (cut) and on the areas where an artery or vein was removed for grafting.

After you leave the ICU, you'll be moved to a less intensive care area of the hospital for 3 to 5 days before going home.

Recovery at Home

Your doctor will give you specific instructions for recovering at home, especially concerning:

- How to care for your healing incisions

- How to recognize signs of infection or other complications

- When to call the doctor right away

- When to make followup appointments

You also may get instructions on how to deal with common side effects from surgery. Side effects often go away within 4 to 6 weeks after surgery, but may include:

- Discomfort or itching from healing incisions

- Swelling of the area where an artery or vein was removed for grafting

- Muscle pain or tightness in the shoulders and upper back

- Fatigue (tiredness), mood swings, or depression

- Problems sleeping or loss of appetite

- Constipation

- Chest pain around the site of the chest bone incision (more frequent with traditional CABG)

Full recovery from traditional CABG may take 6 to 12 weeks or more. Less recovery time is needed for nontraditional CABG.

Your doctor will tell you when you can start physical activity again. It varies from person to person, but there are some typical timeframes. Most people can resume sexual activity within about 4 weeks and driving after 3 to 8 weeks.

Returning to work after 6 weeks is common unless your job involves specific and demanding physical activity. Some people may need to find less physically demanding types of work or work a reduced schedule at first.

Ongoing Care

Care after surgery may include periodic checkups with doctors. During these visits, tests may be done to see how your heart is working. Tests may include EKG (electrocardiogram), stress testing, echocardiography, and cardiac CT.

CABG is not a cure for coronary heart disease (CHD). You and your doctor may develop a treatment plan that includes lifestyle changes to help you stay healthy and reduce the chance of CHD getting worse.

Lifestyle changes may include making changes to your diet, quitting smoking, doing physical activity regularly, and lowering and managing stress.

Your doctor also may refer you to cardiac rehabilitation (rehab). Cardiac rehab is a medically supervised program that helps improve the health and well-being of people who have heart problems.

Rehab programs include exercise training, education on heart healthy living, and counseling to reduce stress and help you return to an active life. Doctors supervise these programs, which may be offered in hospitals and other community facilities. Talk to your doctor about whether cardiac rehab might benefit you.

Taking medicines as prescribed also is an important part of care after surgery. Your doctor may prescribe medicines to manage pain during recovery; lower cholesterol and blood pressure; reduce the risk of blood clots forming; manage diabetes; or treat depression.

What Are the Risks of Coronary Artery Bypass Grafting?

As with any type of surgery, coronary artery bypass grafting (CABG) has risks. The risks of CABG include:

- Wound infection and bleeding
- Reactions to anesthesia

- Fever

- Pain

- Stroke, heart attack, or even death

Some patients have a fever associated with chest pain, irritability, and decreased appetite. This is due to inflammation involving the lung and heart sac.

This complication sometimes occurs after surgeries that involve cutting through the pericardium (the outer covering of the heart). The problem usually is mild, but some patients may develop fluid buildup around the heart that requires treatment.

Memory loss and other issues, such as problems concentrating or thinking clearly, might occur in some people.

These problems are more likely to affect older patients and women. These issues often improve within 6–12 months of surgery.

In general, the risk of complications is higher if CABG is done in an emergency situation (for example, during a heart attack). The risk also is higher if you have other diseases or conditions, such as diabetes, kidney disease, lung disease, or peripheral arterial disease (P.A.D.).

Section 49.5

Stents to Keep Coronary Arteries Open

This section includes text excerpted from "Stents," National Heart, Lung, and Blood Institute (NHLBI), December 17, 2013.

What Is a Stent?

A stent is a small mesh tube that's used to treat narrow or weak arteries. Arteries are blood vessels that carry blood away from your heart to other parts of your body.

A stent is placed in an artery as part of a procedure called percutaneous coronary intervention (PCI), also known as coronary angioplasty. PCI restores blood flow through narrow or blocked arteries. A stent helps support the inner wall of the artery in the months or years after PCI.

Doctors also may place stents in weak arteries to improve blood flow and help prevent the arteries from bursting.

Stents usually are made of metal mesh, but sometimes they're made of fabric. Fabric stents, also called stent grafts, are used in larger arteries.

Some stents are coated with medicine that is slowly and continuously released into the artery. These stents are called drug-eluting stents. The medicine helps prevent the artery from becoming blocked again.

How Are Stents Used?

For the Coronary Arteries

Doctors may use stents to treat coronary heart disease (CHD). CHD is a disease in which a waxy substance called plaque builds up inside the coronary arteries. These arteries supply your heart muscle with oxygen-rich blood.

When plaque builds up in the arteries, the condition is called atherosclerosis.

Plaque narrows the coronary arteries, reducing the flow of oxygen-rich blood to your heart. This can lead to chest pain or discomfort called angina.

The buildup of plaque also makes it more likely that blood clots will form in your coronary arteries. If blood clots block a coronary artery, a heart attack will occur.

Doctors may use percutaneous coronary intervention (PCI), also known as coronary angioplasty, and stents to treat CHD. During PCI, a thin, flexible tube with a balloon or other device on the end is threaded through a blood vessel to the narrow or blocked coronary artery.

Once in place, the balloon is inflated to compress the plaque against the wall of the artery. This restores blood flow through the artery, which reduces angina and other CHD symptoms.

Unless an artery is too small, a stent usually is placed in the treated portion of the artery during PCI. The stent supports the artery's inner wall. It also reduces the chance that the artery will become narrow or blocked again. A stent also can support an artery that was torn or injured during PCI.

Even with a stent, there's about a 10–20 percent chance that an artery will become narrow or blocked again in the first year after PCI. When a stent isn't used, the risk can be as much as 10 times as high.

Research has shown that as time goes by, people who have coronary artery stents are in less danger of risks from the surgery but more prone to the risks of chronic diseases, such as type 2 diabetes and renal failure.

For the Carotid Arteries

Doctors also may use stents to treat carotid artery disease. This is a disease in which plaque builds up in the arteries that run along each side of your neck. These arteries, called carotid arteries, supply oxygen-rich blood to your brain.

The buildup of plaque in the carotid arteries limits blood flow to your brain and puts you at risk for a stroke.

Doctors use stents to help support the carotid arteries after they're widened with PCI. Researchers continue to explore the risks and benefits of carotid artery stenting.

For Other Arteries

Plaque also can narrow other arteries, such as those in the kidneys and limbs. Narrow kidney arteries can affect kidney function and lead to severe high blood pressure.

Narrow arteries in the limbs, a condition called peripheral artery disease (P.A.D.), can cause pain and cramping in the affected arm or leg. Severe narrowing can completely cut off blood flow to a limb, which could require surgery.

To relieve these problems, doctors may do PCI on a narrow kidney, arm, or leg artery. They often will place a stent in the affected artery during the procedure. The stent helps support the artery and keep it open.

For the Aorta in the Abdomen or Chest

The aorta is a major artery that carries oxygen-rich blood from the left side of the heart to the body. This artery runs through the chest and down into the abdomen.

Over time, some areas of the aorta's walls can weaken. These weak areas can cause a bulge in the artery called an aneurysm. An aneurysm in the aorta can burst, leading to serious internal bleeding. When aneurysms occur, they're usually in the abdominal aorta.

To help avoid a burst, doctors may place a fabric stent in the weak area of the abdominal aorta. The stent creates a stronger inner lining for the artery.

Aneurysms also can develop in the part of the aorta that runs through the chest. Doctors also use stents to treat these aneurysms. How well the stents work over the long term still isn't known.

To Close Off Aortic Tears

Another problem that can occur in the aorta is a tear in its inner wall. If blood is forced into the tear, it will widen.

The tear can reduce blood flow to the tissues that the aorta serves. Over time, the tear can block blood flow through the artery or burst. If this happens, it usually occurs in the chest portion of the aorta.

Researchers are developing and testing new kinds of stents that will prevent blood from flowing into aortic tears. A stent placed within the torn area of the aorta might help restore normal blood flow and reduce the risk of a burst aorta.

How Are Stents Placed?

Doctors place stents in arteries as part of a procedure called percutaneous coronary intervention (PCI), also known as coronary angioplasty. To place a stent, your doctor will make a small opening in a blood vessel in your groin (upper thigh), arm, or neck.

Through this opening, your doctor will thread a thin, flexible tube called a catheter. The catheter will have a deflated balloon at its tip.

A stent is placed around the deflated balloon. Your doctor will move the tip of the catheter to the narrow section of the artery or to the aneurysm or aortic tear site.

Special X-ray movies will be taken of the tube as it's threaded through your blood vessel. These movies will help your doctor position the catheter.

For Aortic Aneurysms

The procedure to place a stent in an artery with an aneurysm is very similar to the one described above. However, the stent used to treat an aneurysm is different. It's made out of pleated fabric instead of metal mesh, and it often has one or more tiny hooks.

The stent is expanded to fit tight against the artery wall. The hooks latch on to the wall of the artery, holding the stent in place.

The stent creates a new inner lining for that portion of the artery. Over time, cells in the artery grow to cover the fabric. They create an inner layer that looks like the inside of a normal blood vessel.

What to Expect before a Stent Procedure

Most stent procedures require an overnight stay in a hospital and someone to take you home. Talk with your doctor about:

- When to stop eating and drinking before coming to the hospital
- What medicines you should or shouldn't take on the day of the procedure
- When to come to the hospital and where to go

If you have diabetes, kidney disease, or other conditions, ask your doctor whether you need to take any extra steps during or after the procedure to avoid complications.

Before the procedure, your doctor may talk to you about medicines you'll likely need to take after the stent is placed. These medicines help prevent blood clots from forming in the stent.

What to Expect during a Stent Procedure

For Arteries Narrowed by Plaque

This procedure usually takes about an hour. It might take longer if stents are inserted into more than one artery during the procedure.

Before the procedure starts, you'll get medicine to help you relax. You'll be on your back and awake during the procedure. This allows you to follow your doctor's instructions.

Your doctor will numb the area where the catheter will be inserted. You won't feel the doctor threading the catheter, balloon, or stent inside the artery. You may feel some pain when the balloon is expanded to push the stent into place.

For Aortic Aneurysms

Although this procedure takes only a few hours, it often requires a 2- to 3-day hospital stay.

Before the procedure, you'll be given medicine to help you relax. If your doctor is placing the stent in your abdominal aorta, you may receive medicine to numb your stomach area. However, you'll be awake during the procedure.

If your doctor is placing the stent in the chest portion of your aorta, you'll likely receive medicine to make you sleep during the procedure.

Once you're numb or asleep, your doctor will make a small cut in your groin (upper thigh). He or she will insert a catheter into the blood vessel through this cut.

Sometimes two cuts (one in the groin area of each leg) are needed to place fabric stents that come in two parts. You will not feel the doctor threading the catheter, balloon, or stent into the artery.

What to Expect after a Stent Procedure

Recovery

After either type of stent procedure (for arteries narrowed by plaque or aortic aneurysms), your doctor will remove the catheter from your artery. The site where the catheter was inserted will be bandaged.

A small sandbag or other type of weight may be put on top of the bandage to apply pressure and help prevent bleeding. You'll recover in a special care area, where your movement will be limited.

While you're in recovery, a nurse will check your heart rate and blood pressure regularly. The nurse also will look to see whether you're bleeding from the insertion site.

Eventually, a small bruise and sometimes a small, hard "knot" will appear at the insertion site. This area may feel sore or tender for about a week.

You should let your doctor know if:

- You have a constant or large amount of bleeding at the insertion site that can't be stopped with a small bandage

- You have any unusual pain, swelling, redness, or other signs of infection at or near the insertion site

Common Precautions after a Stent Procedure

Blood Clotting Precautions

After a stent procedure, your doctor will likely recommend that you take aspirin and another anticlotting medicine. These medicines help prevent blood clots from forming in the stent. A blood clot can lead to a heart attack, stroke, or other serious problems.

If you have a metal stent, your doctor may recommend aspirin and another anticlotting medicine for at least 1 month. If your stent is coated with medicine, your doctor may recommend aspirin and another anticlotting medicine for 12 months or more. Your doctor will work with you to decide the best course of treatment.

Your risk of blood clots significantly increases if you stop taking the anticlotting medicine too early. Taking these medicines for as long as your doctor recommends is important. He or she may recommend lifelong treatment with aspirin.

If you're considering surgery for some other reason while you're on these medicines, talk to your doctor about whether it can wait until after you've stopped the medicine. Anticlotting medicines may increase the risk of bleeding.

Also, anticlotting medicines can cause side effects, such as an allergic rash. Talk to your doctor about how to reduce the risk of these side effects.

Other Precautions

You should avoid vigorous exercise and heavy lifting for a short time after the stent procedure. Your doctor will let you know when you can go back to your normal activities.

Metal detectors used in airports and other screening areas don't affect stents. Your stent shouldn't cause metal detectors to go off.

If you have an aortic fabric stent, your doctor will likely recommend followup imaging tests (for example, chest X-ray) within the first year of having the procedure. After the first year, he or she may recommend yearly imaging tests.

Lifestyle Changes

Stents help prevent arteries from becoming narrow or blocked again in the months or years after percutaneous coronary intervention (PCI), also known as coronary angioplasty. However, stents aren't a cure for atherosclerosis or its risk factors.

Making lifestyle changes can help prevent plaque from building up in your arteries again. Talk with your doctor about your risk factors for atherosclerosis and the lifestyle changes you'll need to make.

Lifestyle changes may include changing your diet, quitting smoking, being physically active, losing weight, and reducing stress. You also should take all medicines as your doctor prescribes. Your doctor may suggest taking statins, which are medicines that lower blood cholesterol levels.

What Are the Risks of Having a Stent?

Risks Related to Percutaneous Coronary Intervention

Percutaneous coronary intervention (PCI), the procedure used to place stents, is a medical procedure that is commonly known as coronary angioplasty. PCI carries a small risk of serious complications, such as:

- Bleeding from the site where the catheter was inserted into the skin
- Damage to the blood vessel from the catheter
- Arrhythmias (irregular heartbeats)
- Damage to the kidneys caused by the dye used during the procedure
- An allergic reaction to the dye used during the procedure
- Infection

Another problem that can occur after PCI is too much tissue growth within the treated portion of the artery. This can cause the artery to become narrow or blocked again. When this happens, it's called restenosis.

Using drug-eluting stents can help prevent this problem. These stents are coated with medicine to stop excess tissue growth.

Treating the tissue around the stent with radiation also can delay tissue growth. For this procedure, the doctor threads a wire through a catheter to the stent. The wire releases radiation and stops cells around the stent from growing and blocking the artery.

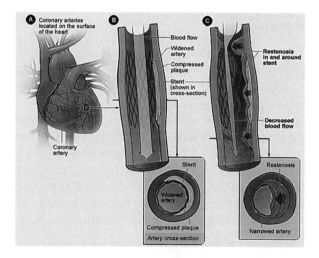

Figure 49.5. *Restenosis of a Stent-Widened Coronary Artery*

(A) shows the coronary arteries located on the surface of the heart. (B) shows a stent-widened artery with normal blood flow. The inset image shows a cross-section of the stent-widened artery. In (C), tissue grows through and around the stent over time. This causes a partial blockage of the artery and abnormal blood flow. The inset image shows a cross-section of the tissue growth around the stent.

Risks Related to Stents

About 1–2 percent of people who have stented arteries develop a blood clot at the stent site. Blood clots can cause a heart attack, stroke, or other serious problems. The risk of blood clots is greatest during the first few months after the stent is placed in the artery.

Your doctor will likely recommend that you take aspirin and another anticlotting medicine, such as clopidogrel, for at least 1 month or up to a year or more after having a stent procedure. These medicines help prevent blood clots.

The length of time you need to take anticlotting medicines depends on the type of stent you have. Your doctor may recommend lifelong treatment with aspirin.

Stents coated with medicine may raise your risk of dangerous blood clots. (These stents often are used to keep clogged heart arteries open.) However, research hasn't proven that these stents increase the chances of having a heart attack or dying, if used as recommended.

Risks Related to Aortic Stents in the Abdomen

Although rare, a few serious problems can occur when surgery or a fabric stent is used to repair an aneurysm in the abdominal aorta. These problems include:

- A burst artery (aneurysm rupture).

- Blocked blood flow to the stomach or lower body.

- Paralysis in the legs due to interruption of blood flow to the spinal cord. This problem is very rare.

Another possible problem is the fabric stent moving further down the aorta. This sometimes happens years after the stent is first placed. The stent movement may require a doctor to place another fabric stent in the area of the aneurysm.

Chapter 50

Procedures to Treat Heart Rhythm Disorders

Chapter Contents

Section 50.1

Cardiac Resynchronization Therapy

This section includes text excerpted from "Medtronic CRT-P and
CRT-D Devices—P010015/S205 and P010031/S381," U.S. Food and
Drug Administration (FDA), January 11, 2016.

What Is Cardiac Resynchronization Therapy?

A cardiac resynchronization therapy (CRT) device is a special
pacemaker designed to treat symptoms of heart failure by sending
specially timed electrical impulses to improve the timing, or resynchronize pumping action of the heart's lower chambers (right and left
ventricles). This improved timing can help control symptoms from
heart failure.

There are two types of implantable CRT devices: one that is only a
pacemaker (CRT-P) and the other that is a combination of a pacemaker
and defibrillator (CRT-D). Defibrillators can shock the heart rhythm
back to normal should dangerously fast rhythms occur.

Each CRT device consists of a pulse generator (containing a battery
and electronic circuitry) connected to insulated wires called leads that
deliver electrical impulses to stimulate the heart. The synchronizing
leads include a right ventricular lead (RV) and a left ventricular (LV)
lead.

A CRT-D combination pacemaker and defibrillator has added features and ability so it is able to detect and treat dangerously fast heart
rhythms. Only some individuals with a damaged heart muscle are
likely enough to develop dangerous heart rhythms to need a defibrillator. A physician can determine whether a CRT-P or CRT-D device
is most appropriate.

How Does It Work?

Both CRT-P and CRT-D devices resynchronize the heart action by
providing electrical impulses to improve timing of the right and left
sides of the heart using RV and LV leads. The leads also carry signals
from the heart to the device. The timing of the impulses is programmed

by the doctor to restore a more natural timing and pumping of the heart muscle which can improve heart failure. The RV leads of CRT-D devices have additional features to deliver high voltage energy to defibrillate the heart should life-threatening, dangerously fast rhythms occur in the ventricles (ventricular arrhythmia).

When Is It Used?

CRT-P and CRT-D devices have been approved for many years for patients with poorly synchronized right and left ventricles to improve their heart failure symptoms. Based on the results of a new clinical study called BLOCK HF, FDA is now expanding who is eligible (or "indicated") for CRT. The new, added patients must have EACH of the following:

- MUST have slow or absent ventricular heart beating (heart block) with symptoms that would traditionally require a conventional pacemaker

- PLUS mild to moderate heart failure symptoms

- PLUS at least mild heart muscle damage

The actual specific indications appear below. After evaluating a patient's degree of heart damage and heart failure symptoms, a doctor can determine whether they fit the new BLOCK HF indication and would benefit from CRT.

CRT-P Device Indications:

- Previously Approved by FDA:
    - Patients with moderate to severe heart failure symptoms (NYHA Functional Class III and IV) despite stable, optimal heart failure medical therapy
    - PLUS severe heart damage (cardiac ejection fraction [LVEF] less than or equal to 35%)
    - PLUS electrocardiogram (EKG) signs of poor synchronization of the ventricles

- New BLOCK HF Indication:
    - slow or absent ventricular heart beating (atrioventricular block [AV block] expected to require a high percentage of ventricular pacing that would traditionally require a conventional pacemaker

- PLUS mild to moderate heart failure symptoms (NYHA Functional Class I, II or III)

- PLUS at least mild heart muscle damage (cardiac ejection fraction [LVEF] less than or equal to 50%)

- NOTE: heart failure medications must be optimized after the device is implanted.

CRT-D Device Indications:

- Previously Approved by FDA:

  - The primary use of a CRT-D system is for automated treatment of life-threatening ventricular arrhythmias. They also provide CRT in heart failure patients on stable, optimal heart failure medical therapy if indicated, and meet any of the following heart failure classifications:

  - Patients with moderate to severe heart failure symptoms (NYHA Functional Class III and IV)

  - PLUS severe heart damage (cardiac ejection fraction [LVEF] less than or equal to 35%)

  - PLUS EKG signs of poor synchronization of the ventricles

OR

- Patients with mild to moderate heart failure symptoms (NYHA Functional Class II)

  - PLUS EKG signs of very poor synchronization of the ventricles (Left bundle branch block (LBBB) with a ventricular stimulation time greater than or equal to130 ms)

  - PLUS severe heart damage (cardiac ejection fraction [LVEF] less than or equal to 30%)

- New BLOCK HF CRT-D Indication:

  - The primary use of a CRT-D system is for automated treatment of life-threatening ventricular arrhythmias. They also provide CRT in heart failure patients on stable, optimal heart failure medical therapy if indicated, and meet any of the following heart failure classifications:

  - slow or absent ventricular heart beating (atrioventricular block [AV block] expected to require a high percentage of ventricular pacing that would traditionally require a conventional pacemaker

- PLUS mild to moderate heart failure symptoms (NYHA Functional Class I, II or III)

- PLUS at least mild heart muscle damage (cardiac ejection fraction [LVEF] less than or equal to 50%)

- NOTE: heart failure medications must be optimized after the device is implanted.

What Will It Accomplish?

Based on the results of the BLOCK HF clinical study, when used in the new population as described above, patients may benefit by experiencing less frequent heart failure worsening or need for urgent treatment.

When Should It Not Be Used?

The contraindications for the CRT-P and CRT-D devices are listed below.

CRT-P Devices

- implantation with another bradycardia device
- implantation with an implantable cardioverter defibrillator

There are no known contraindications for the use of pacing as a therapy to control heart rate. The patient's age and medical condition, however, may determine the particular pacing system, mode of operation, and implant procedure used by the doctor.

- automatic adjustment of pacing rate may be contraindicated in those patients who cannot tolerate pacing rates above the programmed Lower Rate.

- Dual chamber sequential pacing is contraindicated in patients with chronic or persistent supraventricular tachycardias, including atrial fibrillation or flutter.

- Asynchronous pacing is contraindicated in the presence (or likelihood) of competition between paced and intrinsic rhythms.

- Single chamber atrial pacing is contraindicated in patients with an AV conduction disturbance.

- Anti-tachycardia pacing (ATP) therapy is contraindicated in patients with an accessory antegrade pathway

CRT-D Devices

- Patients experiencing tachyarrhythmia with transient or reversible causes including, but not limited to, the following: heart attack (acute myocardial infarction), drug intoxication, drowning, electric shock, electrolyte imbalance, hypoxia, or sepsis.

- Patients who have a unipolar pacemaker implanted.

- Patients with continuous ventricular tachycardia (VT) or ventricular fibrillation (VF).

- Patients whose primary disorder is chronic atrial tachyarrhythmia in the absence of VT or VF. (NOTE: This contraindication does not apply to the Maximo II devices).

Section 50.2

Cardioversion

"Cardioversion," © 2016 Omnigraphics. Reviewed June 2016.

Cardioversion is a medical procedure in which an electrical shock is administered to the heart in order to restore a normal heart rhythm. Although cardioversion is usually performed by placing electrodes on the patient's chest to send electric shocks to the heart, it is sometimes done with medications. Cardioversion is used to treat certain types of arrhythmias, such as atrial fibrillation (A Fib) or atrial flutter (AFL). It restores a normal sinus rhythm in around 90% of patients.

Ordinarily, a heartbeat begins with an electrical signal generated by the sinus node, a group of specialized cells located in the upper right atrium chamber of the heart. This signal travels through the heart to the lower chambers or ventricles, causing the heart muscle to contract and pump blood through the body. When the conduction of the electrical current occurs in a smooth, organized way, it results in a perfectly timed, rhythmic heartbeat. In people with atrial fibrillation, however, the electrical signal travels through the upper chambers in a chaotic, disorganized way. This improper conduction causes the atria to fibrillate or quiver, resulting in an irregular heartbeat.

Cardioversion should not be confused with defibrillation, which is an emergency procedure that delivers much more powerful electrical shocks to the heart. Cardioversion is performed when the heart is beating ineffectively to correct its rhythm. Defibrillation is usually performed when the heart stops beating to restore a heartbeat.

The Cardioversion Procedure

Electrical cardioversion is usually performed in a hospital on an outpatient basis. The patient is placed under anesthesia so they feel no pain from the procedure. Electrodes are attached to the skin of the patient's chest and back. These patches or paddles are connected to a defibrillator machine, which administers a synchronized electrical shock to the patient's heart. The shock disrupts the abnormal electrical conduction for a split second, which allows the sinus node to reset the heartbeat to a normal rhythm. The procedure only takes a few minutes, although the patient will spend a few hours recovering from the anesthesia and being monitored for complications before going home. Repeat procedures are sometimes needed if the irregular heartbeat recurs.

The main complication associated with electrical cardioversion involves blood clots. When the upper chambers of the heart fibrillate irregularly for more than 48 hours, there is a possibility that blood clots may form in the heart. Cardioversion can cause a blood clot to dislodge from the heart and move through the bloodstream to other parts of the body, which can result in a stroke or other dangerous health complications.

To reduce this risk, patients who have experienced symptoms of A fib or AFL for more than 48 hours generally must take blood-thinning medications called anticoagulants for four weeks before undergoing cardioversion. Common anticoagulants include aspirin, heparin, and warfarin. As an alternative, patients may undergo a procedure called a transesophageal echocardiogram (TEE) to check for blood clots prior to cardioversion. During a TEE, a probe is inserted into the patient's esophagus and fed into the chest, enabling the doctor to examine the atria. If no blood clots are found, the cardioversion can proceed.

In chemical cardioversion, the patient receives antiarrhythmic medications to alter the flow of electricity through the heart and restore a normal rhythm. This procedure is sometimes done on an outpatient basis, but it may be performed in the hospital under monitoring in patients with underlying heart disease or severe symptoms. Many patients are prescribed medications to help maintain a normal heart rhythm following cardioversion, as well as blood-thinning medications to prevent new blood clots from forming.

References

1. "Cardioversion," Heart Rhythm Society, 2016.

2. "Cardioversion," Mayo Clinic, 2016.

Section 50.3

Catheter Ablation

"Catheter Ablation," © 2016 Omnigraphics. Reviewed June 2016.

Catheter ablation is a medical procedure in which a narrow, flexible tube is inserted into the heart through a vein or artery to diagnose and treat heart rhythm disorders. Catheter ablation can be used to locate and correct the short circuits in the heart's electrical system that cause several different types of arrhythmias.

Ordinarily, a heartbeat begins with an electrical signal generated by the sinus node, a group of specialized cells located in the upper right atrium chamber of the heart. This signal travels downward to the atrioventricular node, an electrical relay station located between the heart's upper and lower chambers. Finally, the current passes through special fibers into the lower chambers or ventricles. The smooth, constant flow of signals through the heart's electrical system causes the upper and lower chambers of the heart to alternately contract and relax in a perfectly timed rhythm in order to pump blood through the body. If the current is disrupted along the heart's electrical pathway, however, it can create an irregular heartbeat known as an arrhythmia. In a cardiac ablation, energy is delivered to the heart muscle through a catheter to remove the disruption and restore a normal heart rhythm.

When Catheter Ablation Is Used

Catheter ablation can be used to treat many different types of arrhythmias, often taking the place of open-heart surgery. It is particularly helpful for patients whose arrhythmias cannot be controlled with medication, or who cannot tolerate medications designed to control arrhythmias. Some of the conditions catheter ablation can treat successfully include:

- supraventricular tachycardia (SVT), a rapid heartbeat that originates with improper electrical activity above the atrioventricular (AV) node;

- ventricular tachycardia (VT), a rapid, potentially life-threatening heartbeat that originates from electrical impulses in the ventricles;

- atrial fibrillation (A fib) and atrial flutter (AFL), ineffective, quivering heartbeats that originate with extra signals in the atria;

- accessory pathway, a condition in which extra electrical pathways present from birth relay the signals back from the ventricles to the atria; and

- AV nodal reentrant tachycardia (AVNRT), a condition in which an extra pathway near the AV node allows signals to travel in a circle.

How Catheter Ablation Works

A catheter ablation is performed by a specialist called an electrophysiologist in a hospital setting. Before undergoing the procedure, patients should inquire about whether they should continue taking medications. Those on blood thinners like warfarin (Coumadin) and certain other drugs might need to stop taking them or adjust the dosage. Since patients will be receiving anesthesia, they should also avoid eating or drinking anything after midnight the night before the procedure.

After arriving at the hospital, patients will receive an IV to deliver medications to make them drowsy. They will also be connected to monitors for heart rhythm, blood pressure, blood oxygen level, and other vital signs. The insertion site for the catheters—which may be the neck, upper thigh, or arm—will be sterilized and shaved. Then the doctor will numb the insertion site and insert several catheters into a vein or artery through a small incision.

The catheters will be fed through the blood vessels until they reach the heart. A transducer will then be inserted through one of the catheters to allow the doctor to view the heart's internal structures using an intracardiac ultrasound. Next, electrodes at the tip of the catheters will send electrical impulses to enable the doctor to pinpoint the location of the short circuit in the heart's electrical system. Finally, the doctor will send energy through the catheters to either block damaged electrical pathways to prevent faulty signals from getting through, or destroy short circuits to allow electrical signals to flow properly. The energy can take the form of hot (radio frequency waves) or freezing cold (cryoablation).

Once the ablation is complete, the electrophysiologist will observe the electrical signals in the patient's heart to ensure that the arrhythmia was corrected. The entire procedure is likely to last between four and eight hours. Afterward, the catheters will be removed and the patient will remain in bed for several hours to prevent bleeding. Some patients are allowed to return home at this point, while others must remain in the hospital overnight for monitoring.

References

1. "Catheter Ablation," Cleveland Clinic, 2016.

2. "Catheter Ablation," Heart Rhythm Society, 2016.

Section 50.4

Subcutaneous Implantable Defibrillator

This section includes text excerpted from "Subcutaneous Implantable Defibrillator (S-ICD) System—P110042," U.S. Food and Drug Administration (FDA), May 11, 2016.

What Is Subcutaneous Implantable Defibrillator?

The subcutaneous implantable defibrillator (S-ICD) System is a defibrillator that is implanted under the skin (subcutaneous). It provides an electric shock to the heart (defibrillation) for the treatment of an abnormally rapid heartbeat that originates from the lower chambers of the heart (ventricular tachyarrhythmias). The S-ICD System consists of:

- a titanium case containing a battery and electronic circuitry that provides defibrillation therapy and pacing at a rate of 50 beats per minute up to 30 seconds after a shock

- a subcutaneous electrode which has a proximal and distal ring electrode on each side of a 3 inch (8 cm) defibrillation coil electrode.

- accessories include an electrode insertion tool, programmer, telemetry wand, magnet, suture sleeve, torque wrench, and memory card.

How Does It Work?

The S-ICD (pulse generator) is implanted under the skin on the side of the chest below the arm pit. The pulse generator is connected to the electrode which is implanted under the skin from the device pocket along the rib margin to the breastbone with the use of the insertion tool.

The S-ICD monitors cardiac rhythms and delivers defibrillation when ventricular tachyarrhythmias are detected. After delivery of a shock, the S-ICD provides post-shock bradycardia pacing therapy when needed. The S-ICD is programmable as a single or dual zone device which allows the doctor to tailor the therapy for the patient.

When Is It Used?

The S-ICD System is intended to provide defibrillation therapy for the treatment of life-threatening ventricular tachyarrhythmias in patients who do not have symptomatic bradycardia, continual (incessant) ventricular tachycardia, or spontaneous frequently recurring ventricular tachycardia that is reliably terminated with anti-tachycardia pacing.

What Will It Accomplish?

The S-ICD System is effective in providing an electrical shock to the heart to treat life-threatening arrhythmias. In the clinical studies, the S-ICD System was shown to be capable of restoring a normal and stable rhythm thereby supporting life. The subcutaneous lead also eliminates the risks associated with implanting leads on or in the heart (transvenous leads). In addition, the System meets an unmet need for patients who are not suitable for transvenous lead placement.

When Should It Not Be Used?

The S-ICD System should not be used if patients have symptomatic bradycardia, incessant ventricular tachycardia which can be terminated with anti-tachycardia pacing, and/or patients who have unipolar pacemakers.

Section 50.5

Pacemaker

This section includes text excerpted from "Pacemakers," National Heart, Lung, and Blood Institute (NHLBI), February 28, 2012. Reviewed June 2016.

What Is a Pacemaker?

A pacemaker is a small device that's placed in the chest or abdomen to help control abnormal heart rhythms. This device uses electrical pulses to prompt the heart to beat at a normal rate.

Pacemakers are used to treat arrhythmias. Arrhythmias are problems with the rate or rhythm of the heartbeat. During an arrhythmia, the heart can beat too fast, too slow, or with an irregular rhythm.

A heartbeat that's too fast is called tachycardia. A heartbeat that's too slow is called bradycardia.

During an arrhythmia, the heart may not be able to pump enough blood to the body. This can cause symptoms such as fatigue (tiredness), shortness of breath, or fainting. Severe arrhythmias can damage the body's vital organs and may even cause loss of consciousness or death.

A pacemaker can relieve some arrhythmia symptoms, such as fatigue and fainting. A pacemaker also can help a person who has abnormal heart rhythms resume a more active lifestyle.

Understanding the Heart's Electrical System

Your heart has its own internal electrical system that controls the rate and rhythm of your heartbeat. With each heartbeat, an electrical signal spreads from the top of your heart to the bottom. As the signal travels, it causes the heart to contract and pump blood.

Each electrical signal normally begins in a group of cells called the sinus node or sinoatrial (SA) node. As the signal spreads from the top of the heart to the bottom, it coordinates the timing of heart cell activity.

First, the heart's two upper chambers, the atria, contract. This contraction pumps blood into the heart's two lower chambers, the ventricles. The ventricles then contract and pump blood to the rest of the body. The combined contraction of the atria and ventricles is a heartbeat.

Overview

Faulty electrical signaling in the heart causes arrhythmias. Pacemakers use low-energy electrical pulses to overcome this faulty electrical signaling. Pacemakers can:

- Speed up a slow heart rhythm.

- Help control an abnormal or fast heart rhythm.

- Make sure the ventricles contract normally if the atria are quivering instead of beating with a normal rhythm (a condition called atrial fibrillation).

- Coordinate electrical signaling between the upper and lower chambers of the heart.

- Coordinate electrical signaling between the ventricles. Pacemakers that do this are called cardiac resynchronization therapy (CRT) devices. CRT devices are used to treat heart failure.

- Prevent dangerous arrhythmias caused by a disorder called long QT syndrome.

Pacemakers also can monitor and record your heart's electrical activity and heart rhythm. Newer pacemakers can monitor your blood temperature, breathing rate, and other factors. They also can adjust your heart rate to changes in your activity.

Pacemakers can be temporary or permanent. Temporary pacemakers are used to treat short-term heart problems, such as a slow heartbeat that's caused by a heart attack, heart surgery, or an overdose of medicine.

Temporary pacemakers also are used during emergencies. They might be used until your doctor can implant a permanent pacemaker or until a temporary condition goes away. If you have a temporary pacemaker, you'll stay in a hospital as long as the device is in place.

Permanent pacemakers are used to control long-term heart rhythm problems. This article mainly discusses permanent pacemakers, unless stated otherwise.

Doctors also treat arrhythmias with another device called an implantable cardioverter defibrillator (ICD). An ICD is similar to a pacemaker. However, besides using low-energy electrical pulses, an ICD also can use high-energy pulses to treat life-threatening arrhythmias.

Who Needs a Pacemaker?

Doctors recommend pacemakers for many reasons. The most common reasons are bradycardia and heart block.

Bradycardia is a heartbeat that is slower than normal. Heart block is a disorder that occurs if an electrical signal is slowed or disrupted as it moves through the heart.

Heart block can happen as a result of aging, damage to the heart from a heart attack, or other conditions that disrupt the heart's electrical activity. Some nerve and muscle disorders also can cause heart block, including muscular dystrophy.

Your doctor also may recommend a pacemaker if:

- Aging or heart disease damages your sinus node's ability to set the correct pace for your heartbeat. Such damage can cause slower than normal heartbeats or long pauses between heartbeats. The damage also can cause your heart to switch between slow and fast rhythms. This condition is called sick sinus syndrome.

- You've had a medical procedure to treat an arrhythmia called atrial fibrillation. A pacemaker can help regulate your heartbeat after the procedure.

- You need to take certain heart medicines, such as beta blockers. These medicines can slow your heartbeat too much.

- You faint or have other symptoms of a slow heartbeat. For example, this may happen if the main artery in your neck that supplies your brain with blood is sensitive to pressure. Just quickly turning your neck can cause your heart to beat slower than normal. As a result, your brain might not get enough blood flow, causing you to feel faint or collapse.

- You have heart muscle problems that cause electrical signals to travel too slowly through your heart muscle. Your pacemaker may provide cardiac resynchronization therapy (CRT) for this problem. CRT devices coordinate electrical signaling between the heart's lower chambers.

- You have long QT syndrome, which puts you at risk for dangerous arrhythmias.

Doctors also may recommend pacemakers for people who have certain types of congenital heart disease or for people who have had heart transplants. Children, teens, and adults can use pacemakers.

Before recommending a pacemaker, your doctor will consider any arrhythmia symptoms you have, such as dizziness, unexplained fainting, or shortness of breath. He or she also will consider whether you have a history of heart disease, what medicines you're currently taking, and the results of heart tests.

Diagnostic Tests

Many tests are used to detect arrhythmias. You may have one or more of the following tests.

- EKG (Electrocardiogram)

- Holter and Event Monitors

- Echocardiography

- Electrophysiology Study

- Stress Test

How Does a Pacemaker Work?

A pacemaker consists of a battery, a computerized generator, and wires with sensors at their tips. (The sensors are called electrodes.) The battery powers the generator, and both are surrounded by a thin metal box. The wires connect the generator to the heart.

A pacemaker helps monitor and control your heartbeat. The electrodes detect your heart's electrical activity and send data through the wires to the computer in the generator.

If your heart rhythm is abnormal, the computer will direct the generator to send electrical pulses to your heart. The pulses travel through the wires to reach your heart.

Newer pacemakers can monitor your blood temperature, breathing, and other factors. They also can adjust your heart rate to changes in your activity.

The pacemaker's computer also records your heart's electrical activity and heart rhythm. Your doctor will use these recordings to adjust your pacemaker so it works better for you.

Your doctor can program the pacemaker's computer with an external device. He or she doesn't have to use needles or have direct contact with the pacemaker.

Pacemakers have one to three wires that are each placed in different chambers of the heart.

- The wires in a single-chamber pacemaker usually carry pulses from the generator to the right ventricle (the lower right chamber of your heart).

- The wires in a dual-chamber pacemaker carry pulses from the generator to the right atrium (the upper right chamber of your heart) and the right ventricle. The pulses help coordinate the timing of these two chambers' contractions.

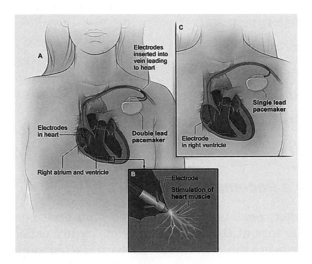

Figure 50.1. *Cross-Section of a Chest with a Pacemaker*

The image shows a cross-section of a chest with a pacemaker. (A) shows the location and general size of a double-lead, or dual-chamber, pacemaker in the upper chest. The wires with electrodes are inserted into the heart's right atrium and ventricle through a vein in the upper chest. (B) shows an electrode electrically stimulating the heart muscle. (C) shows the location and general size of a single-lead, or single-chamber, pacemaker in the upper chest.

- The wires in a biventricular pacemaker carry pulses from the generator to an atrium and both ventricles.

The pulses help coordinate electrical signaling between the two ventricles. This type of pacemaker also is called a cardiac resynchronization therapy (CRT) device.

Types of Pacemaker Programming

The two main types of programming for pacemakers are demand pacing and rate-responsive pacing.

A demand pacemaker monitors your heart rhythm. It only sends electrical pulses to your heart if your heart is beating too slow or if it misses a beat.

A rate-responsive pacemaker will speed up or slow down your heart rate depending on how active you are. To do this, the device monitors your sinus node rate, breathing, blood temperature, and other factors to determine your activity level.

Your doctor will work with you to decide which type of pacemaker is best for you.

A rate-responsive pacemaker will speed up or slow down your heart rate depending on how active you are. To do this, the device monitors your sinus node rate, breathing, blood temperature, and other factors to determine your activity level.

Your doctor will work with you to decide which type of pacemaker is best for you.

What to Expect during Pacemaker Surgery

Placing a pacemaker requires minor surgery. The surgery usually is done in a hospital or special heart treatment laboratory.

Before the surgery, an intravenous (IV) line will be inserted into one of your veins. You will receive medicine through the IV line to help you relax. The medicine also might make you sleepy.

Your doctor will numb the area where he or she will put the pacemaker so you don't feel any pain. Your doctor also may give you antibiotics to prevent infection.

First, your doctor will insert a needle into a large vein, usually near the shoulder opposite your dominant hand. Your doctor will then use the needle to thread the pacemaker wires into the vein and to correctly place them in your heart.

An X-ray "movie" of the wires as they pass through your vein and into your heart will help your doctor place them. Once the wires are in place, your doctor will make a small cut into the skin of your chest or abdomen.

He or she will slip the pacemaker's small metal box through the cut, place it just under your skin, and connect it to the wires that lead to your heart. The box contains the pacemaker's battery and generator.

Once the pacemaker is in place, your doctor will test it to make sure it works properly. He or she will then sew up the cut. The entire surgery takes a few hours.

What to Expect after Pacemaker Surgery

Expect to stay in the hospital overnight so your healthcare team can check your heartbeat and make sure your pacemaker is working well. You'll likely have to arrange for a ride to and from the hospital because your doctor may not want you to drive yourself.

For a few days to weeks after surgery, you may have pain, swelling, or tenderness in the area where your pacemaker was placed. The pain usually is mild; over-the-counter medicines often can relieve it. Talk to your doctor before taking any pain medicines.

Your doctor may ask you to avoid vigorous activities and heavy lifting for about a month after pacemaker surgery. Most people return to their normal activities within a few days of having the surgery.

What Are the Risks of Pacemaker Surgery?

Pacemaker surgery generally is safe. If problems do occur, they may include:

- Swelling, bleeding, bruising, or infection in the area where the pacemaker was placed
- Blood vessel or nerve damage
- A collapsed lung
- A bad reaction to the medicine used during the procedure

Talk with your doctor about the benefits and risks of pacemaker surgery.

How Will a Pacemaker Affect My Lifestyle?

Once you have a pacemaker, you have to avoid close or prolonged contact with electrical devices or devices that have strong magnetic fields. Devices that can interfere with a pacemaker include:

- Cell phones and MP3 players (for example, iPods)
- Household appliances, such as microwave ovens
- High-tension wires
- Metal detectors
- Industrial welders
- Electrical generators

These devices can disrupt the electrical signaling of your pacemaker and stop it from working properly. You may not be able to tell whether your pacemaker has been affected.

How likely a device is to disrupt your pacemaker depends on how long you're exposed to it and how close it is to your pacemaker.

To be safe, some experts recommend not putting your cell phone or MP3 player in a shirt pocket over your pacemaker (if the devices are turned on).

You may want to hold your cell phone up to the ear that's opposite the site where your pacemaker is implanted. If you strap your MP3 player to your arm while listening to it, put it on the arm that's farther from your pacemaker.

You can still use household appliances, but avoid close and prolonged exposure, as it may interfere with your pacemaker.

You can walk through security system metal detectors at your normal pace. Security staff can check you with a metal detector wand as long as it isn't held for too long over your pacemaker site. You should avoid sitting or standing close to a security system metal detector. Notify security staff if you have a pacemaker.

Also, stay at least 2 feet away from industrial welders and electrical generators.

Some medical procedures can disrupt your pacemaker. These procedures include:

- Magnetic resonance imaging, or MRI
- Shock-wave lithotripsy to get rid of kidney stones
- Electrocauterization to stop bleeding during surgery

Let all of your doctors, dentists, and medical technicians know that you have a pacemaker. Your doctor can give you a card that states what kind of pacemaker you have. Carry this card in your wallet. You may want to wear a medical ID bracelet or necklace that states that you have a pacemaker.

Physical Activity

In most cases, having a pacemaker won't limit you from doing sports and exercise, including strenuous activities.

You may need to avoid full-contact sports, such as football. Such contact could damage your pacemaker or shake loose the wires in your heart. Ask your doctor how much and what kinds of physical activity are safe for you.

Battery Replacement

Pacemaker batteries last between 5 and 15 years (average 6 to 7 years), depending on how active the pacemaker is. Your doctor will replace the generator along with the battery before the battery starts to run down.

Replacing the generator and battery is less-involved surgery than the original surgery to implant the pacemaker. Your pacemaker wires also may need to be replaced eventually.

Your doctor can tell you whether your pacemaker or its wires need to be replaced when you see him or her for followup visits.

Chapter 51

Procedures to Treat Heart Valve Problems

How Is Heart Valve Disease Treated?

Currently, no medicines can cure heart valve disease. However, lifestyle changes and medicines often can treat symptoms successfully and delay problems for many years. Eventually, though, you may need surgery to repair or replace a faulty heart valve.

The goals of treating heart valve disease might include:

- Medicines

- Repairing or replacing faulty valves

- Lifestyle changes to treat other related heart conditions

Medicines

In addition to heart-healthy lifestyle changes, your doctor may prescribe medicines to:

- Lower high blood pressure or high blood cholesterol.

- Prevent arrhythmias (irregular heartbeats).

This chapter includes text excerpted from "Heart Valve Disease," National Heart, Lung, and Blood Institute (NHLBI), October 30, 2015.

- Thin the blood and prevent clots (if you have a man-made replacement valve). Doctors also prescribe these medicines for mitral stenosis or other valve defects that raise the risk of blood clots.

- Treat coronary heart disease. Medicines for coronary heart disease can reduce your heart's workload and relieve symptoms.

- Treat heart failure. Heart failure medicines widen blood vessels and rid the body of excess fluid.

Repairing or Replacing Heart Valves

Your doctor may recommend repairing or replacing your heart valve(s), even if your heart valve disease isn't causing symptoms. Repairing or replacing a valve can prevent lasting damage to your heart and sudden death.

The decision to repair or replace heart valves depends on many factors, including:

- The severity of your valve disease

- Whether you need heart surgery for other conditions, such as bypass surgery to treat coronary heart disease. Bypass surgery and valve surgery can be performed at the same time.

- Your age and general health

When possible, heart valve repair is preferred over heart valve replacement. Valve repair preserves the strength and function of the heart muscle. People who have valve repair also have a lower risk of infective endocarditis after the surgery, and they don't need to take blood-thinning medicines for the rest of their lives.

However, heart valve repair surgery is harder to do than valve replacement. Also, not all valves can be repaired. Mitral valves often can be repaired. Aortic and pulmonary valves often have to be replaced.

Repairing Heart Valves

Heart surgeons can repair heart valves by:

- Adding tissue to patch holes or tears or to increase the support at the base of the valve

- Removing or reshaping tissue so the valve can close tighter

- Separating fused valve flaps

Sometimes cardiologists repair heart valves using cardiac catheterization. Although catheter procedures are less invasive than surgery, they may not work as well for some patients. Work with your doctor to decide whether repair is appropriate. If so, your doctor can advise you on the best procedure.

Heart valves that cannot open fully (stenosis) can be repaired with surgery or with a less invasive catheter procedure called balloon valvuloplasty. This procedure also is called balloon valvotomy.

During the procedure, a catheter (thin tube) with a balloon at its tip is threaded through a blood vessel to the faulty valve in your heart. The balloon is inflated to help widen the opening of the valve. Your doctor then deflates the balloon and removes both it and the tube. You're awake during the procedure, which usually requires an overnight stay in a hospital.

Balloon valvuloplasty relieves many symptoms of heart valve disease, but may not cure it. The condition can worsen over time. You still may need medicines to treat symptoms or surgery to repair or replace the faulty valve. Balloon valvuloplasty has a shorter recovery time than surgery. The procedure may work as well as surgery for some patients who have mitral valve stenosis. For these people, balloon valvuloplasty often is preferred over surgical repair or replacement.

Balloon valvuloplasty doesn't work as well as surgery for adults who have aortic valve stenosis. Doctors often use balloon valvuloplasty to repair valve stenosis in infants and children.

Replacing Heart Valves

Sometimes heart valves can't be repaired and must be replaced. This surgery involves removing the faulty valve and replacing it with a man-made or biological valve.

Biological valves are made from pig, cow, or human heart tissue and may have man-made parts as well. These valves are specially treated, so you won't need medicines to stop your body from rejecting the valve.

Man-made valves last longer than biological valves and usually don't have to be replaced. Biological valves usually have to be replaced after about 10 years, although newer ones may last 15 years or longer. Unlike biological valves, however, man-made valves require you to take blood-thinning medicines for the rest of your life. These medicines prevent blood clots from forming on the valve. Blood clots can cause a heart attack or stroke. Man-made valves also raise your risk of infective endocarditis.

You and your doctor will decide together whether you should have a man-made or biological replacement valve.

If you're a woman of childbearing age or if you're athletic, you may prefer a biological valve so you don't have to take blood-thinning medicines. If you're elderly, you also may prefer a biological valve, as it will likely last for the rest of your life.

Ross Procedure

Doctors also can treat faulty aortic valves with the Ross procedure. During this surgery, your doctor removes your faulty aortic valve and replaces it with your pulmonary valve. Your pulmonary valve is then replaced with a pulmonary valve from a deceased human donor.

This is more involved surgery than typical valve replacement, and it has a greater risk of complications. The Ross procedure may be especially useful for children because the surgically replaced valves continue to grow with the child. Also, lifelong treatment with blood-thinning medicines isn't required. But in some patients, one or both valves fail to work well within a few years of the surgery. Researchers continue to study the use of this procedure.

Other Approaches for Repairing and Replacing Heart Valves

Some forms of heart valve repair and replacement surgery are less invasive than traditional surgery. These procedures use smaller incisions (cuts) to reach the heart valves. Hospital stays for these newer types of surgery usually are 3 to 5 days, compared with a 5-day stay for traditional heart valve surgery.

New surgeries tend to cause less pain and have a lower risk of infection. Recovery time also tends to be shorter—2 to 4 weeks versus 6 to 8 weeks for traditional surgery.

Transcatheter Valve Therapy

Interventional cardiologists perform procedures that involve threading clips or other devices to repair faulty heart valves using a catheter (tube) inserted through a large blood vessel. The clips or devices are used to reshape the valves and stop the backflow of blood. People who receive these clips recover more easily than people who have surgery. However, the clips may not treat backflow as well as surgery.

Doctors also may use a catheter to replace faulty aortic valves. This procedure is called transcatheter aortic valve replacement (TAVR). For this procedure, the catheter usually is inserted into an artery in the groin (upper thigh) and threaded to the heart. A deflated balloon with a folded replacement valve around it is at the end of the catheter.

Once the replacement valve is placed properly, the balloon is used to expand the new valve so it fits securely within the old valve. The balloon is then deflated, and the balloon and catheter are removed.

A replacement valve also can be inserted in an existing replacement valve that is failing. This is called a valve-in-valve procedure.

Lifestyle Changes to Treat Other Related Heart

To help treat heart conditions related to heart valve disease, your doctor may advise you to make heart-healthy lifestyle changes, such as:

- Heart-healthy eating
- Maintaining a healthy weight
- Managing stress
- Physical activity
- Quitting smoking

Heart-Healthy Eating

Your doctor may recommend heart-healthy eating, which should include:

- Fat-free or low-fat dairy products, such as skim milk
- Fish high in omega-3 fatty acids, such as salmon, tuna, and trout, about twice a week
- Fruits, such as apples, bananas, oranges, pears, and prunes
- Legumes, such as kidney beans, lentils, chickpeas, black-eyed peas, and lima beans
- Vegetables, such as broccoli, cabbage, and carrots
- Whole grains, such as oatmeal, brown rice, and corn tortillas

When following a heart-healthy diet, you should avoid eating:

- A lot of red meat
- Palm and coconut oils
- Sugary foods and beverages

Two nutrients in your diet make blood cholesterol levels rise:

- Saturated fat—found mostly in foods that come from animals

- *Trans* fat (*trans* fatty acids)—found in foods made with hydrogenated oils and fats, such as stick margarine; baked goods, such as cookies, cakes, and pies; crackers; frostings; and coffee creamers. Some *trans* fats also occur naturally in animal fats and meats.

Saturated fat raises your blood cholesterol more than anything else in your diet. When you follow a heart-healthy eating plan, only 5 percent to 6 percent of your daily calories should come from saturated fat. Food labels list the amounts of saturated fat. To help you stay on track, here are some examples:

Table 51.1. Healthy Amounts of Daily Saturated Fat

If you eat:	Try to eat no more than:
1,200 calories a day	8 grams of saturated fat a day
1,500 calories a day	10 grams of saturated fat a day
1,800 calories a day	12 grams of saturated fat a day
2,000 calories a day	13 grams of saturated fat a day
2,500 calories a day	17 grams of saturated fat a day

Not all fats are bad. Monounsaturated and polyunsaturated fats actually help lower blood cholesterol levels. Some sources of monounsaturated and polyunsaturated fats are:

- Corn, sunflower, and soybean oils

- Nuts and seeds, such as walnuts

- Olive, canola, peanut, safflower, and sesame oils

- Peanut butter

- Salmon and trout

- Tofu

Sodium

You should try to limit the amount of sodium that you eat. This means choosing and preparing foods that are lower in salt and sodium. Try to use low-sodium and "no added salt" foods and seasonings at the table or while cooking. Food labels tell you what you need to know about choosing foods that are lower in sodium. Try to eat no more than

2,300 milligrams of sodium a day. If you have high blood pressure, you may need to restrict your sodium intake even more.

Dietary Approaches to Stop Hypertension

Your doctor may recommend the Dietary Approaches to Stop Hypertension (DASH) eating plan if you have high blood pressure. The DASH eating plan focuses on fruits, vegetables, whole grains, and other foods that are heart healthy and low in fat, cholesterol, and sodium and salt.

The DASH eating plan is a good heart-healthy eating plan, even for those who don't have high blood pressure.

Alcohol

Try to limit alcohol intake. Too much alcohol can raise your blood pressure and triglyceride levels, a type of fat found in the blood. Alcohol also adds extra calories, which may cause weight gain.

Men should have no more than two drinks containing alcohol a day. Women should have no more than one drink containing alcohol a day. One drink is:

- 12 ounces of beer

- 5 ounces of wine

- 1½ ounces of liquor

Maintaining a Healthy Weight

Maintaining a healthy weight is important for overall health and can lower your risk for heart valve disease. Aim for a healthy weight by following a heart-healthy eating plan and keeping physically active.

Knowing your body mass index (BMI) helps you find out if you're a healthy weight in relation to your height and gives an estimate of your total body fat. A BMI:

- Below 18.5 is a sign that you are underweight.

- Between 18.5 and 24.9 is in the normal range.

- Between 25.0 and 29.9 is considered overweight.

- Of 30.0 or higher is considered obese.

A general goal to aim for is a BMI of less than 25. Your doctor or health care provider can help you set an appropriate BMI goal.

Measuring waist circumference helps screen for possible health risks. If most of your fat is around your waist rather than at your hips, you're at a higher risk for heart disease and type 2 diabetes. This risk may be higher with a waist size that is greater than 35 inches for women or greater than 40 inches for men. To learn how to measure your waist, visit Assessing Your Weight and Health Risk.

If you're overweight or obese, try to lose weight. A loss of just 3 percent to 5 percent of your current weight can lower your triglycerides, blood glucose, and the risk of developing type 2 diabetes. Greater amounts of weight loss can improve blood pressure readings, lower LDL cholesterol, and increase HDL cholesterol.

Managing Stress

Learning how to manage stress, relax, and cope with problems can improve your emotional and physical health. Consider healthy stress-reducing activities, such as:

- A stress management program
- Meditation
- Physical activity
- Relaxation therapy
- Talking things out with friends or family

Physical Activity

Regular physical activity can lower many heart valve disease risk factors.

Everyone should try to participate in moderate-intensity aerobic exercise at least 2 hours and 30 minutes per week or vigorous aerobic exercise for 1 hour and 15 minutes per week. Aerobic exercise, such as brisk walking, is any exercise in which your heart beats faster and you use more oxygen than usual. The more active you are, the more you will benefit. Participate in aerobic exercise for at least 10 minutes at a time spread throughout the week.

Quitting Smoking

If you smoke or use tobacco, quit. Smoking can damage and tighten blood vessels and raise your risk for atherosclerosis and other health problems. Talk with your doctor about programs and products that can help you quit. Also, try to avoid secondhand smoke. If you have trouble quitting smoking on your own, consider joining a support group. Many hospitals, workplaces, and community groups offer classes to help people quit smoking.

Chapter 52

Treating Aneurysms

How Is an Aneurysm Treated?

Aortic aneurysms are treated with medicines and surgery. Small aneurysms that are found early and aren't causing symptoms may not need treatment. Other aneurysms need to be treated.

The goals of treatment may include:

- Preventing the aneurysm from growing

- Preventing or reversing damage to other body structures

- Preventing or treating a rupture or dissection

- Allowing you to continue doing your normal daily activities

Treatment for an aortic aneurysm is based on its size. Your doctor may recommend routine testing to make sure an aneurysm isn't getting bigger. This method usually is used for aneurysms that are smaller than 5 centimeters (about 2 inches) across.

How often you need testing (for example, every few months or every year) is based on the size of the aneurysm and how fast it's growing. The larger it is and the faster it's growing, the more often you may need to be checked.

This chapter includes text excerpted from "Aneurysm," National Heart, Lung, and Blood Institute (NHLBI), April 1, 2011. Reviewed June 2016.

Medicines

If you have an aortic aneurysm, your doctor may prescribe medicines before surgery or instead of surgery. Medicines are used to lower blood pressure, relax blood vessels, and lower the risk that the aneurysm will rupture (burst). Beta blockers and calcium channel blockers are the medicines most commonly used.

Surgery

Your doctor may recommend surgery if your aneurysm is growing quickly or is at risk of rupture or dissection.

The two main types of surgery to repair aortic aneurysms are open abdominal or open chest repair and endovascular repair.

1. Open Abdominal or Open Chest Repair

The standard and most common type of surgery for aortic aneurysms is open abdominal or open chest repair. This surgery involves a major incision (cut) in the abdomen or chest.

General anesthesia is used during this procedure. The term "anesthesia" refers to a loss of feeling and awareness. General anesthesia temporarily puts you to sleep.

During the surgery, the aneurysm is removed. Then, the section of aorta is replaced with a graft made of material such as Dacron® or Teflon®. The surgery takes 3 to 6 hours; you'll remain in the hospital for 5 to 8 days.

If needed, repair of the aortic heart valve also may be done during open abdominal or open chest surgery.

It often takes a month to recover from open abdominal or open chest surgery and return to full activity. Most patients make a full recovery.

2. Endovascular Repair

In endovascular repair, the aneurysm isn't removed. Instead, a graft is inserted into the aorta to strengthen it. Surgeons do this type of surgery using catheters (tubes) inserted into the arteries; it doesn't require surgically opening the chest or abdomen. General anesthesia is used during this procedure.

The surgeon first inserts a catheter into an artery in the groin (upper thigh) and threads it to the aneurysm. Then, using an X-ray to see the artery, the surgeon threads the graft (also called a stent graft) into the aorta to the aneurysm.

The graft is then expanded inside the aorta and fastened in place to form a stable channel for blood flow. The graft reinforces the weakened section of the aorta. This helps prevent the aneurysm from rupturing.

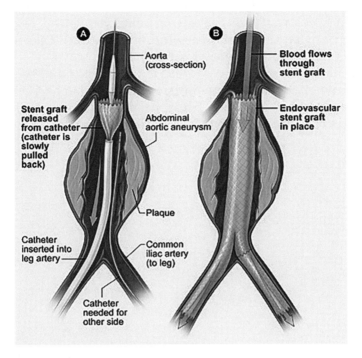

Figure 52.1. *Endovascular Repair*

The illustration shows the placement of a stent graft in an aortic aneurysm. In (A), a catheter is inserted into an artery in the groin (upper thigh). The catheter is threaded to the abdominal aorta, and the stent graft is released from the catheter. In (B), the stent graft allows blood to flow through the aneurysm.

The recovery time for endovascular repair is less than the recovery time for open abdominal or open chest repair. However, doctors can't repair all aortic aneurysms with endovascular repair. The location or size of an aneurysm may prevent the use of a stent graft.

Living with an Aneurysm

If you have an aortic aneurysm, following your treatment plan and having ongoing medical care are important. Early diagnosis and treatment can help prevent rupture and dissection.

Your doctor may advise you to avoid heavy lifting or physical exertion. If your job requires heavy lifting, you may be advised to change jobs.

Also, try to avoid emotional crises. Strong emotions can cause blood pressure to rise, which increases the risk of rupture or dissection. Call your doctor if an emotional crisis occurs.

Your doctor may prescribe medicines to treat your aneurysm. Medicines can lower your blood pressure, relax your blood vessels, and lower the risk that the aneurysm will rupture (burst). Take all of your medicines exactly as your doctor prescribes.

If you have a small aneurysm that isn't causing pain, you may not need treatment. However, aneurysms can develop and grow large before causing any symptoms. Thus, people who are at high risk for aneurysms may benefit from early, routine screening.

Chapter 53

Treating Congenital Heart Defect

How Are Congenital Heart Defects Treated?

Although many children who have congenital heart defects don't need treatment, some do. Doctors repair congenital heart defects with catheter procedures or surgery.

Sometimes doctors combine catheter and surgical procedures to repair complex heart defects, which may involve several kinds of defects.

The treatment your child receives depends on the type and severity of his or her heart defect. Other factors include your child's age, size, and general health.

Some children who have complex congenital heart defects may need several catheter or surgical procedures over a period of years, or they may need to take medicines for years.

Catheter Procedures

Catheter procedures are much easier on patients than surgery. They involve only a needle puncture in the skin where the catheter (thin, flexible tube) is inserted into a vein or an artery.

This chapter include text excerpted from "How Are Congenital Heart Defects Treated?" National Heart, Lung, and Blood Institute (NHLBI), July 1, 2011. Reviewed June 2016.

Doctors don't have to surgically open the chest or operate directly on the heart to repair the defect(s). This means that recovery may be easier and quicker.

The use of catheter procedures has increased a lot in the past 20 years. They have become the preferred way to repair many simple heart defects, such as atrial septal defect (ASD) and pulmonary valve stenosis.

For ASD repair, the doctor inserts a catheter into a vein in the groin (upper thigh). He or she threads the tube to the heart's septum. A device made up of two small disks or an umbrella-like device is attached to the catheter.

When the catheter reaches the septum, the device is pushed out of the catheter. The device is placed so that it plugs the hole between the atria. It's secured in place and the catheter is withdrawn from the body.

Within 6 months, normal tissue grows in and over the device. The closure device does not need to be replaced as the child grows.

For pulmonary valve stenosis, the doctor inserts a catheter into a vein and threads it to the heart's pulmonary valve. A tiny balloon at the end of the catheter is quickly inflated to push apart the leaflets, or "doors," of the valve.

Then, the balloon is deflated and the catheter and ballon are withdrawn. This procedure can be used to repair any narrowed valve in the heart.

To help guide the catheter, doctors often use echocardiography (echo), transesophageal echo (TEE), and coronary angiography.

TEE is a special type of echo that takes pictures of the heart through the esophagus. The esophagus is the passage leading from the mouth to the stomach. Doctors also use TEE to examine complex heart defects.

Surgery

A child may need open-heart surgery if his or her heart defect can't be fixed using a catheter procedure. Sometimes one surgery can repair the defect completely. If that's not possible, the child may need more surgeries over months or years to fix the problem.

Cardiac surgeons may use open-heart surgery to:

- Close holes in the heart with stitches or a patch

- Repair or replace heart valves

- Widen arteries or openings to heart valves

- Repair complex defects, such as problems with the location of blood vessels near the heart or how they are formed

Rarely, babies are born with multiple defects that are too complex to repair. These babies may need heart transplants. In this procedure, the child's heart is replaced with a healthy heart from a deceased child. The heart has been donated by the deceased child's family.

Chapter 54

Total Artificial Heart

What Is a Total Artificial Heart?

A total artificial heart (TAH) is a device that replaces the two lower chambers of the heart. These chambers are called ventricles. You might benefit from a TAH if both of your ventricles don't work due to end-stage heart failure.

Heart failure is a condition in which the heart can't pump enough blood to meet the body's needs. "End stage" means the condition has become so severe that all treatments, except heart transplant, have failed. (A heart transplant is surgery to remove a person's diseased heart and replace it with a healthy heart from a deceased donor.)

Overview

You might need a TAH for one of two reasons:

- To keep you alive while you wait for a heart transplant

- If you're not eligible for a heart transplant, but you have end-stage heart failure in both ventricles

The TAH is attached to your heart's upper chambers—the atria. Between the TAH and the atria are mechanical valves that work

This chapter includes text excerpted from "Total Artificial Heart," National Heart, Lung, and Blood Institute (NHLBI), February 1, 2016.

like the heart's own valves. Valves control the flow of blood in the heart. Currently, the two types of TAHs are the CardioWest and the AbioCor. The main difference between these TAHs is that the CardioWest is connected to an outside power source and the AbioCor isn't.

The CardioWest has tubes that, through holes in the abdomen, run from inside the chest to an outside power source.

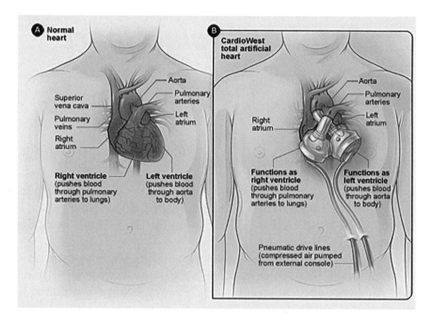

Figure 54.1. *Normal Heart and CardioWest Total Artificial Heart*

(A) shows the normal structure and location of the heart. (B) shows a CardioWest TAH. Tubes exit the body and connect to a machine that powers the TAH and controls how it works.

The AbioCor TAH is completely contained inside the chest. A battery powers this TAH. The battery is charged through the skin with a special magnetic charger.

Energy from the external charger reaches the internal battery through an energy transfer device called transcutaneous energy transmission, or TET.

An implanted TET device is connected to the implanted battery. An external TET coil is connected to the external charger. Also, an implanted controller monitors and controls the pumping speed of the heart.

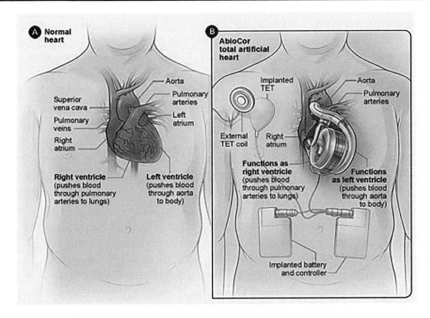

Figure 54.2. *Normal Heart and AbioCor Total Artificial Heart*

(A) shows the normal structure and location of the heart. (B) shows an AbioCor TAH and the internal devices that control how it works.

Outlook

A TAH usually extends life for months beyond what is expected with end-stage heart failure. If you're waiting for a heart transplant, a TAH can keep you alive while you wait for a donor heart. A TAH also can improve your quality of life. However, a TAH is a very complex device. It's challenging for surgeons to implant, and it can cause complications.

Currently, TAHs are used only in a small number of people. Researchers are working to make even better TAHs that will allow people to live longer and have fewer complications.

Other Names for a Total Artificial Heart

- Artificial heart
- AbioCor
- CardioWest

Who Needs a Total Artificial Heart?

You might benefit from a total artificial heart (TAH) if both of your ventricles don't work due to end-stage heart failure.

If you're waiting for a heart transplant, a TAH can help you survive longer. It also can improve your quality of life. If your life expectancy is less than 30 days and you're not eligible for a heart transplant, a TAH may extend your life beyond the expected 30 days.

A TAH is a "last resort" device. This means only people who have tried every other type of treatment, except heart transplant, can get it. TAHs aren't used for people who may benefit from medicines or other procedures.

TAHs also have a size limit. These devices are fairly large and can only fit into large chest areas. Currently, no TAHs are available that can fit into children's chests. However, researchers are trying to make smaller models.

The U.S. Food and Drug Administration (FDA) has approved the TAH for certain types of patients. Your doctor will discuss with you whether you meet the conditions for getting a TAH.

If you and your doctor decide that a TAH is a good option for you, you also will discuss which of the two types of TAH will work best for you.

What to Expect before Total Artificial Heart Surgery

Before you get a total artificial heart (TAH), you'll likely spend at least a week in the hospital to prepare for the surgery. You might already be in the hospital getting treatment for heart failure.

During this time, you'll learn about the TAH and how to live with it. You and your loved ones will spend time with your surgeons, cardiologist (heart specialist), and nurses to make sure you have all the information you need before surgery. You can ask to see what the device looks like and how it will be attached inside your body.

Your doctors will make sure that your body is strong enough for the surgery. If they think your body is too weak, you may need to get extra nutrition through a feeding tube before the surgery.

You also will have tests to make sure you're ready for the surgery. These tests include:

- **A chest CT scan.** This test is used to make sure the TAH, which is fairly large, will fit in your chest. Before you have surgery, your doctor will make sure there's enough room in your chest for the device.

- **Blood tests.** These tests are used to check how well your liver and kidneys are working. Blood tests also are used to check the levels of blood cells and important chemicals in your blood.

- **Chest X-ray.** This test is used to create pictures of the inside of your chest to help your doctors prepare for surgery.

- **EKG (electrocardiogram).** This test is used to check how well your heart is working before the ventricles are replaced by the TAH.

What to Expect during Total Artificial Heart Surgery

Total artificial heart (TAH) surgery is complex and can take between 5 and 9 hours. It requires many experts and assistants. As many as 15 people might be in the operating room during surgery.

The team for TAH surgery includes:

- Surgeons who do the operation

- Surgical nurses who assist the surgeons

- Anesthesiologists who are in charge of the medicine that makes you sleep during surgery

- Perfusionists who are in charge of the heart-lung bypass machine that keeps blood flowing through your body while the TAH is put in your chest

- Engineers who are trained to assemble the TAH and make sure it's working well

Before the surgery, you're given medicine to make you sleep. During the surgery, the anesthesiologist checks your heartbeat, blood pressure, oxygen levels, and breathing.

A breathing tube is placed in your windpipe through your throat. This tube is connected to a ventilator (a machine that supports breathing).

A cut is made down the center of your chest. The chest bone is then cut and your ribcage is opened so the surgeon can reach your heart.

Medicines are used to stop your heart. This allows the surgeons to operate on your heart while it's still. A heart-lung bypass machine keeps oxygen-rich blood moving through your body during surgery.

The surgeons remove your heart's ventricles and attach the TAH to the upper chambers of your heart. When everything is properly attached, the heart-lung bypass machine is switched off and the TAH starts pumping.

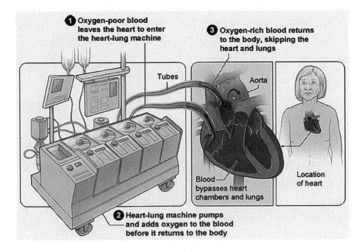

Figure 54.3. *Heart-Lung Bypass Machine*

The image shows how a heart-lung bypass machine works during surgery.

What to Expect after Total Artificial Heart Surgery

Recovery in the Hospital

Recovery time after total artificial heart (TAH) surgery depends a lot on your condition before the surgery.

If you had severe heart failure for a while before getting the TAH, your body may be weak and your lungs may not work very well. Thus, you may still need a ventilator (a machine that supports breathing) after surgery. You also may need to continue getting nutrition through a feeding tube.

Your hospital stay could last a month or longer after TAH surgery.

Right after surgery, you'll be in the hospital's intensive care unit. An intravenous (IV) line will be inserted into a vein in your arm to give you fluids and nutrition. You'll also have a tube in your bladder to drain urine.

After a few days or more, depending on how quickly your body recovers, you'll move to a regular hospital room. Nurses who have experience with TAHs and similar devices will take care of you.

The nurses will help you get out of bed, sit, and walk around. As you get stronger, the feeding and urine tubes will be removed. You'll be able to go to the bathroom on your own and have a regular diet. You'll also be able to take a shower. You'll learn how to do this while taking care of your TAH device.

Nurses and physical therapists will help you gain your strength through a slow increase in activity. You'll also learn how to care for your TAH device at home.

Having family or friends visit you at the hospital can be very helpful. They can help you with various activities. They also can learn about caring for the TAH device so they can help you when you go home.

Going Home

Activity Level

When you go home after TAH surgery, you'll likely be able to do more activities than you could before. You'll probably be able to get out of bed, get dressed, and move around the house. You may even be able to drive. Your healthcare team will advise you on the level of activity that's safe for you.

Bathing

If you have an AbioCor TAH, you can shower or swim, as long as the device is charged.

If you have a CardioWest TAH, you'll have tubes connected to a power source outside of your body. The tubes go through an opening in your skin. This opening can let in bacteria and increase your risk of infections.

You'll need to take special steps before you bathe to make sure the tubes going through your abdomen don't get wet. Your healthcare team will explain how to do this.

Caring for the TAH

If you have an AbioCor TAH, you'll need to keep it charged with its magnetic charger. When it's charged, you can do activities that feel comfortable to you (as your doctor advises).

If you have a CardioWest TAH, it will be attached to an external power source, also called a driver. The driver is portable, so you'll be able to walk around and do activities.

Nutrition and Exercise

While you recover from TAH surgery, it's very important to get good nutrition. Talk with your healthcare team about following a proper eating plan for recovery.

Your healthcare team may recommend a supervised exercise program. Exercise can give your body the strength it needs to recover.

During the months or years when your heart wasn't working well (before surgery), the muscles in your body weakened. Building up the muscles again will allow you to do more activities and feel less tired.

Ongoing Care

You'll have regular checkups with your healthcare team. The team will want to check your progress and make sure your TAH is working well.

If you have an AbioCor TAH, your healthcare team can check it remotely. This means that if you think something is wrong, you can hook up the device to a computer with Internet access.

The computer will transfer data to your healthcare team so they can see how your TAH is working. Certain problems may require you to see your doctor in person.

The CardioWest TAH can't be checked remotely.

Your healthcare team will explain warning signs to watch for. If these signs occur, or if you start feeling sick, you'll need to see your doctor right away.

Cardiac Rehab

Your healthcare team may recommend cardiac rehabilitation (rehab). This is a medically supervised program that helps improve the health and well-being of people who have heart problems.

Rehab programs include exercise training, education on heart healthy living, and counseling to reduce stress and help you return to a more active life.

Medicines

You'll need to take medicine to prevent dangerous blood clots for as long as you have a TAH. Regular blood tests will show whether the medicine is working.

You also will need to take medicine to try to prevent infections. Your doctor may ask you to take your temperature every day to make sure you don't have a fever. A fever can be a warning sign of infection.

Make sure to take all your medicines as prescribed and report any side effects to your doctor.

Heart Transplant

If you're on the waiting list for a heart transplant, you'll likely be in close contact with the transplant center. Most donor hearts must be transplanted within 4 hours after removal from the donor.

The transplant center staff may give you a pager so they can contact you at any time. You need to be prepared to arrive at the hospital within 2 hours of being notified about a donor heart.

Emotional Issues

Getting a TAH may cause fear, anxiety, and stress. If you're waiting for a heart transplant, you may worry that the TAH won't keep you alive long enough to get a new heart. You may feel overwhelmed or depressed.

All of these feelings are normal for someone going through major heart surgery. Talk about how you feel with your healthcare team. Talking to a professional counselor also can help. If you're very depressed, your doctor may recommend medicines or other treatments that can improve your quality of life.

What Are the Risks of a Total Artificial Heart?

Getting a total artificial heart (TAH) involves some serious risks. These risks include blood clots, bleeding, infection, and device malfunctions. Because of these risks, only a small number of people currently have TAHs.

There's a small risk of dying during TAH surgery. There's also a small risk that your body may respond poorly to the medicine used to put you to sleep during the surgery. However, most patients survive and recover from TAH surgery.

If you're eligible for a TAH, you'll work with your doctor to decide whether the benefits of the device outweigh the risks.

Researchers are working to improve TAHs and lessen the risks of using these devices.

Blood Clots

When your blood comes in contact with something that isn't a natural part of your body, such as a TAH, it tends to clot more than normal. Blood clots can disrupt blood flow and may block blood vessels leading to important organs in the body.

Blood clots can lead to severe complications or even death. For this reason, you need to take anticlotting medicine for as long as you have a TAH.

Bleeding

The surgery to implant a TAH is very complex. Bleeding can occur in your chest during and after the surgery.

Anticlotting medicine also raises your risk of bleeding because it thins your blood. Balancing the anticlotting medicine with the risk of bleeding can be hard. Make sure to take your medicine exactly as your doctor prescribes.

Infection

One of the two available TAHs, the CardioWest, attaches to a power source outside your body through holes in your abdomen. These holes increase the risk of bacteria getting in and causing an infection.

With permanent tubes running through your skin, the risk of infection is serious. You'll need to take medicine to try to prevent infections.

Your healthcare team will watch you very closely if you have any signs of infection, such as a fever. You may need to check your temperature several times a day as part of your ongoing care.

With both types of TAH, you're at risk for infection after surgery. Your doctor will prescribe medicine to reduce the risk.

Device Malfunctions

Because TAHs are so complex, they can malfunction (not work properly) in different ways. A TAH's:

- Pumping action may not be exactly right

- Power may fail

- Parts may stop working well

This doesn't mean a TAH is bound to fail. In fact, TAHs that have been implanted in people in recent years have generally worked very well. However, problems with the device can occur.

Chapter 55

Heart Transplant

What Is a Heart Transplant?

A heart transplant is surgery to remove a person's diseased heart and replace it with a healthy heart from a deceased donor. Most heart transplants are done on patients who have end-stage heart failure.

Heart failure is a condition in which the heart is damaged or weak. As a result, it can't pump enough blood to meet the body's needs. "End-stage" means the condition is so severe that all treatments, other than a heart transplant, have failed.

Overview

Heart transplants are done as a life-saving measure for end-stage heart failure.

Because donor hearts are in short supply, patients who need heart transplants go through a careful selection process. They must be sick enough to need a new heart, yet healthy enough to receive it.

Survival rates for people receiving heart transplants have improved, especially in the first year after the transplant.

About 88 percent of patients survive the first year after transplant surgery, and 75 percent survive for 5 years. The 10-year survival rate is about 56 percent.

This chapter includes text excerpted from "Heart Transplant," National Heart, Lung, and Blood Institute (NHLBI), January 3, 2012. Reviewed June 2016.

After the surgery, most heart transplant patients can return to their normal levels of activity. However, less than 30 percent return to work for many different reasons.

The Heart Transplant Process

The heart transplant process starts when doctors refer a patient who has end-stage heart failure to a heart transplant center.

Staff members at the center assess whether the patient is eligible for the surgery. If the patient is eligible, he or she is placed on a waiting list for a donor heart.

Heart transplant surgery is done in a hospital when a suitable donor heart is found. After the transplant, the patient is started on a lifelong healthcare plan. The plan involves multiple medicines and frequent medical checkups.

Who Needs a Heart Transplant?

Most patients referred to heart transplant centers have end-stage heart failure. Their heart failure might have been caused by:

- Coronary heart disease.

- Hereditary conditions.

- Viral infections of the heart.

- Damaged heart valves and muscles. (Alcohol, pregnancy, and certain medicines can damage the heart valves and muscles.)

Most patients considered for heart transplants have tried other, less drastic treatments. They also have been hospitalized many times for heart failure.

Who Is Eligible for a Heart Transplant?

The specialists at the heart transplant center will assess whether a patient is eligible for a transplant. Specialists often include a:

- Cardiologist (a doctor who specializes in diagnosing and treating heart problems)

- Cardiovascular surgeon (a doctor who does the transplant surgery)

- Transplant coordinator (a person who arranges aspects of the surgery, such as transportation of the donor heart)

- Social worker

- Dietitian

- Psychiatrist

In general, patients selected for heart transplants have severe end-stage heart failure, but are healthy enough to have the transplant. Heart failure is considered "end stage" when all possible treatments—such as medicines, implanted devices, and surgery—have failed.

Certain conditions and factors make it less likely that a heart transplant will work well. Examples include:

- Advanced age. There is no widely accepted upper age limit for a heart transplant. However, most transplant surgeries are done on patients younger than 70 years old.

- Poor blood circulation throughout the body, including the brain.

- Kidney, lung, or liver diseases that can't be reversed.

- A history of cancer or malignant tumors.

- Inability or unwillingness to follow a lifelong care plan after a transplant.

- Pulmonary hypertension (high blood pressure in the lungs) that can't be reversed.

- Active infection throughout the body.

- Diabetes with end organ damage (damage of major organs).

Patients who have one or more of the above conditions might not be eligible for heart transplant surgery.

What to Expect before a Heart Transplant

The Heart Transplant Waiting List

Patients who are eligible for a heart transplant are added to a waiting list for a donor heart. This waiting list is part of a national allocation system for donor organs. The Organ Procurement and Transplantation Network (OPTN) runs this system.

OPTN has policies in place to make sure donor hearts are given out fairly. These policies are based on urgency of need, available organs, and the location of the patient who is receiving the heart (the recipient).

Organs are matched for blood type and size of donor and recipient.

The Donor Heart

Guidelines for how a donor heart is selected require that the donor meet the legal requirement for brain death and that the correct consent forms are signed.

Guidelines suggest that the donor should be younger than 65 years old, have little or no history of heart disease or trauma to the chest, and not be exposed to hepatitis or HIV.

The guidelines recommend that the donor heart should not be without blood circulation for more than 4 hours.

Waiting Times

About 3,000 people in the United States are on the waiting list for a heart transplant on any given day. About 2,000 donor hearts are available each year. Wait times vary from days to several months and will depend on a recipient's blood type and condition.

A person might be taken off the list for some time if he or she has a serious medical event, such as a stroke, infection, or kidney failure.

Time spent on the waiting list plays a part in who receives a donor heart. For example, if two patients have equal need, the one who has been waiting longer will likely get the first available donor heart.

Ongoing Medical Treatment

Patients on the waiting list for a donor heart get ongoing treatment for heart failure and other medical conditions.

For example, doctors may treat them for arrhythmias (irregular heartbeats). Arrhythmias can cause sudden cardiac arrest in people who have heart failure.

The doctors at the transplant centers may place implantable cardioverter defibrillators (ICDs) in patients before surgery. ICDs are small devices that are placed in the chest or abdomen. They help control life-threatening arrhythmias.

Another possible treatment for waiting list patients is a ventricular assist device (VAD). A VAD is a mechanical pump that helps support heart function and blood flow.

Routine outpatient care for waiting list patients may include frequent exercise testing, testing the strength of the heartbeat, and right cardiac catheterization (a test to measure blood pressure in the right side of the heart).

You also might start a cardiac rehabilitation (rehab) program. Cardiac rehab is a medically supervised program that helps improve the health and well-being of people who have heart problems.

The program can help improve your physical condition before the transplant. Also, you will learn the types of exercises used in the program, which will help you take part in cardiac rehab after the transplant.

Contact with the Transplant Center during the Wait

Patients on the waiting list often are in close contact with their transplant centers. Most donor hearts must be transplanted within 4 hours after removal from the donor.

At some heart transplant centers, patients get a pager so the center can contact them at any time. They're asked to tell the transplant center staff if they're going out of town. Patients often need to be prepared to arrive at the hospital within 2 hours of being notified about a donor heart.

Not all patients who are called to the hospital will get a heart transplant. Sometimes, at the last minute, doctors find that a donor heart isn't suitable for a patient. Other times, patients from the waiting list are called to come in as possible backups, in case something happens with the selected recipient.

What to Expect during a Heart Transplant

Just before heart transplant surgery, the patient will get general anesthesia. The term "anesthesia" refers to a loss of feeling and awareness. General anesthesia temporarily puts you to sleep.

Surgeons use open-heart surgery to do heart transplants. The surgeon will make a large incision (cut) in the patient's chest to open the rib cage and operate on the heart.

A heart-lung bypass machine is hooked up to the heart's arteries and veins. The machine pumps blood through the patient's lungs and body during the surgery.

The surgeon removes the patient's diseased heart and sews the healthy donor heart into place. The patient's aorta and pulmonary arteries are not replaced as part of the surgery.

Heart transplant surgery usually takes about 4 hours. Patients often spend the first days after surgery in the intensive care unit of the hospital.

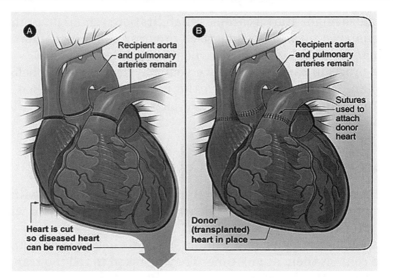

Figure 55.1. *Heart Transplant*

(A) shows where the diseased heart is cut for removal. (B) shows where the healthy donor heart is sutured (stitched) to the recipient's arteries and veins.

What to Expect after a Heart Transplant

Staying in the Hospital

The amount of time a heart transplant recipient spends in the hospital varies. Recovery often involves 1 to 2 weeks in the hospital and 3 months of monitoring by the transplant team at the heart transplant center.

Monitoring may include frequent blood tests, lung function tests, EKGs (electrocardiograms), echocardiograms, and biopsies of the heart tissue.

A heart biopsy is a standard test that can show whether your body is rejecting the new heart. This test is often done in the weeks after a transplant.

During a heart biopsy, a tiny grabbing device is inserted into a vein in the neck or groin (upper thigh). The device is threaded through the vein to the right atrium of the new heart to take a small tissue sample. The tissue sample is checked for signs of rejection.

While in the hospital, your healthcare team may suggest that you start a cardiac rehabilitation (rehab) program. Cardiac rehab is a medically supervised program that helps improve the health and well-being of people who have heart problems.

Cardiac rehab includes counseling, education, and exercise training to help you recover. Rehab may start with a member of the rehab team helping you sit up in a chair or take a few steps. Over time, you'll increase your activity level.

Watching for Signs of Rejection

Your body will regard your new heart as a foreign object. You'll need medicine to prevent your immune system from attacking the heart.

You and the transplant team will work together to protect the new heart. You'll watch for signs and symptoms that your body is rejecting the organ. These signs and symptoms include:

- Shortness of breath

- Fever

- Fatigue (tiredness)

- Weight gain (retaining fluid in the body)

- Reduced amounts of urine (problems in the kidneys can cause this sign)

You and the team also will work together to manage the transplant medicines and their side effects, prevent infections, and continue treatment of ongoing medical conditions.

Your doctors may ask you to check your temperature, blood pressure, and pulse when you go home.

Preventing Rejection

You'll need to take medicine to suppress your immune system so that it doesn't reject the new heart. These medicines are called immunosuppressants.

Immunosuppressants are a combination of medicines that are tailored to your situation. Often, they include cyclosporine, tacrolimus, MMF (mycophenolate mofetil), and steroids (such as prednisone).

Your doctors may need to change or adjust your transplant medicines if they aren't working well or if you have too many side effects.

Managing Transplant Medicines and Their Side Effects

You'll have to manage multiple medicines after having a heart transplant. It's helpful to set up a routine for taking medicines at the same time each day and for refilling prescriptions. It's crucial to never run out of medicine. Always using the same pharmacy may help.

Keep a list of all your medicines with you at all times in case of an accident. When traveling, keep extra doses of medicine with you (not packed in your luggage). Bring your medicines with you to all doctor visits.

Side effects from medicines can be serious. Side effects include risk of infection, diabetes, osteoporosis (thinning of the bones), high blood pressure, kidney disease, and cancer—especially lymphoma and skin cancer.

Discuss any side effects of the medicines with your transplant team. Your doctors may change or adjust your medicines if you're having problems. Make sure your doctors know all of the medicines you're taking.

Preventing Infection

Some transplant medicines can increase your risk of infection. You may be asked to watch for signs of infection, including fever, sore throat, cold sores, and flu-like symptoms.

Signs of possible chest or lung infections include shortness of breath, cough, and a change in the color of sputum (spit).

Watching closely for these signs is important because transplant medicines can sometimes mask them. Also, pay close attention to signs of infection at the site of your incision (cut). These signs can include redness, swelling, or drainage.

Ask your doctor what steps you should take to reduce your risk of infection. For example, your doctor may suggest that you avoid contact with animals or crowds of people in the first few months after your transplant.

Regular dental care also is important. Your doctor or dentist may prescribe antibiotics before any dental work to prevent infections.

Pregnancy

Many successful pregnancies have occurred after heart transplant surgeries; however, special care is needed. If you've had a heart transplant, talk with your doctor before planning a pregnancy.

Emotional Issues and Support

Having a heart transplant may cause fear, anxiety, and stress. While you're waiting for a heart transplant, you may worry that you won't live long enough to get a new heart. After surgery, you may feel overwhelmed, depressed, or worried about complications.

All of these feelings are normal for someone going through major heart surgery. Talk about how you feel with your healthcare team. Talking to a professional counselor also can help.

If you're very depressed, your doctor may recommend medicines or other treatments that can improve your quality of life.

Joining a patient support group may help you adjust to life after a heart transplant. You can see how other people who have had the surgery have coped with it. Talk with your doctor about local support groups or check with an area medical center.

Support from family and friends also can help relieve stress and anxiety. Let your loved ones know how you feel and what they can do to help you.

What Are the Risks of a Heart Transplant?

Although heart transplant surgery is a life-saving measure, it has many risks. Careful monitoring, treatment, and regular medical care can prevent or help manage some of these risks.

The risks of having a heart transplant include:

- Failure of the donor heart
- Complications from medicines
- Infection
- Cancer
- Problems that arise from not following a lifelong care plan after surgery

Failure of the Donor Heart

Over time, the new heart may fail due to the same reasons that caused the original heart to fail. Failure of the donor heart also can occur if your body rejects the donor heart or if cardiac allograft vasculopathy (CAV) develops. CAV is a blood vessel disease.

Patients who have a heart transplant that fails can be considered for another transplant (called a retransplant).

Primary Graft Dysfunction

The most frequent cause of death in the first 30 days after transplant is primary graft dysfunction. This occurs if the new donor heart fails and isn't able to function.

Factors such as shock or trauma to the donor heart or narrow blood vessels in the recipient's lungs can cause primary graft dysfunction. Doctors may prescribe medicines (for example, inhaled nitric oxide and intravenous nitrates) to treat this condition.

Rejection of the Donor Heart

Rejection is one of the leading causes of death in the first year after transplant. The recipient's immune system sees the new heart as a foreign object and attacks it.

During the first year, heart transplant patients have an average of one to three episodes of rejection. Rejection is most likely to occur within 6 months of the transplant surgery.

Cardiac Allograft Vasculopathy

CAV is a chronic (ongoing) disease in which the walls of the coronary arteries in the new heart become thick, hard, and less stretchy. CAV can destroy blood circulation in the new heart and cause serious damage.

CAV is a leading cause of donor heart failure and death in the years following transplant surgery. CAV can cause heart attack, heart failure, dangerous arrhythmias, and sudden cardiac arrest.

To detect CAV, your doctor may recommend coronary angiography yearly and other tests, such as stress echocardiography or intravascular ultrasound.

Complications from Medicines

Taking daily medicines that stop the immune system from attacking the new heart is crucial, even though the medicines have serious side effects.

Cyclosporine and other medicines can cause kidney damage. Kidney damage affects more than 25 percent of patients in the first year after transplant.

Infection

When the immune system—the body's defense system—is suppressed, the risk of infection increases. Infection is a major cause of hospital admission for heart transplant patients. It also is a leading cause of death in the first year after transplant.

Cancer

Suppressing the immune system leaves patients at risk for cancers and malignancies. Malignancies are a major cause of late death in heart transplant patients.

The most common malignancies are tumors of the skin and lips (patients at highest risk are older, male, and fair-skinned) and malignancies in the lymph system, such as non-Hodgkin's lymphoma.

Other Complications

High blood pressure develops in more than 70 percent of heart transplant patients in the first year after transplant and in nearly 95 percent of patients within 5 years.

High levels of cholesterol and triglycerides in the blood develop in more than 50 percent of heart transplant patients in the first year after transplant and in 84 percent of patients within 5 years.

Osteoporosis can develop or worsen in heart transplant patients. This condition thins and weakens the bones.

Complications from Not Following a Lifelong Care Plan

Not following a lifelong care plan increases the risk of all heart transplant complications. Heart transplant patients are asked to closely follow their doctors' instructions and check their own health status throughout their lives.

Lifelong healthcare includes taking multiple medicines on a strict schedule, watching for signs and symptoms of complications, going to all medical checkups, and making healthy lifestyle changes (such as quitting smoking).

Chapter 56

Stem Cell Therapy

Stem Cell Therapy Rebuilds Heart Muscle in Primates

Scientists used human embryonic stem cells to regenerate damaged primate hearts. The strategy might one day be used to repair human hearts, but challenges still need to be overcome.

Damage to the heart—such as that caused by a heart attack—isn't easy to mend. The heart's muscle cells, called cardiomyocytes, don't readily replenish themselves. After a typical heart attack, an estimated billion cardiomyocytes die. This jeopardizes heart function and can lead to chronic heart failure and possibly death.

Scientists have been searching for innovative ways to replenish damaged heart tissue. Human embryonic stem cells have proven promising in small animal models. These cells have the potential to develop into any cell type in the body. Derivatives of the cells are already being tested in people for retinal diseases and spinal cord injury. However, cardiac repair requires much larger numbers of cells. The approaches developed in small animals also need to be tested in larger, more clinically relevant animals.

A research team led by Dr. Charles Murry at the University of Washington set out to test whether an approach they were developing could be scaled up and used in a large animal model. Their work was funded in part by NIH's National Heart, Lung, and Blood Institute

This chapter includes text excerpted from "Stem Cell Therapy Rebuilds Heart Muscle in Primates," National Institutes of Health (NIH), May 12, 2014.

(NHLBI) and National Institute of General Medical Sciences (NIGMS). Results appeared online on April 30, 2014, in *Nature*.

The team first created cardiomyocytes from human embryonic stem cells that were genetically engineered to produce a fluorescent calcium indicator. This indicator allowed the researchers to track the calcium waves that mark the electrical activity of a beating heart. Pigtail macaques (*Macaca nemestrina*) with heart damage were treated to suppress their immune systems. Five days later, the cardiomyocytes were delivered in a surgical procedure to the damaged regions and surrounding border zones.

Over a 3-month period, the grafted cells infiltrated damaged heart muscle, matured, and organized into muscle fibers in all the monkeys who received the treatment. On average, the grafts replaced 40% of damaged tissue. Three-dimensional imaging showed that arteries and veins integrated into the grafts, suggesting the grafts could be long lasting. There was no evidence of graft rejection by the animals' immune systems.

Calcium activity revealed that the grafts were electrically active and coupled to activity of the host heart. Grafts beat along with host muscle at rates of up to 240 beats per minute, the highest rate tested.

All the macaques that received the grafts showed transient arrhythmias—problems with the rate or rhythm of the heartbeat—that subsided by 4 weeks post-transplantation. The animals remained conscious and in no distress during periods of arrhythmia, but this problem will need to be addressed before the approach could be tested in humans.

"Before this study, it was not known if it is possible to produce sufficient numbers of these cells and successfully use them to remuscularize damaged hearts in a large animal whose heart size and physiology is similar to that of the human heart," Murry says.

While several obstacles still need to be addressed, these experiments support the idea that human cardiomyocyte transplantation therapy may be feasible.

Chapter 57

Rehabilitation after Heart Attack or Stroke

Chapter Contents

Section 57.1

Cardiac Rehabilitation

This section contains text excerpted from the following sources:
Text beginning with the heading "What Is Cardiac Rehabilitation?"
is excerpted from "Cardiac Rehabilitation," National Heart, Lung,
and Blood Institute (NHLBI), December 24, 2013; Text beginning
with the heading "Cardiac Rehabilitation Programs," is excerpted
from "Cardiac Rehabilitation Programs," Medicare.gov, Centers for
Medicare and Medicaid Services (CMS), January 7, 2015.

What Is Cardiac Rehabilitation?

Cardiac rehabilitation (rehab) is a medically supervised program
that helps improve the health and well-being of people who have heart
problems.

Rehab programs include exercise training, education on heart
healthy living, and counseling to reduce stress and help you return
to an active life.

Cardiac rehab can help you:

- Recover after a heart attack or heart surgery.

- Prevent future hospital stays, heart problems, and death related
  to heart problems.

- Address risk factors that can lead to coronary heart disease
  and other heart problems. These risk factors include high blood
  pressure, high blood cholesterol, overweight or obesity, diabetes, smoking, lack of physical activity, and depression and other
  emotional health concerns.

- Adopt healthy lifestyle changes. These changes may include following a heart healthy diet, being physically active, and learning
  how to manage stress.

- Improve your health and quality of life.

Your cardiac rehab program will be designed to meet your needs.

The Cardiac Rehabilitation Team

Cardiac rehab involves a long-term commitment from the patient and a team of healthcare providers.

The cardiac rehab team may include doctors (such as a family doctor, a heart specialist, and a surgeon), nurses, exercise specialists, physical and occupational therapists, dietitians or nutritionists, and psychologists or other mental health specialists. Sometimes a case manager will help track your care.

Working with the team is an important part of cardiac rehab. You should share questions and concerns with the team. This will help you reach your goals.

Who Needs Cardiac Rehabilitation?

People of all ages and ethnic backgrounds and both sexes can benefit from cardiac rehabilitation (rehab). Rehab can help people who have had:

- A heart attack
- Percutaneous coronary intervention (PCI), sometimes referred to as angioplasty for coronary heart disease
- Coronary artery bypass grafting for coronary heart disease
- Heart valve repair or replacement
- A heart transplant or a lung transplant
- Stable angina
- Heart failure

Cardiac rehab can improve your overall health and prevent future heart problems and even death.

What to Expect When Starting Cardiac Rehabilitation

Your doctor may refer you to cardiac rehabilitation (rehab) during an office visit or while you're in the hospital recovering from a heart attack or heart surgery. If your doctor doesn't mention it, ask him or her whether cardiac rehab might benefit you.

Rehab activities will vary depending on your condition. If you're recovering from major heart surgery, rehab will likely start with a member of the rehab team helping you sit up in a chair or take a few steps.

You'll work on range-of-motion exercises, such as moving your fingers, hands, arms, legs, and feet. Over time, you'll increase your activity level.

Once you leave the hospital, rehab will continue in a rehab center. The rehab center might be part of the hospital or located elsewhere.

Try to find a center close to home that offers services at a convenient time. If no centers are near your home, or if it's too hard to get to them, ask your doctor about home-based rehab.

For the first 2–3 months, you'll go to rehab regularly to learn how to reduce risk factors and start an exercise program. After that, your rehab team may recommend less frequent visits.

Overall, you may work with the rehab team for 3 months or longer. The length of time you continue cardiac rehab depends on your situation.

Health Assessment

Before you start cardiac rehab, your rehab team will assess your health. This includes taking your medical history and doing a physical exam and tests.

Medical History

A doctor or nurse will ask you about previous heart problems, heart surgery, and any heart-related symptoms you have. He or she also will ask whether you've had medical procedures or other health problems (such as diabetes or kidney disease).

The doctor or nurse may ask:

- Whether your family has a history of heart disease.

- What medicines you take, including over-the-counter medicines and dietary supplements (such as vitamins and herbal remedies). Describe how much, how often, and when you take each medicine.

- Whether you smoke and how much.

- How you check your blood sugar level, and how often you do it (if you have diabetes).

- Whether you've ever had hypoglycemia, which is low blood sugar. This condition can occur in people who take medicine to control their blood sugar levels.

Your answers to these questions will help your rehab team assess your quality of life and well-being

Physical Exam

A doctor or nurse will do a physical exam to check your overall health, including your heart rate, blood pressure, reflexes, and breathing.

Tests

Your doctor might recommend tests to check your heart.

An EKG (electrocardiogram) is a simple test that detects and records your heart's electrical activity. The test shows how fast your heart is beating and its rhythm (steady or irregular). An EKG also shows the strength and timing of electrical signals as they pass through your heart.

An exercise test on a treadmill or stationary bike is often done before starting cardiac rehab to measure your fitness level and determine whether you can handle an exercise program. Sometimes cardiac imaging tests may be ordered to provide additional information on your heart's structure and function.

You also might have tests to measure your cholesterol and blood sugar levels. If you have diabetes, staff will do an HbA1C test to check your blood sugar control. This test shows how well your diabetes has been managed over time.

What to Expect during Cardiac Rehabilitation

During cardiac rehabilitation (rehab), you'll learn how to:

- Increase your physical activity level and exercise safely

- Follow a heart healthy diet

- Reduce risk factors for future heart problems

- Improve your emotional health

Your rehab team will work with you to create a plan that meets your needs. Each part of cardiac rehab will help lower your risk for future heart problems.

Over time, the lifestyle changes you make during rehab will become routine. They will help you maintain a reduced risk for heart disease.

Support from your family can help make cardiac rehab easier. For example, family members can help you plan healthy meals and be physically active. The healthy lifestyle changes you learn during cardiac rehab can benefit your entire family.

Increase Physical Activity and Exercise Safely

Physical activity is an important part of a healthy lifestyle. It can strengthen your heart muscle, reduce your risk for heart disease, and improve your muscle strength, flexibility, and endurance.

Your rehab team will assess your physical activity level to learn how active you are at home, at work, and during recreation. If your job includes heavy labor, the team may recreate your workplace conditions to help you practice in a safe setting.

You'll work with the team to find ways to safely add physical activity to your daily routine. For example, you may decide to park farther from building entrances, walk up two or more flights of stairs, or walk for 15 minutes during your lunch break.

Your rehab team also will work with you to create a safe, easy-to-follow exercise plan. It will include a warmup, flexibility exercises, and cooling down.

Your plan also might include aerobic exercise and muscle-strengthening activities. Aerobic exercise is any exercise in which your heart beats harder and you use more oxygen than usual.

Typically, your rehab team will ask you to do aerobic exercise 3–5 days per week for 20–45 minutes. Examples of aerobic exercise are walking (outside or on a treadmill), cycling, rowing, or climbing stairs.

Your rehab team will likely ask you to do muscle-strengthening activities 2 or 3 days per week. Your exercise plan will list each exercise and how many times you should repeat it.

Examples of muscle-strengthening activities are lifting weights (hand weights, free weights, or weight machines), using a wall pulley, or using elastic bands to stretch and condition your muscles.

You're more likely to make exercise a habit if you enjoy the activity. Work with the rehab team to find the activities that you enjoy and that are safe for you. If you prefer to exercise with other people, join a group or ask a friend to join you.

Exercise training as part of cardiac rehab may not be safe for all patients. For example, if you have very high blood pressure or severe heart disease, you may not be ready for exercise training. Or, you may be able to handle only very light conditioning exercises. The rehab team will determine what level of exercise is safe for you.

Exercise at the Rehab Center and at Home

When you start cardiac rehab, you'll exercise at the rehab center. Members of your rehab team will carefully watch you to make sure you're exercising safely.

A team member will check your blood pressure several times during exercise training. You also might have an EKG (electrocardiogram) to check your heart's electrical activity during exercise. This test shows how fast your heart is beating and whether its rhythm is steady or irregular.

Your exercise program will change as your health improves. After awhile, you'll add at-home exercises to your plan.

Follow a Heart Healthy Diet

Your rehab team will help you create and follow a heart healthy diet. The diet will help you reach your rehab goals, which may include managing your weight, cholesterol levels, blood pressure, diabetes, kidney disease, heart failure, or other health problems that your diet can affect.

You'll learn how to plan meals that meet your calorie needs and are low in saturated and trans fats, cholesterol, and sodium (salt).

Your rehab team also may advise you to limit alcohol and other substances. Alcohol can raise your blood pressure and harm your liver, brain, and heart.

Reduce Risk Factors for Future Heart Problems

Your cardiac rehab team will work with you to control your risk factors for heart problems. Risk factors include high blood pressure, high blood cholesterol, overweight or obesity, diabetes, and smoking.

High Blood Pressure

Your rehab team will work with you to reach the blood pressure goal your doctor sets. This goal will depend on factors such as your age and whether you have heart failure, diabetes, or kidney disease.

Lifestyle changes, such as being physically active and following a heart healthy diet, can help you lower your blood pressure. If lifestyle changes aren't enough, your doctor may prescribe medicine to lower your blood pressure.

High Blood Cholesterol

Too much cholesterol in the blood is a risk factor for heart disease. Your rehab team will work with you to lower high blood cholesterol.

They may recommend lifestyle changes, such as following a heart healthy diet, losing weight, being physically active, quitting smoking, and limiting how much alcohol you drink. (Physical activity also can raise HDL cholesterol, which is the good type of cholesterol.)

Your doctor may prescribe medicine to lower your cholesterol if lifestyle changes aren't enough.

Overweight and Obesity

If you're overweight or obese, your rehab team will help you set short- and long-term weight-loss goals. You can reach these goals by following the diet and exercise plans that the team creates for you.

Diabetes

If you have diabetes, your rehab team will work with you to control your blood sugar level. Following a heart healthy diet, losing weight, and being physically active can lower your blood sugar level.

Your doctor may suggest that you test your blood sugar before and after exercising to watch for numbers that are too high or too low. Your doctors will tell you what numbers to look for.

Your doctor might prescribe medicine to lower your blood sugar level if lifestyle changes aren't enough.

Smoking

Smoking is a risk factor for heart disease. If you smoke, quitting can help you avoid future heart problems. Quitting can lower your blood pressure and keep your cholesterol levels healthy.

If you have trouble quitting smoking on your own, consider joining a support group. Many hospitals, workplaces, and community groups offer classes that help people quit smoking.

Improve Emotional Health

Psychological factors can increase the risk of developing heart disease or making it worse. Depression and anxiety are common among people who have heart disease or have had a heart attack or heart surgery.

If you feel sad, anxious, angry, or isolated, talk with your doctor. These feelings can affect your physical recovery. Depression is linked to complications such as irregular heartbeats, chest pain, a longer recovery time, the need to return to the hospital, and even an increased risk of death.

Treating emotional issues can improve your well-being and might lower your risk for a future heart attack or death. Treatment also may motivate you to exercise and help you relax and learn how to reduce stress.

The rehab team may include a mental health specialist. If not, someone from the team can refer you to one. Without help from a professional, these problems may not go away.

Some communities have support groups for people who have had heart attacks or heart surgery. They also may have walking groups or exercise classes. Help with basic needs and transportation also might be available.

Counseling for Sexual Dysfunction

People who have heart problems sometimes have sexual problems. The most common problem is less interest or no interest in sex. Impotence or premature or delayed ejaculation might occur in men.

Depression, medicines, fear of causing a heart attack, or diabetes can contribute to sexual problems.

Sexual activity often is safe for low-risk patients. The maximum heart rate during usual sexual activity is similar to other daily activities, such as walking up one or two flights of stairs.

Talk to your doctor if you're having sexual problems or to find out whether sexual activity is safe for you.

What Are the Benefits and Risks of Cardiac Rehabilitation?

Benefits

Cardiac rehabilitation (rehab) has many benefits. It can:

- Reduce your overall risk of dying, the risk of future heart problems, and the risk of dying from a heart attack

- Decrease pain and the need for medicines to treat heart or chest pain

- Lessen the chance that you'll have to go back to the hospital or emergency room for a heart problem

- Improve your overall health by reducing your risk factors for heart problems

- Improve your quality of life and make it easier for you to work, take part in social activities, and exercise

Going to cardiac rehab regularly also can reduce stress, improve your ability to move around, and help you stay independent.

People who get help for their emotional health and also start an exercise program can improve their overall health. They can lower their blood pressure and heart rate and control their cholesterol levels. These people are less likely to die or have another heart attack.

Treatment for emotional health also can help some people quit smoking.

Risks

The lifestyle changes that you make during cardiac rehab have few risks.

At first, physical activity is safer in the rehab setting than at home. Members of the rehab team are trained and have experience teaching people who have heart problems how to exercise.

Your rehab team will watch you to make sure you're safe. They'll check your blood pressure several times during your exercise training. They also may use an EKG (electrocardiogram) to see how your heart reacts and adapts to exercise. After some training, most people learn to exercise safely at home.

Very rarely, physical activity during rehab causes serious problems. These problems can include injuries to your muscles and bones or heart rhythm problems that can lead to a heart attack or death.

Your rehab team will tell you about signs and symptoms of possible problems to watch for while exercising at home. If you notice these signs and symptoms, you should stop the activity and contact your doctor.

Cardiac Rehabilitation Programs

How Often Is It Covered?

Medicare Part B (Medical Insurance) covers comprehensive cardiac rehabilitation (CR) programs that include exercise, education, and counseling. Part B also covers intensive cardiac rehabilitation (ICR) programs that, like regular CR programs, include exercise, education, and counseling. ICR programs are typically more rigorous or more intense that CR programs. These programs may be provided in a hospital outpatient setting (including a critical access hospital) or in a doctor's office.

Who's Eligible?

People with Part B are covered. You must be referred by your doctor and have had any of these:

- A heart attack in the last 12 months
- Coronary artery bypass surgery
- Current stable angina pectoris
- A heart valve repair or replacement
- A coronary angioplasty or coronary stent
- A heart or heart-lung transplant
- Stable chronic heart failure

Intensive Cardiac Rehabilitation (ICR) programs are also covered if your doctor orders it or if you have had any of the conditions listed above, with the exception of stable chronic heart failure, which applies only to CR programs.

Your Costs in Original Medicare

You pay 20% of the Medicare-approved amount if you get the services in a doctor's office. In a hospital outpatient setting, you pay the hospital a copayment. The Part B deductible applies.

Section 57.2

Stroke Rehabilitation

This section contains text excerpted from the following sources:
Text beginning with the heading "What Is Stroke Rehabilitation?"
is excerpted from "Stroke Rehabilitation Information," National
Institute of Neurological Disorders and Stroke (NINDS), March 29,
2016; Text beginning with the heading "Post-Stroke Rehabilitation"
is excerpted from "Post-Stroke Rehabilitation," National Institute of
Neurological Disorders and Stroke (NINDS), September 2014.

What Is Stroke Rehabilitation?

Stroke is the third leading cause of death and the leading cause
of long-term disability in the United States. There are approximately 4 million Americans living with the effects of stroke. In
addition, there are millions of husbands, wives, children and friends
who care for stroke survivors and whose own lives are personally
affected.

According to the National Stroke Association:

- 10% of stroke survivors recover almost completely

- 25% recover with minor impairments

- 40% experience moderate to severe impairments that require
  special care

- 10% require care in a nursing home or other long-term facility

- 15% die shortly after the stroke

- Approximately 14% of stroke survivors experience a second
  stroke in the first year following a stroke.

Successful rehabilitation depends on:

- Amount of damage to the brain

- Skill on the part of the rehabilitation team

- Cooperation of family and friends. Caring family/friends can be
  one of the most important factors in rehabilitation

- Timing of rehabilitation—the earlier it begins the more likely survivors are to regain lost abilities and skills

The goal of rehabilitation is to enable an individual who has experienced a stroke to reach the highest possible level of independence and be as productive as possible. Because stroke survivors often have complex rehabilitation needs, progress and recovery are unique for each person. Although a majority of functional abilities may be restored soon after a stroke, recovery is an ongoing process.

Effects of a Stroke

1. Weakness (hemiparesis) or paralysis (hemiplegia) on one side of the body that may affect the whole side or just the arm or leg. The weakness or paralysis is on the side of the body opposite the side of the brain affected by the stroke.

2. Spasticity, stiffness in muscles, painful muscle spasms

3. Problems with balance and/or coordination

4. Problems using language, including having difficulty understanding speech or writing (aphasia); and knowing the right words but having trouble saying them clearly (dysarthria)

5. Being unaware of or ignoring sensations on one side of the body (bodily neglect or inattention)

6. Pain, numbness or odd sensations

7. Problems with memory, thinking, attention or learning

8. Being unaware of the effects of a stroke

9. Trouble swallowing (dysphagia)

10. Problems with bowel or bladder control

11. Fatigue

12. Difficulty controlling emotions (emotional lability)

13. Depression

14. Difficulties with daily tasks

Types of Rehabilitation Programs

- Hospital programs: in an acute care facility or a rehabilitation hospital

- Long-term care facility with therapy and skilled nursing care
- Outpatient programs
- Home-based programs

Rehabilitation Specialists

- **Physicians:** physiatrists (specialists in physical medicine and rehabilitation), neurologists, internists, geriatricians (specialists in the elderly), family practice
- **Rehabilitation nurses:** specialize in nursing care for people with disabilities
- **Physical therapists:** help to restore physical functioning by evaluating and treating problems with movement, balance, and coordination
- **Occupational therapists:** provide exercises and practice to help patient perform activities of daily living.
- **Speech-language pathologists:** to help improve language skills
- **Social workers:** assist with financial decisions and plan the return to the home or a new living place
- **Psychologists:** concerned with the mental and emotional health of patients
- **Therapeutic recreation specialists:** help patients return to activities they enjoyed before the stroke.

Preventing Another Stroke

- People who have had a stroke are at an increased risk of having another one, especially during the first year following the original stroke.
- The following factors increase the risk of having another stroke:
- High blood pressure (hypertension)
- Cigarette smoking
- Diabetes
- Having had a TIA (transient ischemic attack)

- Heart disease

- Older age

- High cholesterol

- Obesity

- Sedentary lifestyle

Although some risk factors for stroke cannot be changed (e.g. age) others such as high blood pressure and smoking can be altered. Patients and families should seek guidance from their physician about lifestyle changes to help prevent another stroke.

Post-Stroke Rehabilitation

In the United States, more than 700,000 people suffer a stroke* each year, and approximately two-thirds of these individuals survive and require rehabilitation. The goals of rehabilitation are to help survivors become as independent as possible and to attain the best possible quality of life. Even though rehabilitation does not "cure" the effects of stroke in that it does not reverse brain damage, rehabilitation can substantially help people achieve the best possible long-term outcome.

An ischemic stroke or "brain attack" occurs when brain cells die because of inadequate blood flow. When blood flow is interrupted, brain cells are robbed of vital supplies of oxygen and nutrients. About 80 percent of strokes are caused by the blockage of an artery in the neck or brain. A hemorrhagic stroke is caused by a burst blood vessel in the brain that causes bleeding into or around the brain.

What Is Post-Stroke Rehabilitation?

Rehabilitation helps stroke survivors relearn skills that are lost when part of the brain is damaged. For example, these skills can include coordinating leg movements in order to walk or carrying out the steps involved in any complex activity. Rehabilitation also teaches survivors new ways of performing tasks to circumvent or compensate for any residual disabilities. Individuals may need to learn how to bathe and dress using only one hand, or how to communicate effectively when their ability to use language has been compromised. There is a strong consensus among rehabilitation experts that the most important element in any rehabilitation program is carefully directed, well-focused, repetitive practice—the same kind of practice used by all people when they learn a new skill, such as playing the piano or pitching a baseball.

Rehabilitative therapy begins in the acute-care hospital after the person's overall condition has been stabilized, often within 24 to 48 hours after the stroke. The first steps involve promoting independent movement because many individuals are paralyzed or seriously weakened. Patients are prompted to change positions frequently while lying in bed and to engage in passive or active range of motion exercises to strengthen their stroke-impaired limbs. ("Passive" range-of-motion exercises are those in which the therapist actively helps the patient move a limb repeatedly, whereas "active" exercises are performed by the patient with no physical assistance from the therapist.) Depending on many factors—including the extent of the initial injury—patients may progress from sitting up and being moved between the bed and a chair to standing, bearing their own weight, and walking, with or without assistance. Rehabilitation nurses and therapists help patients who are able to perform progressively more complex and demanding tasks, such as bathing, dressing, and using a toilet, and they encourage patients to begin using their stroke-impaired limbs while engaging in those tasks. Beginning to reacquire the ability to carry out these basic activities of daily living represents the first stage in a stroke survivor's return to independence.

For some stroke survivors, rehabilitation will be an ongoing process to maintain and refine skills and could involve working with specialists for months or years after the stroke.

What Disabilities Can Result from a Stroke?

The types and degrees of disability that follow a stroke depend upon which area of the brain is damaged. Generally, stroke can cause five types of disabilities: paralysis or problems controlling movement; sensory disturbances including pain; problems using or understanding language; problems with thinking and memory; and emotional disturbances.

Paralysis or Problems Controlling Movement (Motor Control)

Paralysis is one of the most common disabilities resulting from stroke. The paralysis is usually on the side of the body opposite the side of the brain damaged by stroke, and may affect the face, an arm, a leg, or the entire side of the body. This one-sided paralysis is called hemiplegia (one-sided weakness is called hemiparesis). Stroke patients with hemiparesis or hemiplegia may have difficulty with everyday activities such as walking or grasping objects. Some stroke patients have problems with swallowing, called dysphagia, due to damage to the part of the brain that controls the muscles for swallowing. Damage to a lower part of the brain, the cerebellum, can affect the body's ability to coordinate movement, a disability called ataxia, leading to problems with body posture, walking, and balance.

Sensory Disturbances including Pain

Stroke patients may lose the ability to feel touch, pain, temperature, or position. Sensory deficits also may hinder the ability to recognize objects that patients are holding and can even be severe enough to cause loss of recognition of one's own limb. Some stroke patients experience pain, numbness or odd sensations of tingling or prickling in paralyzed or weakened limbs, a symptom known as paresthesias.

The loss of urinary continence is fairly common immediately after a stroke and often results from a combination of sensory and motor deficits. Stroke survivors may lose the ability to sense the need to urinate or the ability to control bladder muscles. Some may lack enough mobility to reach a toilet in time. Loss of bowel control or constipation also may occur. Permanent incontinence after a stroke is uncommon, but even a temporary loss of bowel or bladder control can be emotionally difficult for stroke survivors.

Stroke survivors frequently have a variety of chronic pain syndromes resulting from stroke-induced damage to the nervous system (neuropathic pain). In some stroke patients, pathways for sensation in the brain are damaged, causing the transmission of false signals that result in the sensation of pain in a limb or side of the body that has the sensory deficit. The most common of these pain syndromes is called "thalamic pain syndrome" (caused by a stroke to the thalamus, which processes sensory information from the body to the brain), which can be difficult to treat even with medications. Finally, some pain that occurs after stroke is not due to nervous system damage, but rather to mechanical problems caused by the weakness from the stroke. Patients who have a seriously weakened or paralyzed arm commonly experience moderate to severe pain that radiates outward from the shoulder. Most often, the pain results from lack of movement in a joint that has been immobilized for a prolonged period of time (such as having your arm or shoulder in a cast for weeks) and the tendons and ligaments around the joint become fixed in one position. This is commonly called a "frozen" joint; "passive" movement (the joint is gently moved or flexed by a therapist or caregiver rather than by the individual) at the joint in a paralyzed limb is essential to prevent painful "freezing" and to allow easy movement if and when voluntary motor strength returns.

Problems Using or Understanding Language (Aphasia)

At least one-fourth of all stroke survivors experience language impairments, involving the ability to speak, write, and understand spoken and written language. A stroke-induced injury to any of the brain's language-control centers can severely impair verbal communication. The dominant centers for language are in the left side of the brain for right-handed individuals and many left-handers as well. Damage to a language center located on the dominant side of the brain, known as Broca's area, causes expressive aphasia. People with this type of aphasia have difficulty conveying their thoughts through words or writing. They lose the ability to speak the words they are thinking and to put words together in coherent, grammatically correct sentences. In contrast, damage to a language center located in a rear portion of the brain, called Wernicke's area, results in receptive aphasia. People with this condition have difficulty understanding spoken or written language and often have incoherent speech. Although they can form grammatically correct sentences, their utterances are often devoid of meaning. The most severe form of aphasia, global aphasia, is caused by extensive damage to several areas of the brain involved in language function. People with global aphasia lose nearly all their linguistic abilities; they cannot understand language or use it to convey thought.

Problems with Thinking and Memory

Stroke can cause damage to parts of the brain responsible for memory, learning, and awareness. Stroke survivors may have dramatically shortened attention spans or may experience deficits in short-term memory. Individuals also may lose their ability to make plans, comprehend meaning, learn new tasks, or engage in other complex mental activities. Two fairly common deficits resulting from stroke are anosognosia, an inability to acknowledge the reality of the physical impairments resulting from stroke, and neglect, the loss of the ability to respond to objects or sensory stimuli located on the stroke-impaired side. Stroke survivors who develop apraxia (loss of ability to carry out a learned purposeful movement) cannot plan the steps involved in a complex task and act on them in the proper sequence. Stroke survivors with apraxia also may have problems following a set of instructions. Apraxia appears to be caused by a disruption of the subtle connections that exist between thought and action.

Emotional Disturbances

Many people who survive a stroke feel fear, anxiety, frustration, anger, sadness, and a sense of grief for their physical and mental losses. These feelings are a natural response to the psychological trauma of stroke. Some emotional disturbances and personality changes are caused by the physical effects of brain damage. Clinical depression, which is a sense of hopelessness that disrupts an individual's ability to function, appears to be the emotional disorder most commonly experienced by stroke survivors. Signs of clinical depression include sleep disturbances, a radical change in eating patterns that may lead to sudden weight loss or gain, lethargy, social withdrawal, irritability, fatigue, self-loathing, and suicidal thoughts. Post-stroke depression can be treated with antidepressant medications and psychological counseling.

What Medical Professionals Specialize in Post-Stroke Rehabilitation?

Post-stroke rehabilitation involves physicians; rehabilitation nurses; physical, occupational, recreational, speech-language, and vocational therapists; and mental health professionals.

Physicians

Physicians have the primary responsibility for managing and coordinating the long-term care of stroke survivors, including recommending which rehabilitation programs will best address individual needs. Physicians also are responsible for caring for the stroke survivor's general health and providing guidance aimed at preventing a second stroke, such as controlling high blood pressure or diabetes and eliminating risk factors such as cigarette smoking, excessive weight, a high-cholesterol diet, and high alcohol consumption.

Neurologists usually lead acute-care stroke teams and direct patient care during hospitalization. They sometimes participate on the long-term rehabilitation team. Other subspecialists often lead the rehabilitation stage of care, especially physiatrists, who specialize in physical medicine and rehabilitation.

Rehabilitation Nurses

Nurses specializing in rehabilitation help survivors relearn how to carry out the basic activities of daily living. They also educate survivors about routine healthcare, such as how to follow a medication schedule, how to care for the skin, how to move out of a bed and into a wheelchair, and special needs for people with diabetes. Rehabilitation nurses also work with survivors to reduce risk factors that may lead to a second stroke, and provide training for caregivers.

Nurses are closely involved in helping stroke survivors manage personal care issues, such as bathing and controlling incontinence. Most stroke survivors regain their ability to maintain continence, often with the help of strategies learned during rehabilitation. These strategies include strengthening pelvic muscles through special exercises and following a timed voiding schedule. If problems with incontinence continue, nurses can help caregivers learn to insert and manage catheters and to take special hygienic measures to prevent other incontinence-related health problems from developing.

Physical Therapists

Physical therapists specialize in treating disabilities related to motor and sensory impairments. They are trained in all aspects of anatomy and physiology related to normal function, with an emphasis on movement. They assess the stroke survivor's strength, endurance, range of motion, gait abnormalities, and sensory deficits to design individualized rehabilitation programs aimed at regaining control over motor functions.

Physical therapists help survivors regain the use of stroke-impaired limbs, teach compensatory strategies to reduce the effect of remaining deficits, and establish ongoing exercise programs to help people retain their newly learned skills. Disabled people tend to avoid using impaired limbs, a behavior called learned non-use. However, the repetitive use of impaired limbs encourages brain plasticity** and helps reduce disabilities.

Strategies used by physical therapists to encourage the use of impaired limbs include selective sensory stimulation such as tapping or stroking, active and passive range-of-motion exercises, and temporary restraint of healthy limbs while practicing motor tasks.

In general, physical therapy emphasizes practicing isolated movements, repeatedly changing from one kind of movement to another, and rehearsing complex movements that require a great deal of coordination and balance, such as walking up or down stairs or moving safely between obstacles. People too weak to bear their own weight can still practice repetitive movements during hydrotherapy (in which water provides sensory stimulation as well as weight support) or while being partially supported by a harness. A recent trend in physical therapy emphasizes the effectiveness of engaging in goal-directed activities, such as playing games, to promote coordination. Physical therapists frequently employ selective sensory stimulation to encourage use of impaired limbs and to help survivors with neglect regain awareness of stimuli on the neglected side of the body.

**Functions compromised when a specific region of the brain is damaged by stroke can sometimes be taken over by other parts of the brain. This ability to adapt and change is known as neuroplasticity.

Occupational and Recreational Therapists

Like physical therapists, occupational therapists are concerned with improving motor and sensory abilities, and ensuring patient safety in the post-stroke period. They help survivors relearn skills needed for performing self-directed activities (also called occupations) such as personal grooming, preparing meals, and housecleaning. Therapists can teach some survivors how to adapt to driving and provide on-road training. They often teach people to divide a complex activity into its component parts, practice each part, and then perform the whole sequence of actions. This strategy can improve coordination and may help people with apraxia relearn how to carry out planned actions.

Occupational therapists also teach people how to develop compensatory strategies and change elements of their environment that limit activities of daily living. For example, people with the use of only one hand can substitute hook and loop fasteners (such as Velcro) for buttons on clothing. Occupational therapists also help people make changes in their homes to increase safety, remove barriers, and facilitate physical functioning, such as installing grab bars in bathrooms.

Recreational therapists help people with a variety of disabilities to develop and use their leisure time to enhance their health, independence, and quality of life.

Speech-Language Pathologists

Speech-language pathologists help stroke survivors with aphasia relearn how to use language or develop alternative means of communication. They also help people improve their ability to swallow, and they work with patients to develop problem-solving and social skills needed to cope with the after-effects of a stroke.

Many specialized therapeutic techniques have been developed to assist people with aphasia. Some forms of short-term therapy can improve comprehension rapidly. Intensive exercises such as repeating the therapist's words, practicing following directions, and doing reading or writing exercises form the cornerstone of language rehabilitation. Conversational coaching and rehearsal, as well as the development of prompts or cues to help people remember specific words, are sometimes beneficial. Speech-language pathologists also help stroke survivors develop strategies for circumventing language disabilities. These strategies can include the use of symbol boards or sign language. Recent advances in computer technology have spurred the development of new types of equipment to enhance communication.

Speech-language pathologists use special types of imaging techniques to study swallowing patterns of stroke survivors and identify the exact source of their impairment. Difficulties with swallowing have many possible causes, including a delayed swallowing reflex, an inability to manipulate food with the tongue, or an inability to detect food remaining lodged in the cheeks after swallowing. When the cause has been pinpointed, speech-language pathologists work with the individual to devise strategies to overcome or minimize the deficit. Sometimes, simply changing body position and improving posture during eating can bring about improvement. The texture of foods can be modified to make swallowing easier; for example, thin liquids, which often cause choking, can be thickened. Changing eating habits by taking small bites and chewing slowly can also help alleviate dysphagia.

Vocational Therapists

Approximately one-fourth of all strokes occur in people between the ages of 45 and 65. For most people in this age group, returning to work is a major concern. Vocational therapists perform many of the same functions that ordinary career counselors do. They can help people with residual disabilities identify vocational strengths and develop résumés that highlight those strengths. They also can help identify potential employers, assist in specific job searches, and provide referrals to stroke vocational rehabilitation agencies.

Most important, vocational therapists educate disabled individuals about their rights and protections as defined by the Americans with Disabilities Act of 1990. This law requires employers to make "reasonable accommodations" for disabled employees. Vocational therapists frequently act as mediators between employers and employees to negotiate the provision of reasonable accommodations in the workplace.

When Can a Stroke Patient Begin Rehabilitation?

Rehabilitation should begin as soon as a stroke patient is stable, sometimes within 24 to 48 hours after a stroke. This first stage of rehabilitation can occur within an acute-care hospital; however, it is very dependent on the unique circumstances of the individual patient.

Recently, in the largest stroke rehabilitation study in the United States, researchers compared two common techniques to help stroke patients improve their walking. Both methods—training on a body-weight supported treadmill or working on strength and balance exercises at home with a physical therapist—resulted in equal improvements in the individual's ability to walk by the end of one year. Researchers found that functional improvements could be seen as late as one year after the stroke, which goes against the conventional wisdom that most recovery is complete by 6 months. The trial showed that 52 percent of the participants made significant improvements in walking, everyday function and quality of life, regardless of how severe their impairment was, or whether they started the training at 2 or 6 months after the stroke.

Where Can a Stroke Patient Get Rehabilitation?

At the time of discharge from the hospital, the stroke patient and family coordinate with hospital social workers to locate a suitable living arrangement. Many stroke survivors return home, but some move into some type of medical facility.

Inpatient Rehabilitation Units

Inpatient facilities may be freestanding or part of larger hospital complexes. Patients stay in the facility, usually for 2 to 3 weeks, and engage in a coordinated, intensive program of rehabilitation. Such programs often involve at least 3 hours of active therapy a day, 5 or 6 days a week. Inpatient facilities offer a comprehensive range of medical services, including full-time physician supervision and access to the full range of therapists specializing in post-stroke rehabilitation.

Outpatient Units

Outpatient facilities are often part of a larger hospital complex and provide access to physicians and the full range of therapists specializing in stroke rehabilitation. Patients typically spend several hours, often 3 days each week, at the facility taking part in coordinated therapy sessions and return home at night. Comprehensive outpatient facilities frequently offer treatment programs as intense as those of inpatient facilities, but they also can offer less demanding regimens, depending on the patient's physical capacity.

Nursing Facilities

Rehabilitative services available at nursing facilities are more variable than are those at inpatient and outpatient units. Skilled nursing facilities usually place a greater emphasis on rehabilitation, whereas traditional nursing homes emphasize residential care. In addition, fewer hours of therapy are offered compared to outpatient and inpatient rehabilitation units.

Home-Based Rehabilitation Programs

Home rehabilitation allows for great flexibility so that patients can tailor their program of rehabilitation and follow individual schedules. Stroke survivors may participate in an intensive level of therapy several hours per week or follow a less demanding regimen. These arrangements are often best suited for people who require treatment by only one type of rehabilitation therapist. Patients dependent on Medicare coverage for their rehabilitation must meet Medicare's "homebound" requirements to qualify for such services; at this time lack of transportation is not a valid reason for home therapy. The major disadvantage of home-based rehabilitation programs is the lack of specialized equipment. However, undergoing treatment at home gives people the advantage of practicing skills and developing compensatory strategies in the context of their own living environment. In the recent stroke rehabilitation trial, intensive balance and strength rehabilitation in the home was equivalent to treadmill training at a rehabilitation facility in improving walking.

Part Seven

Preventing Cardiovascular Disorders

Chapter 58

Reduce Heart Health Risks

Know Your Numbers

Cardiovascular disease is the number one cause of death across the globe, according to the World Health Organization (WHO). The good news is that your risk for heart disease can often be reduced with preventative screenings and by modifying your diet, weight, physical activity level, and/or tobacco and alcohol use.

Be Good to Your Heart

Here are six things you can do today to improve your heart health:

1. Eat more fruits and vegetables

2. Exercise regularly

3. Manage stress with relaxation techniques, positive thinking, and enjoyable activities

4. Skip the salt

5. Limit alcohol consumption

6. Quit smoking

This chapter includes text excerpted from "Drawing a Blank? Knowing Your Health Numbers Can Reduce Heart Health Risks," Federal Occupational Health (FOH), February 2, 2016.

Numbers to Live By

The Centers for Disease Control and Prevention (CDC) recommends tracking your body mass index (BMI), blood pressure, blood sugar levels, cholesterol, and physical activity to know where you stand regarding your risk for heart disease, high blood pressure (or hypertension), diabetes, and other medical disorders.

Body Mass Index

BMI numbers can provide the average person a good idea of his or her overall health status. You can use the BMI calculator to the right to find out your index, as a ratio of your height and weight.

Blood Pressure

Blood pressure is the force of blood against the heart. It can be a quick and easy measure of your heart and vascular health. Knowing these numbers can be a lifesaver. Systolic pressure is the measure of pressure when the heart beats. It's usually the higher number. Diastolic is the measure of the pressure when the heart is relaxed. Check your blood pressure at least every two years—more often, depending on your healthcare provider's recommendations—because high blood pressure usually has no symptoms.

Table 58.1. Systolic and Diastolic Pressure

	Systolic	Diastolic
Desirable	less than 120 mmHG	less than 80 mmHG
At risk (pre-hypertension)	120-139 mmHG	80-89 mmHG
High	140 mmHG or higher	90 mmHG or higher

Cholesterol and Other Blood Lipids

Cholesterol is a waxy substance produced by your liver transported to and from cells by lipoproteins. Some types of cholesterol can facilitate healthy blood flow, while other types can start building up on the walls of your blood vessels and restrict the flow of blood to your heart and other organs.

Your cholesterol levels are another important indicator of heart health. A simple blood test can measure the different amounts of cholesterol and triglycerides in your blood. Your healthcare provider can then determine what steps should be taken to lower them, if they're elevated.

Table 58.2. Desirable Amounts of Cholesterol and Triglycerides in Blood

	Desirable Levels
Total cholesterol	Less than 200 mg/dL
LDL ("bad" cholesterol)	Less than 100 mg/dL
HDL ("good" cholesterol)	60 mg/dL or higher
Triglycerides	Less than 150 mg/dL

Blood Sugar

A test of your blood sugar levels after going eight hours or more without eating (a fasting glucose test) can give your healthcare provider an idea if you're at risk for diabetes or may already be showing signs of the disease. Simply losing 5 to 7 percent of your total body weight and eating healthier can often help you delay or possibly prevent type 2 diabetes if you are at risk for the disease. Uncontrolled diabetes can raise your risk for heart disease.

Table 58.3. Blood Sugar Levels and Diabetes

Desirable	99 mg/dL or lower
At risk (pre-diabetes)	100 to 125
Diabetes	126 or above

Get the Pulse on Your Health

The wellness profile (or HRA) is a short survey—about 20 minutes—that you can take to review your daily lifestyle practices. Combined with results from your blood screening, it will help map out potential health risks, including those affecting your heart. This information can empower you to take a more active role in your health and lower your risk of heart disease.

Unlock a Healthier You

Lower your risk for heart disease by:

Being More Active

A good place to start is with at least 30 minutes a day of moderately intense physical activity, such as taking a long, brisk walk. This can be broken down into smaller segments (for example, three segments of ten minutes each) as long as they add up to 30 minutes or more per day. Find some physical activity that you enjoy, so that you'll look forward to exercising and can reap the many health benefits of "getting physical."

Achieving and Maintaining a Healthy Weight

Use the body mass index (BMI) calculator to get your BMI. The desirable BMI range for the average person is between 18.5 and 24.9. If your BMI is above 25, start taking steps to lose weight today.

Not Smoking

Smoking is one of the single greatest health risk factors for heart disease. Quitting is not easy, but there are many smoking cessation programs available. Your agency may provide free one-on-one support to help you quit.

Limiting Alcohol Consumption

If you drink alcohol, do so in moderation. A general rule of thumb for better health is to limit yourself to one drink or fewer per day if you're a woman and two drinks or fewer per day if you're a man.

In some cases, making these simple lifestyle changes may not be enough to significantly lower the risk for heart disease, so be sure to also talk with your healthcare provider.

Start Now

Now is the best time to start making positive changes to lower your risk for heart disease. Often, all it takes are some simple—and consistent—lifestyle tweaks. Enjoy your new life and share your secrets with others to encourage them to stay healthy, too.

Chapter 59

Controlling High Blood Pressure

How Is High Blood Pressure Treated?

Based on your diagnosis, healthcare providers develop treatment plans for high blood pressure that include lifelong lifestyle changes and medicines to control high blood pressure; lifestyle changes such as weight loss can be highly effective in treating high blood pressure.

Treatment Plans

Healthcare providers work with you to develop a treatment plan based on whether you were diagnosed with primary or secondary high blood pressure and if there is a suspected or known cause. Treatment plans may evolve until blood pressure control is achieved.

If your healthcare provider diagnoses you with secondary high blood pressure, he or she will work to treat the other condition or change the medicine suspected of causing your high blood pressure. If high blood pressure persists or is first diagnosed as primary high blood pressure, your treatment plan will include lifestyle changes. When lifestyle changes alone do not control or lower blood pressure, your healthcare provider may change or update your treatment plan

This chapter includes text excerpted from "High Blood Pressure," National Heart, Lung, and Blood Institute (NHLBI), September 10, 2015.

657

by prescribing medicines to treat the disease. Healthcare providers prescribe children and teens medicines at special doses that are safe and effective in children.

If your healthcare provider prescribes medicines as a part of your treatment plan, keep up your healthy lifestyle habits. The combination of the medicines and the healthy lifestyle habits helps control and lower your high blood pressure.

Some people develop "resistant" or uncontrolled high blood pressure. This can happen when the medications they are taking do not work well for them or another medical condition is leading to uncontrolled blood pressure. Healthcare providers treat resistant or uncontrolled high blood pressure with an intensive treatment plan that can include a different set of blood pressure medications or other special treatments.

To achieve the best control of your blood pressure, follow your treatment plan and take all medications as prescribed. Following your prescribed treatment plan is important because it can prevent or delay complications that high blood pressure can cause and can lower your risk for other related problems.

Healthy Lifestyle Changes

Healthy lifestyle habits can help you control high blood pressure. These habits include:

- Healthy eating
- Being physically active
- Maintaining a healthy weight
- Limiting alcohol intake
- Managing and coping with stress

To help make lifelong lifestyle changes, try making one healthy lifestyle change at a time and add another change when you feel that you have successfully adopted the earlier changes. When you practice several healthy lifestyle habits, you are more likely to lower your blood pressure and maintain normal blood pressure readings.

Healthy Eating

To help treat high blood pressure, healthcare providers recommend that you limit sodium and salt intake, increase potassium, and eat foods that are heart healthy.

Limiting Sodium and Salt

A low-sodium diet can help you manage your blood pressure. You should try to limit the amount of sodium that you eat. This means choosing and preparing foods that are lower in salt and sodium. Try to use low-sodium and "no added salt" foods and seasonings at the table or while cooking. Food labels tell you what you need to know about choosing foods that are lower in sodium. Try to eat no more than 2,300 mg sodium a day. If you have high blood pressure, you may need to restrict your sodium intake even more.

Your healthcare provider may recommend the Dietary Approaches to Stop Hypertension (DASH) eating plan if you have high blood pressure. The DASH eating plan focuses on fruits, vegetables, whole grains, and other foods that are heart healthy and low in fat, cholesterol, and salt.

The DASH eating plan is a good heart-healthy eating plan, even for those who don't have high blood pressure.

Heart-Healthy Eating

Your healthcare provider also may recommend heart-healthy eating, which should include:

- Whole grains
- Fruits, such as apples, bananas, oranges, pears, and prunes
- Vegetables, such as broccoli, cabbage, and carrots
- Legumes, such as kidney beans, lentils, chick peas, black-eyed peas, and lima beans
- Fat-free or low-fat dairy products, such as skim milk
- Fish high in omega-3 fatty acids, such as salmon, tuna, and trout, about twice a week

When following a heart-healthy diet, you should avoid eating:

- A lot of red meat
- Palm and coconut oils
- Sugary foods and beverages

Being Physically Active

Routine physical activity can lower high blood pressure and reduce your risk for other health problems. Talk with your healthcare provider

659

before you start a new exercise plan. Ask him or her how much and what kinds of physical activity are safe for you.

Everyone should try to participate in moderate-intensity aerobic exercise at least 2 hours and 30 minutes per week, or vigorous-intensity aerobic exercise for 1 hour and 15 minutes per week. Aerobic exercise, such as brisk walking, is any exercise in which your heart beats harder and you use more oxygen than usual. The more active you are, the more you will benefit. Participate in aerobic exercise for at least 10 minutes at a time, spread throughout the week.

Maintaining a Healthy Weight

Maintaining a healthy weight can help you control high blood pressure and reduce your risk for other health problems. If you're overweight or obese, try to lose weight. A loss of just 3 to 5 percent can lower your risk for health problems. Greater amounts of weight loss can improve blood pressure readings, lower LDL cholesterol, and increase HDL cholesterol. However, research shows that no matter your weight, it is important to control high blood pressure to maintain good health.

A useful measure of overweight and obesity is body mass index (BMI). BMI measures your weight in relation to your height. A BMI:

- Below 18.5 is a sign that you are underweight.

- Between 18.5 and 24.9 is in the healthy range.

- Between 25 and 29.9 is considered overweight.

- Of 30 or more is considered obese.

A general goal to aim for is a BMI below 25. Your healthcare provider can help you set an appropriate BMI goal.

Measuring waist circumference helps screen for possible health risks. If most of your fat is around your waist rather than at your hips, you're at a higher risk for heart disease and type 2 diabetes. This risk may be high with a waist size that is greater than 35 inches for women or greater than 40 inches for men.

Limiting Alcohol Intake

Limit alcohol intake. Too much alcohol will raise your blood pressure and triglyceride levels, a type of fat found in the blood. Alcohol also adds extra calories, which may cause weight gain.

Men should have no more than two drinks containing alcohol a day. Women should have no more than one drink containing alcohol a day. One drink is:

- 12 ounces of beer

- 5 ounces of wine

- 1½ ounces of liquor

Managing and Coping With Stress

Learning how to manage stress, relax, and cope with problems can improve your emotional and physical health and can lower high blood pressure. Stress management techniques include:

- Being physically active

- Listening to music or focusing on something calm or peaceful

- Performing yoga or tai chi

- Meditating

Medicines

Blood pressure medicines work in different ways to stop or slow some of the body's functions that cause high blood pressure. Medicines to lower blood pressure include:

- **Diuretics (Water or Fluid Pills):** Flush excess sodium from your body, which reduces the amount of fluid in your blood and helps to lower your blood pressure. Diuretics are often used with other high blood pressure medicines, sometimes in one combined pill.

- **Beta Blockers:** Help your heart beat slower and with less force. As a result, your heart pumps less blood through your blood vessels, which can help to lower your blood pressure.

- **Angiotensin-Converting Enzyme (ACE) Inhibitors:** Angiotensin-II is a hormone that narrows blood vessels, increasing blood pressure. ACE converts Angiotensin I to Angiotensin II. ACE inhibitors block this process, which stops the production of Angiotensin II, lowering blood pressure.

- **Angiotensin II Receptor Blockers (ARBs):** Block angiotensin II hormone from binding with receptors in the blood vessels.

When angiotensin II is blocked, the blood vessels do not constrict or narrow, which can lower your blood pressure.

- **Calcium Channel Blockers:** Keep calcium from entering the muscle cells of your heart and blood vessels. This allows blood vessels to relax, which can lower your blood pressure.

- **Alpha Blockers:** Reduce nerve impulses that tighten blood vessels. This allows blood to flow more freely, causing blood pressure to go down.

- **Alpha-Beta Blockers:** Reduce nerve impulses the same way alpha blockers do. However, like beta blockers, they also slow the heartbeat. As a result, blood pressure goes down.

- **Central Acting Agents:** Act in the brain to decrease nerve signals that narrow blood vessels, which can lower blood pressure.

- **Vasodilators:** Relax the muscles in blood vessel walls, which can lower blood pressure.

To lower and control blood pressure, many people take two or more medicines. If you have side effects from your medicines, don't stop taking your medicines. Instead, talk with your healthcare provider about the side effects to see if the dose can be changed or a new medicine prescribed.

Future Treatments

Scientists, doctors, and researchers continue to study the changes that cause high blood pressure, to develop new medicines and treatments to control high blood pressure. Possible future treatments under investigation include new combination medicines, vaccines, and interventions aimed at the sympathetic nervous system, such as kidney nerve ablation.

Chapter 60

Controlling High Cholesterol

How Is High Blood Cholesterol Treated?

High blood cholesterol is treated with lifestyle changes and medi-cines. The main goal of treatment is to lower your low-density lipopro-tein (LDL) cholesterol level enough to reduce your risk for coronary heart disease, heart attack, and other related health problems.

Your risk for heart disease and heart attack goes up as your LDL cholesterol level rises and your number of heart disease risk factors increases.

Some people are at high risk for heart attacks because they already have heart disease. Other people are at high risk for heart disease because they have diabetes or more than one heart disease risk factor.

Talk with your doctor about lowering your cholesterol and your risk for heart disease. Also, check the list to find out whether you have risk factors that affect your LDL cholesterol goal:

- Cigarette smoking

- High blood pressure (140/90 mmHg or higher), or you're on med-icine to treat high blood pressure

- Low high-density lipoprotein (HDL) cholesterol (less than 40 mg/dL)

This chapter includes text excerpted from "High Blood Cholesterol," National Heart, Lung, and Blood Institute (NHLBI), March 30, 2016.

- Family history of early heart disease (heart disease in father or brother before age 55; heart disease in mother or sister before age 65)

- Age (men 45 years or older; women 55 years or older)

Based on your medical history, number of risk factors, and risk score, figure out your risk of getting heart disease or having a heart attack using the table below.

Table 60.1. Risk of Getting Heart Disease or Having a Heart Attack

If You Have	You Are in Category	Your LDL Goal Is
Heart disease, diabetes, or a risk score higher than 20%	I. High risk*	Less than 100 mg/dL
Two or more risk factors and a risk score of 10–20%	II. Moderately high risk	Less than 130 mg/dL
Two or more risk factors and a risk score lower than 10%	III. Moderate risk	Less than 130 mg/dL
One or no risk factors	IV. Low to moderate risk	Less than 160 mg/dL

*Some people in this category are at very high risk because they've just had a heart attack or they have diabetes and heart disease, severe risk factors, or metabolic syndrome. If you're at very high risk, your doctor may set your LDL goal even lower, to less than 70 mg/dL. Your doctor also may set your LDL goal at this lower level if you have heart disease alone.

After following the above steps, you should have an idea about your risk for heart disease and heart attack. The two main ways to lower your cholesterol (and, thus, your heart disease risk) include:

- **Therapeutic Lifestyle Changes (TLC).** TLC is a three-part program that includes a healthy diet, weight management, and physical activity. TLC is for anyone whose LDL cholesterol level is above goal.

- **Medicines.** If cholesterol-lowering medicines are needed, they're used with the TLC program to help lower your LDL cholesterol level.

Your doctor will set your LDL goal. The higher your risk for heart disease, the lower he or she will set your LDL goal. Using the following guide, you and your doctor can create a plan for treating your high blood cholesterol.

Table 60.2. Category I, high risk, your LDL goal is less than 100 mg/dL*

Your LDL Level	Treatment
If your LDL level is 100 or higher	You will need to begin the TLC diet and take medicines as prescribed.
Even if your LDL level is below 100	You should follow the TLC diet to keep your LDL level as low as possible.

Your LDL goal may be set even lower, to less than 70 mg/dL, if you're at very high risk or if you have heart disease. If you have this lower goal and your LDL is 70 mg/dL or higher, you'll need to begin the TLC diet and take medicines as prescribed.

Table 60.3. Category II, moderately high risk, your LDL goal is less than 130 mg/dL

Your LDL Level	Treatment
If your LDL level is 130 mg/dL or higher	You will need to begin the TLC diet.
If your LDL level is 130 mg/dL or higher after 3 months on the TLC diet	You may need medicines along with the TLC diet.
If your LDL level is less than 130 mg/dL	You will need to follow a heart healthy diet.

Table 60.4. Category III, moderate risk, your LDL goal is less than 130 mg/dL

Your LDL Level	Treatment
If your LDL level is 130 mg/dL or higher	You will need to begin the TLC diet.
If your LDL level is 160 mg/dL or higher after 3 months on the TLC diet	You may need medicines along with the TLC diet.
If your LDL level is less than 130 mg/dL	You will need to follow a heart healthy diet.

Table 60.5. Category IV, low to moderate risk, your LDL goal is less than 160 mg/dL

Your LDL Level	Treatment
If your LDL level is 160 mg/dL or higher	You will need to begin the TLC diet.
If your LDL level is 160 mg/dL or higher after 3 months on the TLC diet	You may need medicines along with the TLC diet.
If your LDL level is less than 160 mg/dL	You will need to follow a heart healthy diet.

Lowering Cholesterol Using Therapeutic Lifestyle Changes

TLC is a set of lifestyle changes that can help you lower your LDL cholesterol. The main parts of the TLC program are a healthy diet, weight management, and physical activity.

The TLC Diet

With the TLC diet, less than 7 percent of your daily calories should come from saturated fat. This kind of fat is found in some meats, dairy products, chocolate, baked goods, and deep-fried and processed foods.

No more than 25 to 35 percent of your daily calories should come from all fats, including saturated, trans, monounsaturated, and poly-unsaturated fats.

You also should have less than 200 mg a day of cholesterol. The amounts of cholesterol and the types of fat in prepared foods can be found on the foods' Nutrition Facts labels.

Foods high in soluble fiber also are part of the TLC diet. They help prevent the digestive tract from absorbing cholesterol. These foods include:

- Whole-grain cereals such as oatmeal and oat bran

- Fruits such as apples, bananas, oranges, pears, and prunes

- Legumes such as kidney beans, lentils, chick peas, black-eyed peas, and lima beans

A diet rich in fruits and vegetables can increase important cholesterol-lowering compounds in your diet. These compounds, called plant stanols or sterols, work like soluble fiber.

A healthy diet also includes some types of fish, such as salmon, tuna (canned or fresh), and mackerel. These fish are a good source of omega-3 fatty acids. These acids may help protect the heart from blood clots and inflammation and reduce the risk of heart attack. Try to have about two fish meals every week.

You also should try to limit the amount of sodium (salt) that you eat. This means choosing low-salt and "no added salt" foods and seasonings at the table or while cooking. The Nutrition Facts label on food packaging shows the amount of sodium in the item.

Try to limit drinks with alcohol. Too much alcohol will raise your blood pressure and triglyceride level. (Triglycerides are a type of fat found in the blood.) Alcohol also adds extra calories, which will cause weight gain.

Men should have no more than two drinks containing alcohol a day. Women should have no more than one drink containing alcohol a day. One drink is a glass of wine, beer, or a small amount of hard liquor.

Weight Management

If you're overweight or obese, losing weight can help lower LDL cholesterol. Maintaining a healthy weight is especially important if you have a condition called metabolic syndrome.

Metabolic syndrome is the name for a group of risk factors that raise your risk for heart disease and other health problems, such as diabetes and stroke.

The five metabolic risk factors are a large waistline (abdominal obesity), a high triglyceride level, a low HDL cholesterol level, high blood pressure, and high blood sugar. Metabolic syndrome is diagnosed if you have at least three of these metabolic risk factors.

Physical Activity

Routine physical activity can lower LDL cholesterol and triglycerides and raise your HDL cholesterol level.

People gain health benefits from as little as 60 minutes of moderate-intensity aerobic activity per week. The more active you are, the more you will benefit.

Cholesterol-Lowering Medicines

In addition to lifestyle changes, your doctor may prescribe medicines to help lower your cholesterol. Even with medicines, you should continue the TLC program.

Medicines can help control high blood cholesterol, but they don't cure it. Thus, you must continue taking your medicine to keep your cholesterol level in the recommended range.

The five major types of cholesterol-lowering medicines are statins, bile acid sequestrants, nicotinic acid, fibrates, and ezetimibe.

- **Statins** work well at lowering LDL cholesterol. These medicines are safe for most people. Rare side effects include muscle and liver problems.

- **Bile acid sequestrants** also help lower LDL cholesterol. These medicines usually aren't prescribed as the only medicine to lower cholesterol. Sometimes they're prescribed with statins.

- **Nicotinic acid** lowers LDL cholesterol and triglycerides and raises HDL cholesterol. You should only use this type of medicine with a doctor's supervision.

- **Fibrates** lower triglycerides, and they may raise HDL cholesterol. When used with statins, fibrates may increase the risk of muscle problems.

- **Ezetimibe** lowers LDL cholesterol. This medicine works by blocking the intestine from absorbing cholesterol.

While you're being treated for high blood cholesterol, you'll need ongoing care. Your doctor will want to make sure your cholesterol levels are controlled. He or she also will want to check for other health problems.

If needed, your doctor may prescribe medicines for other health problems. Take all medicines exactly as your doctor prescribes. The combination of medicines may lower your risk for heart disease and heart attack.

While trying to manage your cholesterol, take steps to manage other heart disease risk factors too. For example, if you have high blood pressure, work with your doctor to lower it.

If you smoke, quit. Talk with your doctor about programs and products that can help you quit smoking. Also, try to avoid secondhand smoke. If you're overweight or obese, try to lose weight. Your doctor can help you create a reasonable weight-loss plan

Chapter 61

Steps to Control Diabetes

4 Steps to Manage Your Diabetes for Life

Step 1: Learn about diabetes

What Is Diabetes?

There are three main types of diabetes:

1. **Type 1 diabetes**—Your body does not make insulin. This is a problem because you need insulin to take the sugar (glucose) from the foods you eat and turn it into energy for your body. You need to take insulin every day to live.

2. **Type 2 diabetes**—Your body does not make or use insulin well. You may need to take pills or insulin to help control your diabetes. Type 2 is the most common type of diabetes.

3. **Gestational diabetes**—Some women get this kind of diabetes when they are pregnant. Most of the time, it goes away after the baby is born. But even if it goes away, these women and their children have a greater chance of getting diabetes later in life.

This chapter includes text excerpted from "4 Steps to Manage Your Diabetes for Life," National Institute of Diabetes and Digestive and Kidney Diseases (NIDDK), April 2014.

You Are the most Important Member of Your Healthcare Team

You are the one who manages your diabetes day by day. Talk to your doctor about how you can best care for your diabetes to stay healthy. Some others who can help are:

- entist
- diabetes doctor
- diabetes educator
- dietitian
- eye doctor
- foot doctor

- friends and family
- mental health counselor
- nurse
- nurse practitioner
- pharmacist
- social worker

How to learn more about diabetes.

- Take classes to learn more about living with diabetes. To find a class, check with your healthcare team, hospital, or area health clinic. You can also search online.

- Join a support group—in-person or online—to get peer support with managing your diabetes.

- Read about diabetes online.

Take Diabetes Seriously

You may have heard people say they have "a touch of diabetes" or that their "sugar is a little high." These words suggest that diabetes is not a serious disease. That is **not** correct. Diabetes is **serious**, but you can learn to manage it.

People with diabetes need to make healthy food choices, stay at a healthy weight, move more every day, and take their medicine even when they feel good. It's a lot to do. **It's not easy, but it's worth it!**

Why Take Care of Your Diabetes?

Taking care of yourself and your diabetes can help you feel good today and in the future. When your blood sugar (glucose) is close to normal, you are likely to:

- have more energy
- be less tired and thirsty
- need to pass urine less often

- heal better

- have fewer skin or bladder infections

You will also have less chance of having health problems caused by diabetes such as:

- heart attack or stroke

- eye problems that can lead to trouble seeing or going blind

- pain, tingling, or numbness in your hands and feet, also called nerve damage

- kidney problems that can cause your kidneys to stop working

- teeth and gum problems

Actions You Can Take

- Ask your healthcare team what type of diabetes you have.

- Learn where you can go for support.

- Learn how caring for your diabetes helps you feel good today and in the future.

Step 2: Know your diabetes ABCs

Talk to your healthcare team about how to manage your **A**1C, **B**lood pressure, and **C**holesterol. This can help lower your chances of having a heart attack, stroke, or other diabetes problems.

A for the A1C test (A-one-C)

- **What Is It?**

  The A1C is a blood test that measures your average blood sugar level over the past three months. It is different from the blood sugar checks you do each day.

- **Why Is It Important?**

  You need to know your blood sugar levels over time. You don't want those numbers to get too high. High levels of blood sugar can harm your heart, blood vessels, kidneys, feet, and eyes.

- **What Is The A1C Goal?**

  The A1C goal for many people with diabetes is below 7. It may be different for you. Ask what your goal should be.

B for Blood Pressure

- **What Is It?**

  Blood pressure is the force of your blood against the wall of your blood vessels.

- **Why Is It Important?**

  If your blood pressure gets too high, it makes your heart work too hard. It can cause a heart attack, stroke, and damage your kidneys and eyes.

- **What Is The Blood Pressure Goal?**

  The blood pressure goal for most people with diabetes is below 140/90. It may be different for you. Ask what your goal should be.

C for Cholesterol

- **What Is It?**

  There are two kinds of cholesterol in your blood: LDL and HDL.

  LDL or "bad" cholesterol can build up and clog your blood vessels. It can cause a heart attack or stroke.

  HDL or "good" cholesterol helps remove the "bad" cholesterol from your blood vessels.

- **What Are The LDL and HDL Goals?**

  Ask what your cholesterol numbers should be. Your goals may be different from other people. If you are over 40 years of age, you may need to take a statin drug for heart health.

Actions you can take

- Ask your healthcare team:

- what your A1C, blood pressure, and cholesterol numbers are and what they should be. Your ABC goals will depend on how long you have had diabetes, other health problems, and how hard your diabetes is to manage.

- what you can do to reach your ABC goals

Step 3: Learn How to Live with Diabetes

It is common to feel overwhelmed, sad, or angry when you are living with diabetes. You may know the steps you should take to stay healthy, but have trouble sticking with your plan over time. This section has tips on how to cope with your diabetes, eat well, and be active.

Cope with Your Diabetes

- Stress can raise your blood sugar. Learn ways to lower your stress. Try deep breathing, gardening, taking a walk, meditating, working on your hobby, or listening to your favorite music.

- Ask for help if you feel down. A mental health counselor, support group, member of the clergy, friend, or family member who will listen to your concerns may help you feel better.

Eat Well

- Make a diabetes meal plan with help from your healthcare team.

- Choose foods that are lower in calories, saturated fat, trans fat, sugar, and salt.

- Eat foods with more fiber, such as whole grain cereals, breads, crackers, rice, or pasta.

- Choose foods such as fruits, vegetables, whole grains, bread and cereals, and low-fat or skim milk and cheese.

- Drink water instead of juice and regular soda.

- When eating a meal, fill half of your plate with fruits and vegetables, one quarter with a lean protein, such as beans, or chicken or turkey without the skin, and one quarter with a whole grain, such as brown rice or whole wheat pasta.

Be Active

- Set a goal to be more active most days of the week. Start slow by taking 10 minute walks, 3 times a day.

- Twice a week, work to increase your muscle strength. Use stretch bands, do yoga, heavy gardening (digging and planting with tools), or try push-ups.

- Stay at or get to a healthy weight by using your meal plan and moving more.

Know What to Do Every Day

- Take your medicines for diabetes and any other health problems even when you feel good. Ask your doctor if you need aspirin to prevent a heart attack or stroke. Tell your doctor if you cannot afford your medicines or if you have any side effects.

- Check your feet every day for cuts, blisters, red spots, and swelling. Call your healthcare team right away about any sores that do not go away.

- Brush your teeth and floss every day to keep your mouth, teeth, and gums healthy.

- Stop smoking. Ask for help to quit. Call 1-800-QUITNOW (1-800-784-8669).

- Keep track of your blood sugar. You may want to check it one or more times a day. Check your blood pressure if your doctor advises and keep a record of it.

Talk to Your Healthcare Team

- Ask your doctor if you have any questions about your diabetes.

- Report any changes in your health.

Actions You Can Take

- Ask for a healthy meal plan.

- Ask about ways to be more active.

- Ask how and when to test your blood sugar and how to use the results to manage your diabetes.

- Use these tips to help with your self-care.

- Discuss how your diabetes plan is working for you each time you visit your healthcare team.

Step 4: Get Routine Care to Stay Healthy

See your healthcare team at least twice a year to find and treat any problems early.

At Each Visit, Be Sure You Have a:

- blood pressure check

- foot check

- weight check
- review of your self-care plan

Two Times Each Year, Have an:

- A1C test. It may be checked more often if it is over 7.

Once Each Year, Be Sure You Have a:

- cholesterol test
- complete foot exam
- dental exam to check teeth and gums
- dilated eye exam to check for eye problems
- flu shot
- urine and a blood test to check for kidney problems

At Least Once in Your Lifetime, Get a:

- pneumonia shot
- hepatitis B shot

Medicare and Diabetes

If you have Medicare, check to see how your plan covers diabetes care. Medicare covers some of the costs for:

- diabetes education
- diabetes supplies
- diabetes medicine
- visits with a dietitian
- special shoes, if you need them

Actions You Can Take

- Ask your healthcare team about these and other tests you may need. Ask what your results mean.
- Write down the date and time of your next visit.
- Use the card at the back of this booklet to keep a record of your diabetes care.
- If you have Medicare, check your plan.

Chapter 62

Heart-Healthy Eating

Heart-healthy eating is an important way to lower your risk for heart disease and stroke. Heart disease is the number one cause of death for American women. Stroke is the number three cause of death. To get the most benefit for your heart, you should choose more fruits, vegetables and foods with whole grains and healthy proteins. You also should eat less food with added sugar, calories, and unhealthy fats.

What Foods Should I Eat to Help Lower My Risk for Heart Disease and Stroke?

You should choose these foods most of the time:

- **Fruits and vegetables.** At least half of your plate should be fruits and vegetables.

- **Grains.** At least half of your grains should be whole grains.

- **Fat-free or low-fat dairy products.** These include milk, calcium-fortified soy drinks (soy milk), cheese, yogurt, and other milk products.

- **Seafood, skinless poultry, lean meats, beans, eggs, and unsalted nuts.**

This chapter contains text excerpted from the following sources: Text beginning with the heading "Heart-Healthy Eating" is excerpted from "Heart-Healthy Eating," Office on Women's Health (OWH), U.S. Department of Health and Human Services (HHS), June 30, 2014; Text beginning with the heading "DASH Eating Plan" is excerpted from "DASH Eating Plan," National Heart, Lung, and Blood Institute (NHLBI), September 16, 2015.

What Foods Should I Limit to Lower My Risk of Heart Disease and Stroke?

You should limit:

- **Saturated fats.** These fats are found in foods such as pizza, ice cream, fried chicken, many cakes and cookies, bacon, and hamburgers. Check the Nutrition Facts label for saturated fat. Less than 10% of your daily calories should be from saturated fats.

- **Trans fats.** These fats are found mainly in commercially prepared baked goods, snack foods, fried foods, and margarine. The U.S. Food and Drug Administration is taking action to remove artificial trans fats from our food supply because of their risk to heart health. Check the Nutrition Facts label and choose foods with no trans fats as much as possible.

- **Cholesterol.** Cholesterol is found in foods made from animals, such as bacon, whole milk, cheese made from whole milk, ice cream, full-fat frozen yogurt, and eggs. Fruits and vegetables do not contain cholesterol. You should eat less than 300 milligrams of cholesterol per day. Check the Nutrition Facts label for cholesterol. Foods with 20% or more of the "Daily Value" of cholesterol are high in cholesterol.

- **Sodium.** Sodium is found in salt, but most of the sodium we eat is not from salt that we add while cooking or at the table. Most of our sodium comes from breads and rolls, cold cuts, pizza, hot dogs, cheese, pasta dishes, and condiments (like ketchup and mustard). Limit your daily sodium to less than 2,300 milligrams (equal to a teaspoon), unless your doctor says something else. Check the Nutrition Facts label for sodium. Foods with 20% or more of the "Daily Value" of sodium are high in sodium.

- **Added sugars.** Foods like fruit and dairy prod ucts naturally contain sugar. But you should limit foods that contain added sugars. These foods include sodas, sports drinks, cakes, candy, and ice cream. Check the Nutrition Facts label for added sugars and limit how much food you eat with added sugars.

How Can I Tell What Is in the Foods I Eat?

The Nutrition Facts label on most packaged foods has information about how many calories and how much saturated fat, trans fat, cholesterol, sodium, and added sugars are in each serving.

What Tools Can Help Me Choose Foods That Are Good for My Heart?

The following resources can help you choose heart-healthy foods:

- **ChooseMyPlate** (choosemyplate.gov). This resource is based on the Dietary Guidelines for Americans. You can use the Super-Tracker tool to create a personal daily food plan based on your goals.

- **Dietary Approaches to Stop Hypertension (DASH) eating plan** (www.nhlbi.nih.gov/health/health-topics/topics/dash/). The DASH diet is for people with hypertension to help them lower their blood pressure. But it can also be used to help prevent heart disease.

- **Therapeutic Lifestyle Changes (TLC) diet** (www.nhlbi.nih.gov/health/public/heart/chol/ chol_tlc.pdf). The TLC diet helps people with unhealthy cholesterol levels.

Description of the DASH Eating Plan

DASH is a flexible and balanced eating plan that helps creates a heart-healthy eating style for life.

The DASH eating plan requires no special foods and instead provides daily and weekly nutritional goals. This plan recommends:

- Eating vegetables, fruits, and whole grains

- Including fat-free or low-fat dairy products, fish, poultry, beans, nuts, and vegetable oils

- Limiting foods that are high in saturated fat, such as fatty meats, full-fat dairy products, and tropical oils such as coconut, palm kernel, and palm oils

- Limiting sugar-sweetened beverages and sweets.

Based on these recommendations, the following table shows examples of daily and weekly servings that meet DASH eating plan targets for a 2,000-calorie-a-day diet.

When following the DASH eating plan, it is important to choose foods that are:

- Low in saturated and trans fats

- Rich in potassium, calcium, magnesium, fiber, and protein

- Lower in sodium

Table 62.1. Daily and Weekly DASH Eating Plan Goals for a 2,000-Calorie-a-Day Diet

Food Group	Daily Servings
Grains	6–8
Meats, poultry, and fish	6 or less
Vegetables	4–5
Fruit	4–5
Low-fat or fat-free dairy products	2–3
Fats and oils	2–3
Sodium	2,300 mg*
	Weekly Servings
Nuts, seeds, dry beans, and peas	4–5
Sweets	5 or less

1,500 milligrams (mg) sodium lowers blood pressure even further than 2,300 mg sodium daily.

Health Benefits of the DASH Eating Plan

Three NHLBI-funded trials showed the health benefits of the DASH diet, such as lowering high blood pressure and LDL (bad) cholesterol in the blood, and shaped the final DASH eating plan recommendations.

Study Results

Three NHLBI-funded trials found the following health benefits of the DASH diet.

- **DASH (Dietary Approaches to Stop Hypertension Trial):** The DASH diet lowers blood pressure and LDL (bad) cholesterol compared with a typical American diet alone or a typical American diet with more fruits and vegetables.

- **DASH-Sodium (DASH Diet, Sodium Intake, and Blood Pressure Trial):** The DASH diet lowers blood pressure better than a typical American diet at three daily sodium levels. Combining the DASH diet with sodium reduction gives greater health benefits than the DASH diet alone.

- **PREMIER clinical trial:** People can lose weight and lower their blood pressure by following the DASH eating plan and increasing their physical activity.

DASH Trial

This trial included 459 adults, some with and without confirmed high blood pressure, and compared three diets including 3,000 mg daily sodium:

- Typical American diet
- Typical American diet plus more fruits and vegetables
- DASH diet

None of the plans were vegetarian or used specialty foods. After 2 weeks, participants who added fruits and vegetables to a typical American diet or those on the DASH diet had lower blood pressure than those who followed a typical American diet alone. However, the participants on the DASH diet had the greatest effect of lowering their high blood pressure.

Follow-up reports from the DASH trial showed that in addition to improving blood pressure, the DASH diet also lowered LDL cholesterol levels. High blood pressure and elevated LDL cholesterol are two major risk factors for cardiovascular disease.

DASH-Sodium Trial

This trial randomly assigned 412 participants to a typical American diet or the DASH diet. While on their assigned diet, participants were followed for a month at a high daily sodium level (3,300 mg) and two lower daily sodium levels (2,300 mg and 1,500 mg). Reducing daily sodium lowered blood pressure for participants on either diet. However, blood pressures were lower for participants on the DASH diet versus a typical American diet. Blood pressure decreased with each reduction of sodium. These results showed that lowering sodium intake and eating the DASH diet is more beneficial for lowering blood pressure than following the DASH diet alone.

PREMIER Trial

The PREMIER trial included 810 participants who were placed into three groups to lower blood pressure, lose weight, and improve health. The groups included:

- Advice-only group, did not receive counseling on behavior changes
- Established treatment plan, including counseling for 6 months

- Established treatment plan, plus counseling and use of the DASH diet

After 6 months, blood pressure levels declined in all three groups. The two groups that received counseling and followed a treatment plan had more weight loss than the advice-only group. However, participants in the established treatment plan who followed the DASH diet had the greatest improvement in their blood pressure.

Following the DASH Eating Plan

The DASH eating plan is easy to follow using common foods available in your grocery store. The plan includes daily servings from different food groups. The number of servings you should have depends on your daily calorie (energy) needs.

To figure out your calorie needs, you need to consider your age and physical activity level. If you want to maintain your current weight, you should eat only as many calories as you burn by being physically active. This is called energy balance.

If you need to lose weight, you should eat fewer calories than you burn or increase your activity level to burn more calories than you eat.

Consider your physical activity level. Are you sedentary, moderately active, or active?

- Sedentary means that you do only light physical activity as part of your typical daily routine.

- Moderately active means that you do physical activity equal to walking about 1.5 to 3 miles a day at 3 to 4 miles per hour, plus light physical activity.

- Active means that you do physical activity equal to walking more than 3 miles per day at 3 to 4 miles per hour, plus light physical activity.

Table 62.2. Daily Calorie Needs for Women

Age (years)	Calories Needed for Sedentary Activity Level	Calories Needed for Moderately Active Activity Level	Calories Needed for Active Activity Level
19–30	2000	2,000–2,200	2400
31–50	1800	2000	2200
51	1600	1800	2,000–2,200

Table 62.3. Daily Calorie Needs for Men

Age (years)	Calories Needed for Sedentary Activity Level	Calories Needed for Moderately Active Activity Level	Calories Needed for Active Activity Level
19–30	2400	2,600–2,800	3000
31–50	2200	2,400–2,600	2,800–3,000
51	2000	2,200–2,400	2,400–2,800

After figuring out your daily calorie needs, go to the table below and find the closest calorie level to yours. This table estimates the number of servings from each food group that you should have. Serving quantities are per day, unless otherwise noted.

The DASH Eating Plan as Part of a Heart-Healthy Lifestyle

The DASH eating plan is just one key part of a heart-healthy lifestyle, and combining it with other lifestyle changes such as physical activity can help you control your blood pressure and LDL-cholesterol for life.

To help prevent and control high blood pressure:

- Be physically active.

- Maintain a healthy weight.

- Limit alcohol intake.

- Manage and cope with stress.

Other lifestyle changes can improve your overall health, such as:

- If you smoke, quit.

- Get plenty of sleep.

To help make lifelong lifestyle changes, try making one change at a time and add another when you feel that you have successfully adopted the earlier changes. When you practice several healthy lifestyle habits, you are more likely to achieve and maintain healthy blood pressure and cholesterol levels.

Living with the DASH Eating Plan

Understanding the DASH eating plan will help you start and follow this plan for life.

Table 62.4. DASH Eating Plan—Number of Food Servings by Calorie Level

Food Group	1,200 Cal.	1,400 Cal.	1,600 Cal.	1,800 Cal.	2,000 Cal.	2,600 Cal.	3,100 Cal.
Grains[a]	4–5	5–6	6	6	6–8	10–11	12–13
Vegetables	3–4	3–4	3–4	4–5	4–5	5–6	6
Fruits	3–4	4	4	4–5	4–5	5–6	6
Fat-free or low-fat dairy products[b]	2–3	2–3	2–3	2–3	2–3	3	3–4
Lean meats, poultry, and fish	3 or less	3–4 or less	3–4 or less	6 or less	6 or less	6 or less	6–9
Nuts, seeds, and legumes	3 per week	3 per week	3–4 per week	4 per week	4–5 per week	1	1
Fats and oils[c]	1	1	2	2–3	2–3	3	4
Sweets and added sugars	3 or less per week	3 or less per week	3 or less per week	5 or less per week	5 or less per week	≤2	≤2
Maximum sodium limit[d]	2,300 mg/day	2,300 mg/day	2,300 mg/day	2,300 mg/day	2,300 mg/day	2,300 mg/day	2,300 mg/day

[a]Whole grains are recommended for most grain servings as a good source of fiber and nutrients.

[b]For lactose intolerance, try either lactase enzyme pills with dairy products or lactose-free or lactose-reduced milk.

[c]Fat content changes the serving amount for fats and oils. For example, 1 Tbsp regular salad dressing = one serving; 1 Tbsp low-fat dressing = one-half serving; 1 Tbsp fat-free dressing = zero servings.

[d]The DASH eating plan has a sodium limit of either 2,300 mg or 1,500 mg per day.

Table 62.5. DASH Eating Plan—Serving Sizes, Examples, and Significance

Food Group	Serving Sizes	Examples and Notes	Significance of Each Food Group to the DASH Eating Plan
Grains[a]	1 slice bread 1 oz dry cereal[b] ½ cup cooked rice, pasta, or cereal[b]	Whole-wheat bread and rolls, whole-wheat pasta, English muffin, pita bread, bagel, cereals, grits, oatmeal, brown rice, unsalted pretzels and popcorn	Major sources of energy and fiber
Vegetables	1 cup raw leafy vegetable ½ cup cut-up raw or cooked vegetable ½ cup vegetable juice	Broccoli, carrots, collards, green beans, green peas, kale, lima beans, potatoes, spinach, squash, sweet potatoes, tomatoes	Rich sources of potassium, magnesium, and fiber
Fruits	1 medium fruit ¼ cup dried fruit ½ cup fresh, frozen, or canned fruit ½ cup fruit juice	Apples, apricots, bananas, dates, grapes, oranges, grapefruit, grapefruit juice, mangoes, melons, peaches, pineapples, raisins, strawberries, tangerines	Important sources of potassium, magnesium, and fiber
Fat-free or low-fat dairy products[c]	1 cup milk or yogurt 1½ oz cheese	Fat-free milk or buttermilk; fat-free, low-fat, or reduced-fat cheese; fat-free/low-fat regular or frozen yogurt	Major sources of calcium and protein
Lean meats, poultry, and fish	1 oz cooked meats, poultry, or fish 1 egg	Select only lean; trim away visible fats; broil, roast, or poach; remove skin from poultry	Rich sources of protein and magnesium

Table 62.5. (Continued)

Food Group	Serving Sizes	Examples and Notes	Significance of Each Food Group to the DASH Eating Plan
Nuts, seeds, and legumes	⅓ cup or 1½ oz nuts 2 Tbsp peanut butter 2 Tbsp or ½ oz seeds ½ cup cooked legumes (dried beans, peas)	Almonds, filberts, mixed nuts, peanuts, walnuts, sunflower seeds, peanut butter, kidney beans, lentils, split peas	Rich sources of energy, magnesium, protein, and fiber
Fats and oils[d]	1 tsp soft margarine 1 tsp vegetable oil 1 Tbsp mayonnaise 2 Tbsp salad dressing	Soft margarine, vegetable oil (canola, corn, olive, safflower), low-fat mayonnaise, light salad dressing	The DASH study had 27% of calories as fat, including fat in or added to foods
Sweets and added sugars	1 Tbsp sugar 1 Tbsp jelly or jam ½ cup sorbet, gelatin dessert 1 cup lemonade	Fruit-flavored gelatin, fruit punch, hard candy, jelly, maple syrup, sorbet and ices, sugar	Sweets should be low in fat

[a]*Whole grains are recommended for most grain servings as a good source of fiber and nutrients.*

[b]*Serving sizes vary between ½ cup and 1¼ cups, depending on cereal type. Check the product's Nutrition Facts label.*

[c]*For lactose intolerance, try either lactase enzyme pills with dairy products or lactose-free or lactose-reduced milk.*

[d]*Fat content changes the serving amount for fats and oils. For example, 1 Tbsp regular salad dressing = one serving; 1 Tbsp low-fat dressing = one-half serving; 1 Tbsp fat-free dressing = zero servings.##<TFn>##*

Controlling Daily Sodium and Calories

To benefit from the proven DASH eating plan, it is important to limit daily sodium levels to 2,300 mg, or 1,500 mg if desired, and to consume the appropriate amount of calories to maintain a healthy weight or lose weight if needed.

Ways to Control Sodium Levels

The key to lowering your sodium intake is to make healthier food choices when you're shopping, cooking, and eating out.

Table 62.6. Tips for Lowering Sodium When Shopping, Cooking, and Eating Out

Shopping	Cooking	Eating Out
• Read food labels, and choose items that are lower in sodium and salt, particularly for convenience foods and condiments.* • Choose fresh poultry, fish, and lean meats instead of cured food such as bacon and ham. • Choose fresh or frozen versus canned fruits and vegetables. • Avoid food with added salt, such as pickles, pickled vegetables, olives, and sauerkraut. • Avoid instant or flavored rice and pasta.	• Don't add salt when cooking rice, pasta, and hot cereals. • Flavor your foods with salt-free seasoning blends, fresh or dried herbs and spices, or fresh lemon or lime juice. • Rinse canned foods or foods soaked in brine before using to remove the sodium. • Use less table salt to flavor food.	• Ask that foods be prepared without added salt or MSG, commonly used in Asian foods. • Avoid choosing menu items that have salty ingredients such as bacon, pickles, olives, and cheese. • Avoid choosing menu items that include foods that are pickled, cured, smoked, or made with soy sauce or broth. • Choose fruit or vegetables as a side dish, instead of chips or fries.

Examples of convenience foods are frozen dinners, prepackaged foods, and soups; examples of condiments are mustard, ketchup, soy sauce, barbecue sauce, and salad dressings.

Most of the sodium Americans eat comes from processed and prepared foods, such as breads, cold cuts, pizza, poultry, soups, sandwiches and burgers, cheese, pasta and meat dishes, and salty snacks. Therefore, healthier choices when shopping and eating out are particularly important.

Ways to Control Calories

To benefit from the DASH eating plan, it is important to consume the appropriate amount of calories to maintain a healthy weight. To help, read nutrition labels on food, and plan for success with DASH eating plan sample menus and other heart-healthy recipes.

The DASH eating plan can be used to help you lose weight. To lose weight, follow the DASH eating plan and try to reduce your total daily calories gradually. Find out your daily calorie needs or goals with the Body Weight Planner and calorie chart. Talk with your doctor before beginning any diet or eating plan.

General tips for reducing daily calories include:

- Eat smaller portions more frequently throughout the day.

- Reduce the amount of meat that you eat while increasing the amount of fruits, vegetables, whole grains, or dry beans.

- Substitute low-calorie foods, such as when snacking (choose fruits or vegetables instead of sweets and desserts) or drinking (choose water instead of soda or juice), when possible.

Increasing Daily Potassium

The DASH eating plan is designed to be rich in potassium, with a target of 4,700 mg potassium daily, to enhance the effects of reducing sodium on blood pressure. The following are examples of potassium-rich foods.

Table 62.7. Sample Foods and Potassium Levels

Food	Potassium (mg)
Potato, 1 small	738
Plain yogurt, nonfat or low-fat, 8 ounces	530–570
Sweet potato, 1 medium	542
Orange juice, fresh, 1 cup	496
Lima beans, ½ cup	478
Soybeans, cooked, ½ cup	443
Banana, 1 medium	422
Fish (cod, halibut, rockfish, trout, tuna), 3 ounces	200–400
Tomato sauce, ½ cup	405
Prunes, stewed, ½ cup	398
Skim milk, 1 cup	382

Table 62.7. Continued

Food	Potassium (mg)
Apricots, ¼ cup	378
Pinto beans, cooked, ½ cup	373
Pork tenderloin, 3 ounces	371
Lentils, cooked, ½ cup	365
Kidney beans, cooked, ½ cup	360
Split peas, cooked, ½ cup	360

Meal Planning and Tips

Tips for Lifelong Success

When changing lifestyle habits, it is normal to slip off track occasionally. Follow these tips to get you back on track.

- **Ask yourself why you got off track.** Find out what triggered your sidetrack, and restart the DASH eating plan.

- **Don't worry about a slip.** Everyone slips, especially when learning something new. Remember that changing your lifestyle is a long-term process.

- **Don't change too much at once.** When starting a new lifestyle, try to avoid changing too much at once. Slow changes lead to success.

- **Break down the process.** Break goals into smaller, simpler steps, each of which is attainable.

- **Write it down.** Use the Daily DASH Log to keep track of what you eat and what you're doing while you are eating. You may find that you eat unhealthy foods while watching television. If so, you could start keeping a healthier substitute snack on hand.

- **Celebrate success.** Instead of eating out to celebrate your accomplishments, try a night at the movies, go shopping, visit the library or bookstore, or watch your favorite TV show.

Chapter 63

Complementary and Alternative Therapy to Prevent Cardiovascular Disease

Chapter Contents

Section 63.1

Supplements for the Primary Prevention of Cardiovascular Disease

This section includes text excerpted from "Vitamin, Mineral, and Multivitamin Supplements for the Primary Prevention of Cardiovascular Disease and Cancer," U.S. Preventive Services Task Force (USPSTF), U.S. Department of Health and Human Services (HSS), February 2014.

What Are Vitamin and Mineral Supplements?

Supplements are vitamins or minerals added to the diet. They can be taken in pill, capsule, tablet, or liquid form. A multivitamin is a combination of three or more vitamins and minerals.

Facts about the Use of Vitamin and Mineral Supplements

Vitamin and mineral supplements are commonly used in the United States. About half of adults say they have used at least one dietary supplement and a third say they have used a multivitamin. More women than men use supplements, and older adults are more likely than younger adults use them.

People take vitamin and mineral supplements for many reasons, including maintaining or improving their overall health, preventing illness, and slowing the progress of existing disease. This recommendation is limited to use of supplements specifically to prevent CVD and cancer.

Vitamin and mineral supplements are found in many forms, including multivitamins (a supplement containing three or more vitamins and minerals), paired supplements (a supplement containing two vitamins or minerals, such as vitamin D and calcium), and single supplements (for example, vitamin C or folic acid). Multivitamins are the most commonly used dietary supplement.

Potential Benefits and Harms of Taking Multivitamins to Prevent CVD or Cancer

The Task Force reviewed studies that examined whether taking vitamin and mineral supplements might prevent CVD or cancer. The Task Force looked at these studies because CVD and cancer are leading causes of illness and death in the United States.

The Task Force reviewed studies on multivitamins, paired supplements, and single vitamins and minerals. It found that there was not enough evidence to say whether taking multivitamins, paired vitamin and mineral supplements, or most single vitamins or minerals will help prevent CVD or cancer.

However, the Task Force did find enough evidence to make a recommendation against using two specific vitamin supplements:beta-carotene and vitamin E. The Task Force found that:

- Vitamin E supplements do not help prevent CVD or cancer.

- Beta-carotene supplements do not help prevent CVD or cancer. They also can increase the chance of getting lung cancer in people who are already at risk for lung cancer, such as current smokers.

Should You Take a Vitamin or Mineral Supplement to Prevent CVD or Cancer?

Getting the best health care means making smart decisions about using preventive medications, screening tests, and counseling services. Many people don't get the medications, tests, or counseling they need. Others get medications, tests, or counseling they don't need or that may be harmful to them.

Task Force recommendations can help you learn about preventive medications, screening tests, and counseling services. These medications and services can keep you healthy and prevent disease. The Task Force recommendations do not cover diagnosis (tests to find out why you are sick) or treatment of disease.

Task Force recommendations also apply to some groups of people, but not others. For example, this recommendation does not apply to women who are pregnant or to those who are in a hospital.

Making a Decision about Taking Vitamin and Mineral Supplements

Good nutrition is essential to overall health. For most people, the best way to get the nutrients they need for good health is through a balanced diet. A diet that is rich in vegetables and fruits, whole grains, fat-free and low-fat dairy products, and seafood and that is low in saturated fats, salt, and added sugars has been associated with a reduced risk of CVD and cancer.

When deciding whether to take vitamin and mineral supplements to prevent CVD or cancer, consider your own health and lifestyle. Think about your personal beliefs and preferences for health care. Talk with your health care professional about your risks for CVD and cancer. Be comfortable that all your questions have been answered. And consider scientific recommendations, like this one from the Task Force. Use this information to become fully informed and to decide whether vitamin and mineral supplements are right for you.

Section 63.2

Vitamin E and Coronary Heart Disease

This section includes text excerpted from "Vitamin E," Office of Dietary Supplements, National Institutes of Health (NIH), May 9, 2016.

Vitamin E is found naturally in some foods, added to others, and available as a dietary supplement. "Vitamin E" is the collective name for a group of fat-soluble compounds with distinctive antioxidant activities.

Antioxidants protect cells from the damaging effects of free radicals, which are molecules that contain an unshared electron. Free radicals damage cells and might contribute to the development of cardiovascular disease and cancer. Unshared electrons are highly energetic and react rapidly with oxygen to form reactive oxygen species (ROS). The body forms ROS endogenously when it converts food to energy, and antioxidants might protect cells from the damaging effects of ROS. The body is also exposed to free radicals from environmental exposures, such as cigarette smoke, air pollution, and ultraviolet radiation from the sun. ROS are part of signaling mechanisms among cells.

Vitamin E is a fat-soluble antioxidant that stops the production of ROS formed when fat undergoes oxidation. Scientists are investigating whether, by limiting free-radical production and possibly through other mechanisms, vitamin E might help prevent or delay the chronic diseases associated with free radicals.

In addition to its activities as an antioxidant, vitamin E is involved in immune function and, as shown primarily by *in vitro* studies of cells, cell signaling, regulation of gene expression, and other metabolic processes. Alpha-tocopherol inhibits the activity of protein kinase C, an enzyme involved in cell proliferation and differentiation in smooth muscle cells, platelets, and monocytes. Vitamin-E–replete endothelial cells lining the interior surface of blood vessels are better able to resist blood-cell components adhering to this surface. Vitamin E also increases the expression of two enzymes that suppress arachidonic acid metabolism, thereby increasing the release of prostacyclin from the endothelium, which, in turn, dilates blood vessels and inhibits platelet aggregation.

What Foods Provide Vitamin E?

Vitamin E is found naturally in foods and is added to some fortified foods. You can get recommended amounts of vitamin E by eating a variety of foods including the following:

- Vegetable oils like wheat germ, sunflower, and safflower oils are among the best sources of vitamin E. Corn and soybean oils also provide some vitamin E.

- Nuts (such as peanuts, hazelnuts, and, especially, almonds) and seeds (like sunflower seeds) are also among the best sources of vitamin E.

- Green vegetables, such as spinach and broccoli, provide some vitamin E.

- Food companies add vitamin E to some breakfast cereals, fruit juices, margarines and spreads, and other foods. To find out which ones have vitamin E, check the product labels.

Vitamin E and Coronary Heart Disease

Randomized clinical trials cast doubt on the efficacy of vitamin E supplements to prevent CHD. For example, the Heart Outcomes Prevention Evaluation (HOPE) study, which followed almost 10,000 patients at high risk of heart attack or stroke for 4.5 years, found that participants taking 400 IU/day of natural vitamin E experienced no fewer cardiovascular events or hospitalizations for heart failure or chest pain than participants taking a placebo. In the HOPE-TOO followup study, almost 4,000 of the original participants continued to take vitamin E or placebo for an additional 2.5 years. HOPE-TOO found that vitamin E provided no significant protection against heart attacks, strokes, unstable angina, or deaths from cardiovascular disease or other causes after 7 years of treatment. Participants taking vitamin E, however, were 13% more likely to experience, and 21% more likely to be hospitalized for, heart failure, a statistically significant but unexpected finding not reported in other large studies.

Section 63.3

Omega-3 Fatty Acids for Prevention of Heart Disease

This section includes text excerpted from "5 Things to Know about Omega-3s for Heart Disease," National Center for Complementary and Integrative Health (NCCIH), September 24, 2015.

Omega-3 fatty acids are a group of polyunsaturated fatty acids that are important for a number of functions in the body. They are found in foods such as fatty fish and certain vegetable oils and are also available as dietary supplements. While experts agree that fish rich in omega-3 fatty acids should be included in a heart-healthy diet, there isn't conclusive evidence that shows omega-3s have a protective effect against heart disease.

Experts agree that fish rich in omega-3 fatty acids should be included in a heart-healthy diet. Much research has been done on fish and heart disease, and the results provide strong, though not conclusive evidence that people who eat fish at least once a week are less likely to die of heart disease than those who rarely or never eat fish.

Omega-3s in supplement form have not been shown to protect against heart disease. While there has been a substantial amount of research on omega-3 supplements and heart disease, the findings of individual studies have been inconsistent. In 2012, two combined analyses of the results of these studies did not find convincing evidence that omega-3s protect against heart disease.

Omega-3 supplements may interact with drugs that affect blood clotting. Omega-3 supplements may extend the time it takes for a cut to stop bleeding. People who take drugs such as anticoagulants ("blood thinners") or nonsteroidal anti-inflammatory drugs should discuss the use of omega-3 fatty acid supplements with a healthcare provider.

Fish liver oils (which are not the same as fish oils) contain vitamins A and D as well as omega-3 fatty acids; these vitamins can be toxic in high doses. Fish liver oils contain vitamins A and D as well as omega-3 fatty acids. Both of these vitamins can be toxic in large doses. The amounts of vitamins in fish liver oil supplements vary from one product to another.

Talk to your healthcare provider before using omega-3 supplements. If you are pregnant or nursing a child, if you take medicine that affects blood clotting, if you are allergic to fish or shellfish, or if you are considering giving a child an omega-3 supplement, it is especially important to consult your (or your child's) healthcare provider.

Section 63.4

Tai Chi

This section contains text excerpted from the following sources:
Text begins with excerpts from "Spotlight on a Modality: Tai
Chi," National Center for Complementary and Integrative Health
(NCCIH), November 19, 2015; Text under the heading "5 Tips: What
You Should Know about Tai Chi for Health," is excerpted from "5
Tips: What You Should Know about Tai Chi for Health," National
Center for Complementary and Integrative Health (NCCIH),
September 24, 2015.

Cardiovascular Health

There is only limited, inconsistent evidence available on the effectiveness of tai chi for cardiovascular health. A few studies suggest beneficial effects of tai chi on cardiovascular risk factors, but most of the studies have been small, of short duration, and of poor quality to draw conclusions.

The Evidence Base

The evidence base on efficacy of tai chi for cardiovascular health consists of systematic reviews and meta-analyses of several small studies of low methodological quality.

Efficacy

- A 2015 systematic review and meta-analysis of 20 studies involving 1,868 participants showed that tai chi had beneficial effects on outcomes of cardiovascular function, including blood pressure, heart rate, stroke volume, lung capacity, and V02 peak. However, no definitive conclusions could be drawn due to the low methodological quality of the studies included in the analysis.

- A 2014 Cochrane systematic review of 13 small trials of short duration concluded that because of the limited evidence available, no conclusions can be drawn as the effectiveness of tai chi on cardiovascular disease risk factors.

- A 2015 single-blind randomized controlled trial in patients with a recent myocardial infarction found that after 12 weeks of practicing tai chi, those in the tai chi group had a significant (14%) increase in VO2 peak from baseline, whereas those in the control group had a nonsignificant (5%) decrease in VO2 peak.

Safety

- Tai chi appears to be a safe practice.

- Complaints of musculoskeletal pain after starting tai chi may occur, but have been found to improve with continued practice.

- Women who are pregnant and those with heart conditions should talk with their healthcare providers before beginning tai chi or any other exercise program.

5 Tips: What You Should Know about Tai Chi for Health

Tai chi is a centuries-old, mind and body practice. It involves certain postures and gentle movements with mental focus, breathing, and relaxation. The movements can be adapted or practiced while walking, standing, or sitting. Several clinical trials have evaluated the effects of tai chi in people with various health conditions. Here are five things to know about tai chi for health.

1. Research findings suggest that practicing tai chi may improve balance and stability in older people and reduce the risk of falls. There is also some evidence that tai chi may improve balance impairments in people with mid-to-moderate Parkinson disease.

2. There is some evidence to suggest that practicing tai chi may help people manage chronic pain associated with knee osteoarthritis and help people with fibromyalgia sleep better and cope with pain, fatigue, and depression.

3. Although tai chi has not been shown to have an effect on the disease activity of rheumatoid arthritis (e.g., tender and swollen joints, activities of daily living), there is some evidence that tai chi may improve lower extremity (ankle) range of motion in people with rheumatoid arthritis. It is not known if tai chi improves pain associated with rheumatoid arthritis or quality of life.

4. Tai chi may promote quality of life and mood in people with heart failure and cancer. Tai chi also may offer psychological benefits, such as reducing anxiety. However, differences in how the research on anxiety was conducted make it difficult to draw firm conclusions about this.

5. Take charge of your health—talk with your healthcare providers about any complementary health approaches you use. Together, you can make shared, well-informed decisions.

Chapter 64

How to Prevent and Control Coronary Heart Disease Risk Factors

You can prevent and control many coronary heart disease (CHD) risk factors with heart-healthy lifestyle changes and medicines. Examples of risk factors you can control include high blood cholesterol, high blood pressure, and overweight and obesity. Only a few risk factors—such as age, gender, and family history—can't be controlled.

To reduce your risk of CHD and heart attack, try to control each risk factor you can. The good news is that many lifestyle changes help control several CHD risk factors at the same time. For example, physical activity may lower your blood pressure, help control diabetes and prediabetes, reduce stress, and help control your weight.

Heart-Healthy Lifestyle Changes

A heart-healthy lifestyle can lower the risk of CHD. If you already have CHD, a heart-healthy lifestyle may prevent it from getting worse. Heart-healthy lifestyle changes include:

- Heart-healthy eating
- Maintaining a healthy weight

This chapter includes text excerpted from "Coronary Heart Disease Risk Factors," National Heart, Lung, and Blood Institute (NHLBI), October 23, 2015.

- Managing stress

- Physical activity

- Quitting smoking

Many lifestyle habits begin during childhood. Thus, parents and families should encourage their children to make heart-healthy choices, such as following a healthy diet and being physically active. Make following a healthy lifestyle a family goal. Making lifestyle changes can be hard. But if you make these changes as a family, it may be easier for everyone to prevent or control their CHD risk factors.

Heart-Healthy Eating

Heart-healthy eating is an important part of a heart-healthy lifestyle. Your doctor may recommend heart-healthy eating, which should include:

- Fat-free or low-fat dairy products, such as skim milk

- Fish high in omega-3 fatty acids, such as salmon, tuna, and trout, about twice a week

- Fruits, such as apples, bananas, oranges, pears, and prunes

- Legumes, such as kidney beans, lentils, chickpeas, black-eyed peas, and lima beans

- Vegetables, such as broccoli, cabbage, and carrots

- Whole grains, such as oatmeal, brown rice, and corn tortillas

When following a heart-healthy diet, you should avoid eating:

- A lot of red meat

- Palm and coconut oils

- Sugary foods and beverages

Two nutrients in your diet make blood cholesterol levels rise:

- **Saturated fat**—found mostly in foods that come from animals

- ***Trans* fat (*trans* fatty acids)**—found in foods made with hydrogenated oils and fats, such as stick margarine; baked goods, such as cookies, cakes, and pies; crackers; frostings; and coffee creamers. Some *trans* fats also occur naturally in animal fats and meats.

Saturated fat raises your blood cholesterol more than anything else in your diet. When you follow a heart-healthy eating plan, only 5 percent to 6 percent of your daily calories should come from saturated fat. Food labels list the amounts of saturated fat. To help you stay on track, here are some examples:

Table 64.1. Healthy Amounts of Daily Saturated Fat

If you eat:	Try to eat no more than:
1,200 calories a day	8 grams of saturated fat a day
1,500 calories a day	10 grams of saturated fat a day
1,800 calories a day	12 grams of saturated fat a day
2,000 calories a day	13 grams of saturated fat a day
2,500 calories a day	17 grams of saturated fat a day

Not all fats are bad. Monounsaturated and polyunsaturated fats actually help lower blood cholesterol levels. Some sources of monounsaturated and polyunsaturated fats are:

- Avocados
- Corn, sunflower, and soybean oils
- Nuts and seeds, such as walnuts
- Olive, canola, peanut, safflower, and sesame oils
- Peanut butter
- Salmon and trout
- Tofu

Sodium

You should try to limit the amount of sodium that you eat. This means choosing and preparing foods that are lower in salt and sodium. Try to use low-sodium and "no added salt" foods and seasonings at the table or while cooking. Food labels tell you what you need to know about choosing foods that are lower in sodium. Try to eat no more than 2,300 milligrams of sodium a day. If you have high blood pressure, you may need to restrict your sodium intake even more.

Dietary Approaches to Stop Hypertension (DASH)

Your doctor may recommend the Dietary Approaches to Stop Hypertension (DASH) eating plan if you have high blood pressure. The DASH eating plan focuses on fruits, vegetables, whole grains, and other foods that are heart healthy and low in fat, cholesterol, and sodium and salt.

The DASH eating plan is a good heart-healthy eating plan, even for those who don't have high blood pressure.

Alcohol

Try to limit alcohol intake. Too much alcohol can raise your blood pressure and triglyceride levels, a type of fat found in the blood. Alcohol also adds extra calories, which may cause weight gain.

Men should have no more than two drinks containing alcohol a day. Women should have no more than one drink containing alcohol a day. One drink is:

- 12 ounces of beer

- 5 ounces of wine

- 1½ ounces of liquor

Maintaining a Healthy Weight

Maintaining a healthy weight is important for overall health and can lower your risk for coronary heart disease. Aim for a healthy weight by following a heart-healthy eating plan and keeping physically active.

Knowing your body mass index (BMI) helps you find out if you're a healthy weight in relation to your height and gives an estimate of your total body fat. A BMI:

- Below 18.5 is a sign that you are underweight.

- Between 18.5 and 24.9 is in the healthy range.

- Between 25 and 29.9 is considered overweight.

- Of 30 or more is considered obese.

A general goal to aim for is a BMI below 25. Your healthcare provider can help you set an appropriate BMI goal.

Measuring waist circumference helps screen for possible health risks. If most of your fat is around your waist rather than at your hips, you're at a higher risk for heart disease and type 2 diabetes. This risk may be high with a waist size that is greater than 35 inches for women or greater than 40 inches for men.

If you're overweight or obese, try to lose weight. A loss of just 3 percent to 5 percent of your current weight can lower your triglycerides, blood glucose, and the risk of developing type 2 diabetes. Greater amounts of weight loss can improve blood pressure readings, lower LDL cholesterol, and increase HDL cholesterol.

Managing Stress

Research shows that the most commonly reported "trigger" for a heart attack is an emotionally upsetting event—particularly one involving anger. Also, some of the ways people cope with stress—such as drinking, smoking, or overeating—aren't healthy.

Learning how to manage stress, relax, and cope with problems can improve your emotional and physical health. Consider healthy stress-reducing activities, such as:

- A stress management program.
- Meditation
- Physical activity
- Relaxation therapy
- Talking things out with friends or family

Physical Activity

Routine physical activity can lower many CHD risk factors, including LDL ("bad") cholesterol, high blood pressure, and excess weight. Physical activity also can lower your risk for diabetes and raise your HDL cholesterol level. HDL is the "good" cholesterol that helps prevent CHD.

Everyone should try to participate in moderate-intensity aerobic exercise at least 2 hours and 30 minutes per week, or vigorous aerobic exercise for 1 hour and 15 minutes per week. Aerobic exercise, such as brisk walking, is any exercise in which your heart beats faster and you use more oxygen than usual. The more active you are, the more you will benefit. Participate in aerobic exercise for at least 10 minutes at a time spread throughout the week.

Quitting Smoking

If you smoke, quit. Smoking can raise your risk for coronary heart disease and heart attack and worsen other coronary heart disease risk factors. Talk with your doctor about programs and products that can help you quit smoking. Also, try to avoid secondhand smoke.

If you have trouble quitting smoking on your own, consider joining a support group. Many hospitals, workplaces, and community groups offer classes to help people quit smoking.

Medicines

Sometimes lifestyle changes aren't enough to control your blood cholesterol levels. For example, you may need statin medications to control or lower your cholesterol. By lowering your cholesterol level, you can decrease your chance of having a heart attack or stroke. Doctors usually prescribe statins for people who have:

- Coronary heart disease, peripheral artery disease, or had a prior stroke

- Diabetes

- High LDL cholesterol levels

Doctors may discuss beginning statin treatment with those who have an elevated risk for developing heart disease or having a stroke. Your doctor also may prescribe other medications to:

- Decrease your chance of having a heart attack or dying suddenly.

- Lower your blood pressure.

- Prevent blood clots, which can lead to heart attack or stroke.

- Prevent or delay the need for a procedure or surgery, such as percutaneous coronary intervention or coronary artery bypass grafting.

- Reduce your heart's workload and relieve CHD.

Take all medicines regularly, as your doctor prescribes. Don't change the amount of your medicine or skip a dose unless your doctor tells you to. You should still follow a heart-healthy lifestyle, even if you take medicines to treat your CHD.

Chapter 65

Physical Activity: Key to a Healthy Heart

What Is Physical Activity?

Physical activity is any body movement that works your muscles and requires more energy than resting. Walking, running, dancing, swimming, yoga, and gardening are a few examples of physical activity.

According to the Department of Health and Human Services' *2008 Physical Activity Guidelines for Americans* physical activity generally refers to movement that enhances health.

Exercise is a type of physical activity that's planned and structured. Lifting weights, taking an aerobics class, and playing on a sports team are examples of exercise.

Physical activity is good for many parts of your body. This chapter focuses on the benefits of physical activity for your heart and lungs. It also provides tips for getting started and staying active, and it discusses physical activity as part of a heart healthy lifestyle.

Outlook

Being physically active is one of the best ways to keep your heart and lungs healthy. Following a healthy diet and not smoking are other important ways to keep your heart and lungs healthy.

This chapter includes text excerpted from "Physical Activity and Your Heart," National Heart, Lung, and Blood Institute (NHLBI), October 29, 2015.

Many Americans are not active enough. The good news, though, is that even modest amounts of physical activity are good for your health. The more active you are, the more you will benefit.

Types of Physical Activity

The four main types of physical activity are aerobic, muscle-strengthening, bone-strengthening, and stretching. Aerobic activity is the type that benefits your heart and lungs the most.

Aerobic Activity

Aerobic activity moves your large muscles, such as those in your arms and legs. Running, swimming, walking, bicycling, dancing, and doing jumping jacks are examples of aerobic activity. Aerobic activity also is called endurance activity.

Aerobic activity makes your heart beat faster than usual. You also breathe harder during this type of activity. Over time, regular aerobic activity makes your heart and lungs stronger and able to work better.

Other Types of Physical Activity

The other types of physical activity—muscle-strengthening, bone strengthening, and stretching—benefit your body in other ways.

Muscle-strengthening activities improve the strength, power, and endurance of your muscles. Doing pushups and situps, lifting weights, climbing stairs, and digging in the garden are examples of muscle-strengthening activities.

With bone-strengthening activities, your feet, legs, or arms support your body's weight, and your muscles push against your bones. This helps make your bones strong. Running, walking, jumping rope, and lifting weights are examples of bone-strengthening activities.

Muscle-strengthening and bone-strengthening activities also can be aerobic, depending on whether they make your heart and lungs work harder than usual. For example, running is both an aerobic activity and a bone-strengthening activity.

Stretching helps improve your flexibility and your ability to fully move your joints. Touching your toes, doing side stretches, and doing yoga exercises are examples of stretching.

Levels of Intensity in Aerobic Activity

You can do aerobic activity with light, moderate, or vigorous intensity. Moderate- and vigorous-intensity aerobic activities are better for your heart than light-intensity activities. However, even light-intensity activities are better than no activity at all.

The level of intensity depends on how hard you have to work to do the activity. To do the same activity, people who are less fit usually have to work harder than people who are more fit. So, for example, what is light-intensity activity for one person may be moderate-intensity for another.

Light- and Moderate-Intensity Activities

Light-intensity activities are common daily activities that don't require much effort.

Moderate-intensity activities make your heart, lungs, and muscles work harder than light-intensity activities do.

On a scale of 0 to 10, moderate-intensity activity is a 5 or 6 and produces noticeable increases in breathing and heart rate. A person doing moderate-intensity activity can talk but not sing.

Vigorous-Intensity Activities

Vigorous-intensity activities make your heart, lungs, and muscles work hard. On a scale of 0 to 10, vigorous-intensity activity is a 7 or 8. A person doing vigorous-intensity activity can't say more than a few words without stopping for a breath.

Examples of Aerobic Activities

Below are examples of aerobic activities. Depending on your level of fitness, they can be light, moderate, or vigorous in intensity:

- Pushing a grocery cart around a store
- Gardening, such as digging or hoeing that causes your heart rate to go up
- Walking, hiking, jogging, running
- Water aerobics or swimming laps
- Bicycling, skateboarding, rollerblading, and jumping rope
- Ballroom dancing and aerobic dancing
- Tennis, soccer, hockey, and basketball

Benefits of Physical Activity

Physical activity has many health benefits. These benefits apply to people of all ages and races and both sexes.

For example, physical activity helps you maintain a healthy weight and makes it easier to do daily tasks, such as climbing stairs and shopping.

Physically active adults are at lower risk for depression and declines in cognitive function as they get older. (Cognitive function includes thinking, learning, and judgment skills.) Physically active children and teens may have fewer symptoms of depression than their peers.

Physical activity also lowers your risk for many diseases, such as coronary heart disease (CHD), diabetes, and cancer.

Many studies have shown the clear benefits of physical activity for your heart and lungs.

Physical Activity Strengthens Your Heart and Improves Lung Function

When done regularly, moderate- and vigorous-intensity physical activity strengthens your heart muscle. This improves your heart's ability to pump blood to your lungs and throughout your body. As a result, more blood flows to your muscles, and oxygen levels in your blood rise.

Capillaries, your body's tiny blood vessels, also widen. This allows them to deliver more oxygen to your body and carry away waste products.

Physical Activity Reduces Coronary Heart Disease Risk Factors

When done regularly, moderate- and vigorous-intensity aerobic activity can lower your risk for CHD. CHD is a condition in which a waxy substance called plaque builds up inside your coronary arteries. These arteries supply your heart muscle with oxygen-rich blood.

Plaque narrows the arteries and reduces blood flow to your heart muscle. Eventually, an area of plaque can rupture (break open). This causes a blood clot to form on the surface of the plaque.

If the clot becomes large enough, it can mostly or completely block blood flow through a coronary artery. Blocked blood flow to the heart muscle causes a heart attack.

Certain traits, conditions, or habits may raise your risk for CHD. Physical activity can help control some of these risk factors because it:

- Can lower blood pressure and triglyceride. Triglycerides are a type of fat in the blood.

- Can raise HDL cholesterol levels. HDL sometimes is called "good" cholesterol.

- Helps your body manage blood sugar and insulin levels, which lowers your risk for type 2 diabetes.

- Reduces levels of C-reactive protein (CRP) in your body. This protein is a sign of inflammation. High levels of CRP may suggest an increased risk for CHD.

- Helps reduce overweight and obesity when combined with a reduced-calorie diet. Physical activity also helps you maintain a healthy weight over time once you have lost weight.

- May help you quit smoking. Smoking is a major risk factor for CHD.

Inactive people are more likely to develop CHD than people who are physically active. Studies suggest that inactivity is a major risk factor for CHD, just like high blood pressure, high blood cholesterol, and smoking.

Physical Activity Reduces Heart Attack Risk

For people who have CHD, aerobic activity done regularly helps the heart work better. It also may reduce the risk of a second heart attack in people who already have had heart attacks.

Vigorous aerobic activity may not be safe for people who have CHD. Ask your doctor what types of activity are safe for you.

Risks of Physical Activity

In general, the benefits of regular physical activity far outweigh risks to the heart and lungs.

Rarely, heart problems occur as a result of physical activity. Examples of these problems include arrhythmias, sudden cardiac arrest, and heart attack. These events generally happen to people who already have heart conditions.

The risk of heart problems due to physical activity is higher for youth and young adults who have congenital heart problems. The term "congenital" means the heart problem has been present since birth.

Congenital heart problems include hypertrophic cardiomyopathy, congenital heart defects, and myocarditis. People who have these conditions should ask their doctors what types of physical activity are safe for them.

For middle-aged and older adults, the risk of heart problems due to physical activity is related to coronary heart disease (CHD). People who have CHD are more likely to have a heart attack when they're exercising vigorously than when they're not.

The risk of heart problems due to physical activity is related to your fitness level and the intensity of the activity you're doing. For example, someone who isn't physically fit is at higher risk for a heart attack during vigorous activity than a person who is physically fit.

If you have a heart problem or chronic (ongoing) disease—such as heart disease, diabetes, or high blood pressure—ask your doctor what types of physical activity are safe for you. You also should talk with your doctor about safe physical activities if you have symptoms such as chest pain or dizziness.

Recommendations for Physical Activity

The U.S. Department of Health and Human Services (HHS) has released physical activity guidelines for all Americans aged 6 and older.

The *2008 Physical Activity Guidelines for Americans* explain that regular physical activity improves health. They encourage people to be as active as possible.

The guidelines recommend the types and amounts of physical activity that children, adults, older adults, and other groups should do. The guidelines also provide tips for how to fit physical activity into your daily life.

The information below is based on the HHS guidelines.

Guidelines for Children and Youth

The guidelines advise that:

- Children and youth do 60 minutes or more of physical activity every day. Activities should vary and be a good fit for their age and physical development. Children are naturally active, especially when they're involved in unstructured play (like recess). Any type of activity counts toward the advised 60 minutes or more.

- Most physical activity should be moderate-intensity aerobic activity. Examples include walking, running, skipping, playing on the playground, playing basketball, and biking.

- Vigorous-intensity aerobic activity should be included at least 3 days a week. Examples include running, doing jumping jacks, and fast swimming.

- Muscle-strengthening activities should be included at least 3 days a week. Examples include playing on playground equipment, playing tug-of-war, and doing pushups and pullups.

- Bone-strengthening activities should be included at least 3 days a week. Examples include hopping, skipping, doing jumping jacks, playing volleyball, and working with resistance bands.

Children and youth who have disabilities should work with their doctors to find out what types and amounts of physical activity are safe for them. When possible, these children should meet the recommendations in the guidelines.

Some experts also advise that children and youth reduce screen time because it limits time for physical activity. They recommend that children aged 2 and older should spend no more than 2 hours a day watching television or using a computer (except for school work).

Guidelines for Adults

The guidelines advise that:

- Some physical activity is better than none. Inactive adults should gradually increase their level of activity. People gain health benefits from as little as 60 minutes of moderate-intensity aerobic activity per week.

- For major health benefits, do at least 150 minutes (2 hours and 30 minutes) of moderate-intensity aerobic activity or 75 minutes (1 hour and 15 minutes) of vigorous-intensity aerobic activity each week. Another option is to do a combination of both. A general rule is that 2 minutes of moderate-intensity activity counts the same as 1 minute of vigorous-intensity activity.

- For even more health benefits, do 300 minutes (5 hours) of moderate-intensity aerobic activity or 150 minutes (2 hours and 30 minutes) of vigorous-intensity activity each week (or a combination of both). The more active you are, the more you will benefit.

- When doing aerobic activity, do it for at least 10 minutes at a time. Spread the activity throughout the week. Muscle-strengthening activities that are moderate or vigorous intensity should be included 2 or more days a week. These activities should work all of the major muscle groups (legs, hips, back, chest, abdomen, shoulders, and arms). Examples include lifting weights, working with resistance bands, and doing situps and pushups, yoga, and heavy gardening.

Guidelines for Adults Aged 65 or Older

The guidelines advise that:

- Older adults should be physically active. Older adults who do any amount of physical activity gain some health benefits. If inactive, older adults should gradually increase their activity levels and avoid vigorous activity at first.

- Older adults should follow the guidelines for adults, if possible. Do a variety of activities, including walking. Walking has been shown to provide health benefits and a low risk of injury.

- If you can't do 150 minutes (2 hours and 30 minutes) of activity each week, be as physically active as your abilities and condition allow.

- You should do balance exercises if you're at risk for falls. Examples include walking backward or sideways, standing on one leg, and standing from a sitting position several times in a row.

- If you have a chronic (ongoing) condition—such as heart disease, lung disease, or diabetes—ask your doctor what types and amounts of activity are safe for you.

Guidelines for Women during Pregnancy and Soon after Delivery

The guidelines advise that:

- You should ask your doctor what physical activities are safe to do during pregnancy and after delivery.

- If you're healthy but not already active, do at least 150 minutes (2 hours and 30 minutes) of moderate-intensity aerobic activity each week. If possible, spread this activity across the week.

- If you're already active, you can continue being active as long as you stay healthy and talk with your doctor about your activity level throughout your pregnancy.

- After the first 3 months of pregnancy, you shouldn't do exercises that involve lying on your back.

- You shouldn't do activities in which you might fall or hurt yourself, such as horseback riding, downhill skiing, soccer, and basketball.

Guidelines for Other Groups

The HHS guidelines also have recommendations for other groups, including people who have disabilities and people who have chronic conditions, such as osteoarthritis, diabetes, and cancer.

Getting Started and Staying Active

Physical activity is an important part of a heart healthy lifestyle. To get started and stay active, make physical activity part of your daily routine, keep track of your progress, be active and safe, and talk to your doctor if you have a chronic (ongoing) health condition.

Make Physical Activity Part of Your Daily Routine

You don't have to become a marathon runner to get all of the benefits of physical activity. Do activities that you enjoy, and make them part of your daily routine.

If you haven't been active for a while, start low and build slow. Many people like to start with walking and slowly increase their time and distance. You also can take other steps to make physical activity part of your routine.

Personalize the Benefits

People value different things. Some people may highly value the health benefits from physical activity. Others want to be active because they enjoy recreational activities or they want to look better or sleep better.

Some people want to be active because it helps them lose weight or it gives them a chance to spend time with friends. Identify which physical activity benefits you value. This will help you personalize the benefits of physical activity.

Be Active with Friends and Family

Friends and family can help you stay active. For example, go for a hike with a friend. Take dancing lessons with your spouse, or play ball with your child. The possibilities are endless.

Make Everyday Activities More Active

You can make your daily routine more active. For example, take the stairs instead of the elevator. Instead of sending e-mails, walk down the hall to a coworker's office. Rake the leaves instead of using a leaf blower.

Reward Yourself with Time for Physical Activity

Sometimes, going for a bike ride or a long walk relieves stress after a long day. Think of physical activity as a special time to refresh your body and mind.

Keep Track of Your Progress

Consider keeping a log of your activity. A log can help you track your progress. Many people like to wear a pedometer (a small device that counts your steps) to track how much they walk every day. These tools can help you set goals and stay motivated.

Be Active and Safe

Physical activity is safe for almost everyone. You can take steps to make sure it's safe for you too.

- Be active on a regular basis to raise your fitness level.

- Do activities that fit your health goals and fitness level. Start low and slowly increase your activity level over time. As your fitness improves, you will be able to do physical activities for longer periods and with more intensity.

- Spread out your activity over the week and vary the types of activity you do.

- Use the right gear and equipment to protect yourself. For example, use bicycle helmets, elbow and knee pads, and goggles.

- Be active in safe environments. Pick well-lit and well-maintained places that are clearly separated from car traffic.

- Follow safety rules and policies, such as always wearing a helmet when biking.

- Make sensible choices about when, where, and how to be active. Consider weather conditions, such as how hot or cold it is, and change your plans as needed.

Talk to Your Doctor if Needed

Healthy people who don't have heart problems don't need to check with a doctor before beginning moderate-intensity activities.

If you have a heart problem or chronic disease, such as heart disease, diabetes, or high blood pressure, talk to your doctor about what types of physical activity are safe for you.

You also should talk to your doctor about safe physical activities if you have symptoms such as chest pain or dizziness.

Chapter 66

Managing Stress for a Healthy Heart

Take Time to Unwind...

Stress happens. Sometimes it's unavoidable, at times it's unbearable. That's why taking time for yourself is invaluable. It's healthy to relax, renew, and rejuvenate.

Stress does not merely afflict your mind; it can also affect you on a cellular level. In fact, long-term stress can lead to a wide range of illnesses—from headaches to stomach disorders to depression—and can even increase the risk of serious conditions like stroke and heart disease. Understanding the mind/stress/health connection can help you better manage stress and improve your health and well-being.

The Fight or Flight Response

The sympathetic stress response is a survival mechanism that is hardwired into our nervous systems. This automatic response is necessary for mobilizing quick reflexes when there is imminent danger, such as swerving to avoid a car crash.

This chapter contains text excerpted from the following sources: Text beginning with the heading "Take Time to Unwind..." is excerpted from "Stress Awareness," Federal Occupational Health (FOH), March 26, 2016; Text under the heading "Heart-Healthy Breathing Blows Stress Away" is excerpted from "Heart-Healthy Breathing Blows Stress Away," Military Health System (MHS), February 26, 2016.

When you perceive a threat, stress hormones rush into your bloodstream—increasing heart rate, blood pressure, and glucose levels. Other hormones also suppress functions like digestion and the immune system, which is one of the reasons why chronic stress can leave you more vulnerable to illness.

Danger triggers the stress response. Unfortunately, so can work conflicts, concerns over debt, bad memories, or anxiety in general. Although one bad day at work won't compromise your health, weeks or months of stress can dampen your immune response and raise your risk for disease.

Combat Your Stress

If you suffer from chronic stress and can't influence or change the situation, then you'll need to change your approach. Be willing to be flexible. Remember, you have the ability to choose your response to stressors, and you may have to try various options.

- Recognize when you don't have control, and let it go.

- Don't get anxious about situations that you cannot change.

- Take control of your own reactions and focus your mind on something that makes you feel calm and in control. This may take some practice, but it pays off in peace of mind.

- Develop a vision for healthy living, wellness, and personal growth, and set realistic goals to help you realize your vision.

Relax and Recharge

Be sure to carve out some time to relax and take care of yourself each day—even just 10 to 15 minutes per day can improve your ability to handle life's stressors. Also, remember that exercise is an excellent stress reliever.

Everyone has different ways they like to relax and unwind. Here are a few ideas to get you started:

- Take a walk
- Read a book
- Go for a run
- Have a cup of tea
- Play a sport

- Spend time with a friend or loved one

- Meditate (learn how in the sidebar)

- Do yoga

While you can't avoid stress, you can minimize it by changing how you choose to respond to it. The ultimate reward for your efforts is a healthy, balanced life, with time for work, relationships, relaxation, and fun.

Heart-Healthy Breathing Blows Stress Away

Stress can take its toll on your mental and physical health, including your heart health, but there are breathing techniques to buffer yourself from it! When you're less focused on your breathing, it's typical to breathe erratically—especially when you face the stressors of day-to-day life. In turn, your heart rate can become less rhythmic, causing your heart to not function as well.

But when you have longer, slower exhales—breathing at about 4-second-inhale and 6-second-exhale paces—your heart rate rhythmically fluctuates up and down. This rhythmic variability in heart rate mirrors your inhales and exhales so that you have maximum heart rate *at the end of the inhale* and minimum heart rate *at the end of the exhale*. More importantly, this physiological shift could help you feel less stressed, anxious, or depressed—and experience better heart health.

It's easy to go through the motions of breathing while absorbed in your own thoughts; instead, take notice of your breathing and other body sensations. Regularly tuning in to your body sensations could help you feel more resilient and ready to:

- Adapt to change

- Deal with whatever comes your way

- See the brighter, or funnier, side of problems

- Overcome stress

- Tolerate unpleasant feelings

- Bounce back after illnesses, failures, or other hardships

- Achieve goals despite obstacles

- Stay focused under pressure

- Feel stronger

Chapter 67

Quitting Smoking: Why It Is Important and How to Do It

No matter your age, quitting smoking improves your health. If you quit smoking, you are likely to add years to your life, breathe more easily, and save money. You will also:

- Lower your risk of cancer, heart attack, stroke, and lung disease

- Have better blood circulation

- Improve your sense of taste and smell

- Stop smelling like smoke

- Set a healthy example for your children and grandchildren

Smoking shortens your life. It causes about 1 of every 5 deaths in the United States each year. Smoking makes millions of Americans sick by causing:

- **Lung disease.** Smoking damages your lungs and airways, sometimes causing chronic bronchitis. It can also cause a disease called emphysema that destroys your lungs, making it very hard for you to breathe.

- **Heart disease.** Smoking increases your risk of heart attack and stroke.

This chapter includes text excerpted from "Smoking: It's Never Too Late to Stop," National Institute on Aging (NIA), May 4, 2016.

- **Cancer.** Smoking can lead to cancer of the lung, mouth, larynx (voice box), esophagus, stomach, liver, pancreas, kidney, bladder, and cervix.

- **Respiratory problems.** If you smoke, you are more likely than a nonsmoker to get the flu (influenza), pneumonia, or other infections that can interfere with your breathing.

- **Osteoporosis.** If you smoke, your chance of developing osteoporosis (weak bones) is greater.

Nicotine Is a Drug

Nicotine is the drug in tobacco that makes tobacco products addictive. People become addicted to nicotine. That's one reason why the first few weeks after quitting are the hardest. Some people who give up smoking have withdrawal symptoms. They may feel grumpy, hungry, or tired. Some people have headaches, feel depressed, or have problems sleeping or concentrating. These symptoms fade over time. Some people have no withdrawal symptoms.

Breaking the Addiction

Many people say the first step to stop smoking is to make a firm decision to quit and pick a definite date to stop. Then make a clear plan for how you will stick to it.

Your plan might include:

- Talking with your doctor

- Setting a quit date, when you stop smoking completely

- Developing a plan for dealing with urges to smoke

- Reading self-help information

- Going to individual or group counseling

- Asking a friend for help

- Taking medicine to help with symptoms of nicotine withdrawal

- Calling your state quitline (1-800-784-8669 or 1-800-QUITNOW) or visiting www.smokefree.gov on the internet

Find what works best for you. Using many approaches to quitting may be the answer.

Help with Quitting

When you quit, you may need support to cope with your body's desire for nicotine. Nicotine replacement products help some smokers quit. You can buy gum, patches, or lozenges over-the-counter.

There are also products that require a doctor's prescription. A nicotine nasal spray or inhaler can reduce withdrawal symptoms and make it easier for you to quit smoking.

Other drugs may also help with withdrawal symptoms. Talk to your doctor about what medicines might be best for you.

Cigars, Pipes, Chewing Tobacco, and Snuff Are Not Safe

Some people think smokeless tobacco (chewing tobacco and snuff), pipes, and cigars are safe. They are not. Smokeless tobacco causes cancer of the mouth and pancreas. It also causes pre-cancerous lesions known as oral leukoplakia, gum problems, and nicotine addiction. Pipe and cigar smokers may develop cancer of the mouth, lip, larynx, esophagus, and bladder. Those who inhale are also at increased risk of getting lung cancer.

Secondhand Smoke Is Dangerous

Secondhand smoke created by cigarettes, cigars, and pipes can cause serious health problems for family, friends, and even pets of smokers. Secondhand smoke is especially dangerous for people who already have lung or heart disease. In adults, secondhand smoke can cause heart disease and lung cancer. In babies it can cause Sudden Infant Death Syndrome (SIDS). Children are also more likely to have lung problems, ear infections, and severe asthma if they are around secondhand smoke.

Good News about Quitting

The good news is that after you quit:

- Your lungs, heart, and circulatory system will begin to function better.

- Your chance of having a heart attack or stroke will drop.

- Your breathing will improve.

- Your chance of getting cancer will be lower.

No matter how old you are, all of these health benefits are important reasons to make a plan to stop smoking.

725

Chapter 68

Other Interventions to Help Reduce Risk of Cardiovascular Disease

Chapter Contents

Section 68.1

Aspirin for Reducing Your Risk of Heart Attack and Stroke

This section includes text excerpted from "Aspirin for Reducing Your
Risk of Heart Attack and Stroke: Know the Facts," U.S. Food and
Drug Administration (FDA), February 5, 2014.

Aspirin for Reducing Your Risk of Heart Attack and Stroke

You can walk into any pharmacy, grocery or convenience store and
buy aspirin without a prescription. The *Drug Facts* label on medication
products, will help you choose aspirin for relieving headache, pain,
swelling, or fever. The *Drug Facts* label also gives directions that will
help you use the aspirin so that it is safe and effective.

But what about using aspirin for a different use, time period, or in
a manner that is not listed on the label? For example, using aspirin to
lower the risk of heart attack and clot-related strokes. In these cases,
the labeling information is not there to help you with how to choose
and how to use the medicine safely. **Since you don't have the labeling directions to help you, you need the medical knowledge of
your doctor, nurse practitioner or other health professional.**

You can increase the chance of getting the good effects and decrease
the chance of getting the bad effects of any medicine by choosing and
using it wisely. When it comes to using aspirin to lower the risk of
heart attack and stroke, choosing and using wisely means:

Know the Facts and Work with Your Health Professional

FACT: Daily Use of Aspirin Is Not Right for Everyone

Aspirin has been shown to be helpful when used daily to lower the
risk of heart attack, clot-related strokes and other blood flow problems
in patients who have cardiovascular disease or who have already had
a heart attack or stroke. Many medical professionals prescribe aspirin
for these uses. There may be a benefit to daily aspirin use for you if you

have some kind of heart or blood vessel disease, or if you have evidence of poor blood flow to the brain. However, the risks of long-term aspirin use may be greater than the benefits if there are no signs of, or risk factors for heart or blood vessel disease.

Every prescription and over-the-counter medicine has benefits and risks—even such a common and familiar medicine as aspirin. Aspirin use can result in serious side effects, such as stomach bleeding, bleeding in the brain, kidney failure, and some kinds of strokes. No medicine is completely safe. By carefully reviewing many different factors, your health professional can help you make the best choice for you.

When you don't have the labeling directions to guide you, you need the medical knowledge of your doctor, nurse practitioner, or other health professional.

FACT: Daily Aspirin Can Be Safest When Prescribed by a Medical Health Professional

Before deciding if daily aspirin use is right for you, your health professional will need to consider:

- Your medical history and the history of your family members

- Your use of other medicines, including prescription and over-the-counter

- Your use of other products, such as dietary supplements, including vitamins and herbals

- Your allergies or sensitivities, and anything that affects your ability to use the medicine

- What you have to gain, or the benefits, from the use of the medicine

- Other options and their risks and benefits

- What side effects you may experience

- What dose, and what directions for use are best for you

- How to know when the medicine is working or not working for this use

Make sure to tell your health professional all the medicines (prescription and over-the-counter) and dietary supplements, including vitamins and herbals, that you use—even if only occasionally.

FACT: Aspirin Is a Drug

If you are at risk for heart attack or stroke your doctor may prescribe aspirin to increase blood flow to the heart and brain. But any drug—including aspirin—can have harmful side effects, especially when mixed with other products. In fact, the chance of side effects increases with each new product you use.

New products includes prescription and other over-the-counter medicines, dietary supplements (including vitamins and herbals), and sometimes foods and beverages. For instance, people who already use a prescribed medication to thin the blood should not use aspirin unless recommended by a health professional. There are also dietary supplements known to thin the blood. Using aspirin with alcohol or with another product that also contains aspirin, such as a cough-sinus drug, can increase the chance of side effects.

Your health professional will consider your current state of health. Some medical conditions, such as pregnancy, uncontrolled high blood pressure, bleeding disorders, asthma, peptic (stomach) ulcers, liver and kidney disease, could make aspirin a bad choice for you.

Make sure that all your health professionals are aware that you are using aspirin to reduce your risk of heart attack and clot-related strokes.

FACT: Once Your Doctor Decides That Daily Use of Aspirin Is for You, Safe Use Depends on Following Your Doctor's Directions.

There are no directions on the label for using aspirin to reduce the risk of heart attack or clot-related stroke. You may rely on your health professional to provide the correct information on dose and directions for use. Using aspirin correctly gives you the best chance of getting the greatest benefits with the fewest unwanted side effects. Discuss with your health professional the different forms of aspirin products that might be best suited for you.

Aspirin has been shown to lower the risk of heart attack and stroke in patients who have cardiovascular disease or who have already had a heart attack or stroke, but not all over-the-counter pain and fever reducers do that. Even though the directions on the aspirin label do not apply to this use of aspirin, you still need to read the label to confirm that the product you buy and use contains aspirin at the correct dose. Check the *Drug Facts* label for "active ingredients: aspirin" or "acetyl-salicylic acid" at the dose that your health professional has prescribed.

Remember, if you are using aspirin everyday for weeks, months or years to prevent a heart attack, stroke, or for any use not listed on the label—without the guidance from your health professional—you could be doing your body more harm than good.

Section 68.2

Chelation for Coronary Heart Disease

This section includes text excerpted from "Chelation for Coronary Heart Disease," National Center for Complementary and Integrative Health (NCCIH), March 25, 2016.

Chelation for Coronary Heart Disease

Coronary heart disease is the number-one killer of men and women in the United States. Lifestyle changes (such as quitting smoking), medicines, and medical and surgical procedures are among the mainstays of conventional treatment. Some heart patients also turn to chelation therapy using disodium EDTA (ethylene diamine tetra-acetic acid), a controversial complementary health approach. The use of disodium EDTA for heart disease has not been approved by the U.S. Food and Drug Administration (FDA). Use of this therapy to treat heart disease and other diseases grew, however, in the United States from 2002 to 2007 by nearly 68 percent, to an estimated 111,000 people using it annually.

Chelation is a chemical process in which a substance is used to bind molecules, such as metals or minerals, and hold them tightly so that they can be removed from the body. Chelation has been used to rid the body of excess or toxic metals. It has some uses in conventional medicine, such as treating lead poisoning or iron overload. When used as a complementary treatment for heart disease, a health care provider typically administers a solution of disodium EDTA, a man-made amino acid, in a series of infusions through the veins. A course of treatment can require 30 or more infusions of several hours each, taken weekly until the maintenance phase. Patients also typically take high-dose pills of vitamins and minerals.

To determine whether chelation therapy, with or without high-dose vitamins and minerals, may be useful, NCCIH and the National Heart, Lung, and Blood Institute sponsored the first large-scale, multicenter clinical trial on chelation therapy in people with coronary heart disease. Results of the Trial to Assess Chelation Therapy (TACT) began to be released in 2013.

Bottom Line

- Overall, TACT showed that infusions of EDTA chelation therapy produced a modest reduction in cardiovascular events in EDTA-treated participants. However, further examination of the data showed that chelation therapy benefitted only the patients with diabetes.

- Patients with diabetes, who made up approximately one third of the 1,708 TACT participants, had a 41 percent overall reduction in the risk of any cardiovascular event; a 40 percent reduction in the risk of death from heart disease, nonfatal stroke, or nonfatal heart attack; a 52 percent reduction in recurrent heart attacks; and a 43 percent reduction in death from any cause. In contrast, there was no significant benefit of EDTA treatment in participants who didn't have diabetes.

- The TACT study team also looked at the impact of taking high-dose vitamins and minerals in addition to the chelation therapy. They found that chelation plus high-dose vitamins and minerals produced the greatest reduction in risk of cardiovascular events versus placebo.

- Further research is needed to fully understand the TACT results. Since this is the first clinical trial to show a benefit, these results are not, by themselves, sufficient to support the routine use of chelation as a post-heart attack therapy.

Safety

- In the TACT study, which had extensive safety monitoring, 16 percent of people receiving chelation and 15 percent of people receiving the placebo stopped their infusions because of an adverse event. Four of those events were serious; two were in the chelation group (one death) and two were in the placebo group (one death).

- The most common side effect of EDTA chelation is a burning sensation at the site where EDTA is administered. Rare side effects can include fever, headache, nausea, and vomiting. Even more rare are serious and potentially fatal side effects that can include heart failure, a sudden drop in blood pressure, abnormally low calcium levels in the blood (hypocalcemia), permanent kidney damage, and bone marrow depression (blood cell counts fall). Hypocalcemia and death may occur particularly if disodium EDTA is infused too rapidly. Reversible injury to the kidneys, although infrequent, has been reported with EDTA chelation therapy. Other serious side effects can occur if EDTA is not administered by a trained health professional.

- If you're considering chelation therapy, discuss it first with your cardiologist or other health care provider for your heart care. Seek out and consider information available from scientific studies on the therapy.

- If you decide to use chelation, choose the practitioner carefully. Do not take over-the-counter products marketed for "chelation" purposes.

- Give all your health care providers a full picture of what you do to manage your health. This will help ensure coordinated and safe care.

733

Part Eight

Additional Help and Information

Chapter 69

Glossary of Terms Related to Cardiovascular Disorders

abdomen: The part of the body between the ribs and pelvis that holds the stomach, intestines, liver, and other organs.

acute coronary syndrome: It is a term that includes heart attack and unstable angina.

aerobic exercise: A type of physical activity that burns fat, gets your heart rate going (you will be able to feel it beating faster), and makes your heart muscle stronger.

amniotic fluid: Clear, yellowish liquid that surrounds an unborn baby during pregnancy.

anemia: When the total amount of red blood cells or hemoglobin is below normal. Anemia can cause severe fatigue and other health problems.

anesthesia: A drug that makes you sleepy or can numb a part of your body before surgery so that you don't feel pain.

aneurysm: A thin or weak spot in an artery that balloons out and can burst.

angina: A recurring pain or discomfort in the chest that happens when some part of the heart does not receive enough blood.

This glossary contains terms excerpted from documents produced by several sources deemed reliable.

angioplasty: A medical procedure used to open a blocked artery.

anorexia nervosa: An illness in which people don't eat enough and therefore can't stay at a healthy body weight. Anorexia nervosa can result in life-threatening weight loss and amenorrhea.

antibiotic: Medicine used to fight bacterial infections by killing bacteria or stopping it from growing. Antibiotics can help your body's immune system fight off infections.

antidepressant: Drugs given by your doctor to treat depression.

arrhythmia: An arrhythmia is a problem with the rate or rhythm of the heartbeat. During an arrhythmia, the heart can beat too fast, too slow, or with an irregular rhythm.

artery: Any of the thick-walled blood vessels that carry blood away from the heart to other parts of the body.

atherosclerosis: Atherosclerosis occurs when plaque builds up in the arteries that supply blood to the heart (called coronary arteries).

atrial fibrillation: Atrial fibrillation is a type of arrhythmia that can cause rapid, irregular beating of the heart's upper chambers.

biopsy: When a doctor takes a very small piece of your body, such as some skin, to look at under a microscope.

birth defect: A problem that happens while a baby is forming in the mother's body. Most birth defects happen during the first three months of pregnancy and may affect how the baby's body looks, works, or both.

blood glucose level: The amount of glucose in the blood.

blood pressure: blood pressure is the force of blood against the walls of arteries.

blood test: This is either done by using a finger prick to get a few drops or by inserting a needle into a vein to get a larger amount of blood. Blood tests are used to check for many different diseases and viruses.

blood vessel: A tube-shaped part of the circulatory system which helps blood move through the body.

broken heart syndrome: Broken heart syndrome is a condition in which extreme stress can lead to heart muscle failure.

calorie: When talking about food, a calorie is a measure of the amount of energy you get from eating a certain amount of food. When talking about physical activity, a calorie is a measure of the energy that your body uses in performing the activity.

capillary: Any of the tiny blood vessels that branch through body tissues to deliver oxygen and nutrients and carry away waste products.

cardiac rehabilitation: Cardiac rehabilitation (rehab) is a medically supervised program that helps improve the health and well-being of people who have heart problems.

cardiogenic shock: Cardiogenic shock is a condition in which a suddenly weakened heart isn't able to pump enough blood to meet the body's needs.

cardiomyopathy: Cardiomyopathy occurs when the heart muscle becomes enlarged or stiff. This can lead to inadequate heart pumping (or weak heart pump) or other problems.

cardiovascular diseases: Disease of the heart and blood vessels.

carotid artery disease: Carotid artery disease is a disease in which a waxy substance called plaque builds up inside the carotid arteries.

cerebrovascular disease: Disease of the blood vessels in the brain.

cholesterol: A soft, waxy substance that is present in all parts of the body.

congenital heart defects: Congenital heart defects are problems with the heart that are present at birth. They are the most common type of major birth defect.

coronary heart disease: Coronary heart disease is a disease in which a waxy substance called plaque builds up inside the coronary arteries.

coronary microvascular disease: Coronary microvascular disease is heart disease that affects the tiny coronary (heart) arteries. In coronary MVD, the walls of the heart's tiny arteries are damaged or diseased.

coronary stent: A device used to keep an artery open.

DASH eating plan: DASH is a flexible and balanced eating plan that helps creates a heart-healthy eating style for life.

deep vein thrombosis: Deep vein thrombosis, or DVT, is a blood clot that forms in a vein deep in the body. Blood clots occur when blood thickens and clumps together.

depression: An illness that involves the body, mood, and thoughts. It affects the way a person functions, eats and sleeps, feels about herself, and thinks about things.

electrocardiogram: An external, noninvasive test that records the electrical activity of the heart.

electrolyte imbalance: When the amounts of sodium and potassium in the body become too much or too little.

emphysema: A disease than involves damage to the air sacs (alveoli) in the lungs. The air sacs have trouble deflating once filled with air, so they are unable to fill up again with the fresh air needed to supply the body. Cigarette smoking is the most common cause of emphysema.

endocarditis: Endocarditis is an infection of the inner lining of the heart chambers and valves.

endurance: The measure of your body's ability to keep up an activity without getting tired. The more endurance you have, the longer you can swim, bike, run, or play a sport before tiring out.

fat: A source of energy used by the body to make substances it needs.

fatigue: A feeling of lack of energy, weariness or tiredness.

heart: Your heart is a muscular organ that pumps blood to your body.

heart attack: A heart attack happens when the flow of oxygen-rich blood to a section of heart muscle suddenly becomes blocked and the heart can't get oxygen.

heart block: Heart block is a problem that occurs with the heart's electrical system.

heart failure: Heart failure is a serious condition that occurs when the heart can't pump enough blood to meet the body's needs. It does not mean that the heart has stopped but that muscle is too weak to pump enough blood.

heart murmur: A heart murmur is an extra or unusual sound heard during a heartbeat. Murmurs range from very faint to very loud.

heart valve disease: Heart valve disease occurs if one or more of your heart valves don't work well.

hemochromatosis: Hemochromatosis is a disease in which too much iron builds up in your body (iron overload). Iron is a mineral found in many foods.

high blood pressure: High blood pressure is a common disease in which blood flows through blood vessels (arteries) at higher than normal pressures.

hypotension: Hypotension is abnormally low blood pressure.

Ischemia: decrease in the blood supply to a an organ, tissue, or other part caused by the narrowing or blockage of the blood vessels.

ischemic stroke: A blockage of blood vessels supplying blood to the brain, causing a decrease in blood supply.

Kawasaki disease: Kawasaki disease is a rare childhood disease. This condition involves inflammation of the blood vessels.

long QT syndrome: Long QT syndrome is a disorder of the heart's electrical activity. It can cause sudden, uncontrollable, dangerous arrhythmias in response to exercise or stress.

lupus: One of a type of chronic diseases that causes the immune system to attack healthy tissues in the body. Lupus can affect many body parts including joints, skin, the heart, lungs, kidneys, and the nervous system.

marfan syndrome: Marfan syndrome is a condition in which your body's connective tissue is abnormal.

metabolic syndrome: Metabolic syndrome is the name for a group of risk factors that raises your risk for heart disease and other health problems, such asdiabetes and stroke.

mitral valve prolapse: Mitral valve prolapse is a condition in which the heart's mitral valve doesn't work well. The flaps of the valve are "floppy" and may not close tightly.

obesity: Having too much body fat. Obesity is more extreme than being overweight, which means weighing too much.

palpitations: Palpitations are feelings that your heart is skipping a beat, fluttering, or beating too hard or too fast.

patent ductus arteriosus: Patent ductus arteriosus (PDA) is a heart problem that occurs soon after birth in some babies. In PDA, abnormal blood flow occurs between two of the major arteries connected to the heart.

pericarditis: Pericarditis is a condition in which the membrane, or sac, around your heart is inflamed.

peripheral artery disease: Peripheral arterial disease (PAD) occurs when the arteries that supply blood to the arms and legs (the periphery) become narrow or stiff.

plaque: A buildup of fat, cholesterol and other substances that accumulate in the walls of the arteries.

platelet: Any of the small cells in the blood that play a key role in blood clotting.

pulmonary embolism: Pulmonary embolism, or PE, is a sudden blockage in a lung artery. The blockage usually is caused by a blood clot that travels to the lung from a vein in the leg.

Raynaud's phenomenon: Raynaud's phenomenon is a rare disorder that affects the arteries.

rheumatic heart disease: Rheumatic heart disease is damage to the heart valves caused by a bacterial (streptococcal) infection called rheumatic fever.

stroke: A stroke occurs if the flow of oxygen-rich blood to a portion of the brain is blocked.

sudden cardiac arrest: Sudden cardiac arrest is a condition in which the heart suddenly and unexpectedly stops beating. If this happens, blood stops flowing to the brain and other vital organs.

trans fat: A type of fat, usually made by food manufacturers so that foods last longer on shelves or in cans. Eating transfats increases the risk of some illnesses, like heart disease.

varicose veins: Varicose veins are swollen, twisted veins that you can see just under the surface of the skin.

vasculitis: Vasculitis is a condition that involves inflammation in the blood vessels.

vein: Any of the thin-walled blood vessels that receive blood from capillaries and return it to the heart.

Chapter 70

Directory of Resources Providing Information about Cardiovascular Disorders

Government Agencies That Provide Information about Cardiovascular Disorders

Centers for Disease Control and Prevention
1600 Clifton Rd.
Atlanta, GA 30333
Toll-Free: 800-CDC-INFO
(800-232-4636)
Toll-Free TTY: 888-232-6348
Fax: 770-488-8151
Website: www.cdc.gov
E-mail: cdcinfo@cdc.gov

National Center for Complementary and Alternative Medicine
9000 Rockville Pike
Bethesda, MD 20892
Toll-free: 888-644-6226
Toll-Free TTY: 866-464-3615
Website: www.nccam.nih.gov

National Heart, Lung, and Blood Institute, NHLBI Health Information Center
P.O. Box 30105
Bethesda, MD 20824-0105
Phone: 301-592-8573
Fax: 240-629-3246
Website: www.nhlbi.nih.gov
E-mail: nhlbiinfo@nhlbi.nih.gov

National Human Genome Research Institute, National Institutes of Health
31 Center Dr., MSC 2152
Bldg. 31, Rm. 4B09
Bethesda, MD 20892-2152
Phone: 301-402-0911
Fax: 301-402-2218
Website: www.genome.gov

Resources in this chapter were compiled from several sources deemed reliable; all contact information was verified and updated in June 2016.

**National Institute
of Arthritis and
Musculoskeletal and Skin
Diseases, National Institutes
of Health**
1 AMS Cir.
Bethesda, MD 20892-3675
Toll-Free: 877-22-NIAMS
(877-226-4267)
Phone: 301-495-4484
TTY: 301-565-2966
Fax: 301-718-6366
Website: www.niams.nih.gov
E-mail: NIAMSinfo@mail.nih.
gov

**National Institute of
Diabetes, Digestive, and
Kidney Diseases**
1 Center Dr., MSC 2560
Bldg. 31, Rm. 9A063
Bethesda, MD 20892-2560
Phone: 301-496-3583
Website: www.niddk.nih.gov

**National Institute of
Neurological Disorders and
Stroke, National Institutes
of Health (NIH) Neurological
Institute**
P.O. Box 5801
Bethesda, MD 20824
Toll-Free: 800-352-9424
Phone: 301-496-5751
TTY: 301-468-5981
Website: www.ninds.nih.gov
E-mail: braininfo@ninds.nih.gov

National Institute on Aging
31 Center Dr., MSC 2292
Bldg. 31, Rm. 5C27
Bethesda, MD 20892
Toll-Free: 800-222-2225
Phone: 301-496-1752
Toll-Free TTY: 800-222-4225
Fax: 301-496-1072
Website: www.nia.nih.gov
E-mail: niaic@nia.nih.gov

National Institutes of Health
9000 Rockville Pike
Bethesda, MD 20892
Phone: 301-496-4000
TTY: 301-402-9612
Website: www.nih.gov
E-mail: NIHinfo@od.nih.gov

**Office on Women's Health,
Department of Health and
Human Services**
200 Independence Ave. S.W.
Rm. 712E
Washington, DC 20201
Toll-Free: 800-994-9662
Phone: 202-690-7650
Fax: 202-205-2631
Website: womenshealth.gov

**U.S. Food and Drug
Administration**
10903 New Hampshire Ave.
Silver Spring, MD 20993-0002
Toll-Free: 888-INFO-FDA
(888-463-6332)
Website: www.fda.gov

Private Agencies That Provide Information about Cardiovascular Disorders

About KidsHealth, The Hospital for Sick Children (SickKids)
555 University Ave.
Toronto, ON
M5G 1X8
Canada
Website: www.aboutkids health.ca

American Academy of Family Physicians
P.O. Box 11210
Shawnee Mission, KS
66207-1210
Toll-Free: 800-274-2237
Phone: 913-906-6000
Fax: 913-906-6075
Website: www.aafp.org

American Academy of Pediatrics
141 N.W. Point Blvd.
Elk Grove Village, IL 60007-1098
Toll-Free: 800-433-9016
Phone: 847-434-4000
Fax: 847-434-8000
Website: www.aap.org
E-mail: kidsdocs@aap.org

American Association for Clinical Chemistry
1850 K St. N.W.
Ste. 625
Washington, DC 20006
Toll-Free: 800-892-1400
Fax: 202-887-5093
Website: www.aacc.org
E-mail: custserv@aacc.org

American Association of Cardiovascular and Pulmonary Rehabilitation
330 N. Michigan Ave.
Ste. 2000
Chicago, IL 60611
Phone: 312-321-5146
Fax: 312-673-6924
Website: www.aacvpr.org
E-mail: aacvpr@aacvpr.org

American College of Cardiology, Heart House
2400 N St. N.W.
Washington, DC 20037
Toll-Free: 800-253-4636
Phone: 202-375-6000
Fax: 202-375-7000
Website: www.acc.org
E-mail: resource@aac.org

American College of Chest Physicians
3300 Dundee Rd.
Northbrook, IL 60062-2348
Toll-Free: 800-343-2227
Phone: 847-498-1400
Fax: 847-498-5460
Website: www.chestnet.org

American College of Rheumatology
2200 Lake Blvd. N.E.
Atlanta, GA 30319
Phone: 404-633-3777
Fax: 404-633-1870
Website: www.rheumatology.org
E-mail: acr@rheumatology.org

American Heart Association
7272 Greenville Ave.
Dallas, TX 75231
Toll-Free: 800-AHA-USA-1
(800-242-8721)
Phone: 214-570-5978
Website: www.heart.org
E-mail: info@heart.org

American Society of Echocardiography
2100 Gateway Centre Blvd.
Ste. 310
Morrisville, NC 27560
Phone: 919-861-5574
Fax: 919-882-9900
Website: www.asecho.org
E-mail: ase@asecho.org

American Society of Hypertension
45 Main St.
Ste. 712
Brooklyn, NY 11202
Phone: 212-696-9099
Fax: 347-916-0267
Website: www.ash-us.org
E-mail: ash@ash-us.org

American Stroke Association
7272 Greenville Ave.
Dallas, TX 75231
Toll-Free: 888-4-STROKE
(888-478-7653)
Website: www.strokeassociation.
org

Brain Aneurysm Foundation
269 Hanover St.
Bldg. 3
Hanover, MA 02339
Toll-Free: 888-272-4602
Phone: 781-826-5556
Website: www.bafound.org
E-mail: office@bafound.org

Cardiovascular Research Foundation
111 E. 59th St.
New York, NY 10022-1202
Phone: 646-434-4500
Website: www.crf.org
E-mail: info@crf.org

Center for Prevention of Heart and Vascular Disease
535 Mission Bay Blvd. S.
San Francisco, CA 94143
Phone: 415-353-2873
Fax: 415-353-2528
Website: www.healthyheart.ucsf.
edu
E-mail: info@healthyheart.ucsf.
edu

Children's Cardiomyopathy Foundation
P.O. Box 547
Tenafly, NJ 07670
Phone: 866-808-CURE
(866-808-2873)
Fax: 201-227-7016
Website: www.childrens
cardiomyopathy.org
E-mail: info@
childrenscardiomyopathy.org

Children's Hemiplegia and Stroke Association (CHASA)
4101 W. Green Oaks
Ste. 305
Arlington, TX 76016
Phone: 817-492-4325
Website: www.chasa.org

Cleveland Clinic
9500 Euclid Ave.
Cleveland, OH 44195
Toll-Free: 800-223-2273
Phone: 216-444-2200
TTY: 216-444-0261
Website: www.clevelandclinic.org

Heart and Stroke Foundation of Canada
222 Queen St.
Ste. 1402
Ottawa, ON
K1P 5V9
Canada
Phone: 613-569-4361
Fax: 613-569-3278
Website: www.heartandstroke.com

Heart Failure Society of America
5425 Wisconsin Ave.
Ste. 600
Chevy Chase, MD 20815
Phone: 301-718-4800
Fax: 301-968-2431
Website: www.hfsa.org
E-mail: info@hfsa.org

Heart Rhythm Society
1400 K St. N.W.
Ste. 500
Washington, DC 20005
Phone: 202-464-3400
Fax: 202-464-3401
Website: www.hrsonline.org
E-mail: info@HRSonline.org

Hypertrophic Cardiomyopathy Association
P.O. Box 306
Hibernia, NJ 07842
Phone: 973-983-7429
Fax: 973-983-7870
Website: www.4hcm.org
E-mail: support@4hcm.org

Minneapolis Heart Institute Foundation
920 E. 28th St.
Ste. 100
Minneapolis, MN 55407
Toll-Free: 877-800-2729
Phone: 612-863-3833
Fax: 612-863-3801
Website: www.mplsheart.org
E-mail: info@mhif.org

National Stroke Association
9707 E. Easter Ln.
Ste. B
Centennial, CO 80112
Toll-Free: 800-STROKES
Fax: 303-649-1328
Website: www.stroke.org
E-mail: info@stroke.org

Nemours Foundation
Website: kidshealth.org

Office of Minority Health,
Resource Center
P.O. Box 37337
Washington, DC 20103-7337
Toll-Free: 800-444-6472
Fax: 301-251-2160
Website: https://minorityhealth.
hhs.gov
E-mail: info@minorityhealth.
hhs.gov

Society for Vascular Surgery
633 N. Saint Clair
22nd Fl.
Chicago, IL 60611
Toll-Free: 800-258-7188
Phone: 312-334-2300
Fax: 312-334-2320
Website: www.vascularsociety.
org
E-mail: vascular@
vascularsociety.org

Texas Heart Institute
MC 3-116
P.O. Box 20345
Houston, TX 77225-0345
Phone: 832-355-4011
Website: www.texasheart.org

The Mended Hearts, Inc.
8150 N. Central Expy.
M2248
Dallas, TX 75206
Toll-Free: 888-HEART99
(888-432-7899)
Phone: 214-206-9259
Fax: 214-295-9552
Website: www.mendedhearts.org
E-mail: info@mendedhearts.org

The Society of Thoracic
Surgeons
Phone: 312-202-5800
Fax: 312-202-5801
Website: www.sts.org

Vascular Disease Foundation
550 M Ritchie Hwy
PMB-281
Severna Park, MD 21146
Phone: 443-261-5564
Website: www.vdf.org
E-mail: info@vdf.org

Women's Heart Foundation
P.O. Box 7827
West Trenton, NJ 08628
Phone: 609-771-9600
Website: www.womensheart.org

World Heart Federation
7, rue des Battoirs
Case postale 155
1211 Geneva
Switzerland
Website: www.world-heart-
federation.org
E-mail: info@worldheart.org

Arrhythmias

Heart Rhythm Society
1400 K St. N.W.
Ste. 500
Washington, DC 20005
Phone: 202-464-3400
Fax: 202-464-3401
Website: www.hrsonline.org
E-mail: info@HRSonline.org

Washington Heart Rhythm Associates, LLC
10230 New Hampshire Ave.
Ste. 204
Silver Spring, MD 20903
Phone: 301-408-7890
Fax: 301-408-7892
Website: www.washingtonhra.com

Congenital Disorders

Congenital Heart Information Network
P.O. Box 3397
Margate City, NJ 08402-0397
Phone: 609-823-4507
Website: www.tchin.org

March of Dimes Foundation
1275 Mamaroneck Ave.
White Plains, NY 10605
Phone: 914-997-4488
Website: www.marchofdimes.com

Myocarditis

Myocarditis Foundation
100 W. Main St.
Utica, MN 55979
Toll Free: 866-846-1600
Phone: 732-295-3700
Fax: 732-295-3701
Website: www.myocarditisfoundation.org

Peripheral Arterial Disorders

Erythromelalgia Association
200 Old Castle Ln.
Wallingford, PA 19086
Phone: 610-566-0797
Website: www.erythromelalgia.org
E-mail: memberservices@burningfeet.org

Fibromuscular Dysplasia Society of America
20325 Center Ridge Rd.
Ste. 620
Rocky River, OH 44116
Toll-Free: 888-709-7089
Phone: 216-834-2410
Website: www.fmdsa.org
E-mail: admin@fmdsa.org

Sudden Cardiac Arrest

Sudden Cardiac Arrest Association
12100 Sunset Hills Rd., Ste. 130
Reston, VA 20190
Toll-Free: 866-972-SCAA (866-972-7222)
Website: www.suddencardiacarrest.org
E-mail: info@suddencardiacarrest.org

Sudden Cardiac Arrest Foundation
7500 Brooktree Rd.
Ste. 207
Wexford, PA 15090
Toll Free: 877-722-8641
Website: www.sca-aware.org

Valvular Disorders

The Howard Gilman Institute for Heart Valve Disease
635 Madison Ave.
Third Fl.
New York, NY 10022
Phone: 212-289-7777
Website: www.gilmanheartvalve.
us
E-mail: info@gilmanheartvalve.
us

Vasculitis

Vasculitis Foundation
P.O. Box 28660
Kansas City, MO 64188
Toll-Free: 800-277-9474
Phone: 816-436-8211
Fax: 816-436-8211
Website: www.
vasculitisfoundation.org
E-mail: info@behuman.com

Vasculitis Foundation Canada
425 Hespeler Rd.
Ste. 446
Cambridge, ON
N1R 8J6
Canada
Phone: 877-572-9474
Website: www.vasculitis.ca
E-mail: contact@vasculitis.ca

Index

Index